Strategies in Fracture Treatments

This series provides a clearly structured and comprehensive overview of fracture treatments based on the most recent scientific data. Each book in the series is organized anatomically, so the surgeon can quickly access practical aspects, examples, pearls and pitfalls of specific areas. Trauma and orthopaedic surgeons worldwide who are searching for a current knowledge of new implants, therapeutic strategies and advancements will be able to quickly and efficiently apply the information to their daily clinical practice. The books in the series are written by a group of experts from the Association for the Rationale Treatment of Fractures (ARTOF) who aim to provide an independent, unbiased summary of fracture treatments to improve the clinical and long term outcomes for patients.

More information about this series at: http://www.springer.com/series/13623

Peter Biberthaler
Chlodwig Kirchhoff
James P. Waddell
Editors

Fractures of the Proximal Humerus

Springer

Editors
Peter Biberthaler
Department of Trauma Surgery
Klinikum rechts der Isar Technical
University Munich
Munich
Germany

James P. Waddell
St. Michael's Hospital
Toronto, Ontario
Canada

Chlodwig Kirchhoff
Department of Trauma Surgery
Klinikum rechts der Isar Technical
University Munich
Munich
Germany

ISSN 2364-8295 ISSN 2364-8309 (electronic)
Strategies in Fracture Treatments
ISBN 978-3-319-20299-0 ISBN 978-3-319-20300-3 (eBook)
DOI 10.1007/978-3-319-20300-3

Library of Congress Control Number: 2015954403

Springer Cham Heidelberg New York Dordrecht London

Printed on acid-free paper

Springer International Publishing AG Switzerland is part of Springer Science+Business Media (www.springer.com)

Contents

Contributors

Philipp Ahrens Department of Orthopedics and Sports Medicine, Klinikum rechts der Isar, Technical University of Munich, Munich, Germany

Ingo J. Banke Clinic of Orthopedics and Sports Orthopedics, Department of Orthopedic Sports Medicine, Klinikum rechts der Isar, Technical University of Munich, Munich, Germany

Marc Beirer Department of Trauma Surgery, Klinikum rechts der Isar, Technical University of Munich, Munich, Germany

Peter Biberthaler Department for Trauma Surgery, Klinikum rechts der Isar, Technical University Munich, Munich, Germany

Volker Braunstein Orthoplus, Munich, Germany

Stefan Buchmann Department of Orthopedic Sports Medicine, Klinikum rechts der Isar, Munich, Germany

Moritz Crönlein Department of Trauma Surgery, Klinikum rechts der Isar, Technical University of Munich, Munich, Germany

Thomas R. Duquin, MD Department of Orthopaedic Surgery, University at Buffalo, Buffalo, NY, USA

Hans-Henning Eckstein Department of vascular surgery, Klinikum rechts der Isar, Technical University of Munich, Munich, Germany

Stefan Greiner Shoulder and Elbow Surgery, Sporthopaedicum, Regensburg, Germany

Andrew W. Howard Division of Orthopaedic Surgery, Hospital for Sick Children, Toronto, ON, Canada

Departments of Surgery and Health Policy, Management and Evaluation, University of Toronto, Toronto, ON, Canada

Stefan Huber-Wagner, MD Department for Trauma Surgery, Klinikum rechts der Isar, Technical University Munich, Munich, Germany

Andreas B. Imhoff Department of Sports Orthopaedics, Klinikum rechts der Isar, Technical University of Munich, Munich, Germany

Florian B. Imhoff Department of Trauma Surgery, Klinikum rechts der Isar, Technical University of Munich, Munich, Germany

Ulrich Irlenbusch Orthopaedic Clinic, Marienstift Arnstadt, Arnstadt, Germany

Mohamed Kenawey Lecturer and Consultant of Orthopaedic Surgery, Orthopaedic Surgery Department, Faculty of Medicine, Sohag University, Sohag, Egypt

Chlodwig Kirchhoff Department of Trauma Surgery, Klinikum rechts der Isar, Technical University Munich, Munich, Germany

Gertrud Kirchhoff Institute for Assessment and Occupational Medicine, Munich, Germany

Rainer Kirchhoff DEZEMBA-Deutsches Zentralinstitut für Begutachtungs- und Arbeitsmedizin, Institute for Assessment and Occupational Medicine, Munich, Germany

MEDEX Plus, Diessen-Riederau, Germany

Sonja M. Kirchhoff Department of Clinical Radiology, Munich University Hospital, Downtown Campus, Ludwig Maximilian University of Munich, Munich, Germany

Ashesh Kumar, MD, MSc, FRCSC Division of Orthopaedics, St. Michael's Hospital, Toronto, ON, Canada

Rolf Lefering Institute for Research in Operative Medicine (IFOM), University Witten/Herdecke, Cologne, Germany

Andreas Lenich Department of Sports Orthopaedics, Klinikum rechts der Isar, Technical University of Munich, Munich, Germany

Ulrich Lenze Klinik für Orthopädie und Sportorthopädie, Klinikum rechts der Isar Technische Universität München, Munich, Germany

Dominik Pförringer Department of Trauma Surgery, Klinikum rechts der Isar, Technical University of Munich, Munich, Germany

Florian Pohlig Klinik für Orthopädie und Sportorthopädie, Klinikum rechts der Isar Technische Universität München, Munich, Germany

Lukas K.L. Postl Department of Trauma Surgery, Klinikum rechts der Isar, Technical University of Munich, Munich, Germany

Peter Michael Prodinger Klinik für Orthopädie und Sportorthopädie, Klinikum rechts der Isar, Technical University of Munich, Munich, Germany

Christian Reeps Department of vascular surgery, Klinikum rechts der Isar, Technical University of Munich, Munich, Germany

Gunther H. Sandmann Department of Traumatology, Technical University of Munich, Munich, Germany

Marcus Schmitt-Sody Orthopaedic Department, Medical Park Chiemsee, Bavaria, Germany

Elaine Schubert Institute for Diagnostic and Interventional Radiology, Klinikum rechts der Isar, Technical University Munich, Munich, Germany

Sebastian Siebenlist, MD Department of Trauma Surgery, Klinikum rechts der Isar, Technical University Munich, Munich, Germany

John W. Sperling, MD Department of Orthopaedic Surgery, Mayo Clinic, Rochester, MN, USA

Andreas Toepfer Klinik für Orthopädie und Sportorthopädie, Klinikum rechts der Isar Technische Universität München, Munich, Germany

Arne J. Venjakob Sports Orthopaedics Department, Marienkrankenhaus Kaiserswerth, Duesseldorf, Germany

Helen Vester Department of Trauma Surgery, Klinikum rechts der Isar, Technical University of Munich, Munich, Germany

Rüdiger von Eisenhart-Rothe Klinik für Orthopädie und Sportorthopädie, Klinikum rechts der Isar Technische Universität München, Munich, Germany

James P. Waddell, MD, FRCSC Division of Orthopaedics, St. Michael's Hospital, Toronto, ON, Canada

Ernst Wiedemann Shoulder and Elbow Surgery, OCM Clinic, Munich, Germany

Part I

Basics

1 Epidemiology

Marc Beirer

Introduction

In general epidemiology is the analysis of sickness and health in human study populations [1]. Epidemiologic research provides information about etiology, prevalence, incidence and consequential economic effects of the analysed human populations. These scientific conclusions lead to changes in treatment, reduction of risk-factors, development of intervention strategies and prophylactic arrangements to minimize disease-dependent consequences. Furthermore, findings are included in the calculations of the socioeconomic costs and in the planning of the health care for the elderly [2]. An epidemiologic analysis of fracture incidence in the year 2000 showed an occurrence of fractures in general at an average age of 49 years and a 1:1 female to male gender ratio [3]. The general distribution of fractures is demonstrated in Fig. 1.1. Women showed a considerable increase in fracture incidence at an age >50 years whereas for men a peak in fracture incidence was found in the younger population between 12 and 19 years with a corresponding decrease until the age of 60 years. Henceforward the fracture incidence in the male population rose again, but only of minor character compared to the female population. The reason of the dramatic increase in fracture incidences in the elderly is most likely due to osteoporotic fracture genesis. In conclusion this study showed an increase in osteoporotic fractures emphasizing the need to detect, prevent and treat osteoporosis.

M. Beirer
Department of Trauma Surgery,
Klinikum rechts der Isar,
Technical University of Munich,
Munich, Germany
e-mail: marc.beirer@mri.tum.de

Epidemiology of Proximal Humerus Fractures

Similar to other fractures of the upper extremity, fractures of the proximal humerus compromise the patient's self-supply and might convert fit, elderly independent patients to somewhat social dependant people [4], resulting in leading causes of morbidity and mortality [2]. Fractures of the proximal humerus account for approximately 5 % of all fractures of the human body [3] and rank seventh following fractures of the distal radius, the metacarpal, the proximal femur, phalanges, the ankle and of the metatarsal (see Fig. 1.1). In patients with an age of 65 years or older fractures of the proximal humerus even account for 10 % of all fractures [5]. As the number of elderly increases, proximal humerus fractures will even more intensive contribute to the growing public health problem due to osteoporotic fractures [6, 7].

P. Biberthaler et al. (eds.), *Fractures of the Proximal Humerus*, Strategies in Fracture Treatments,
DOI 10.1007/978-3-319-20300-3_1

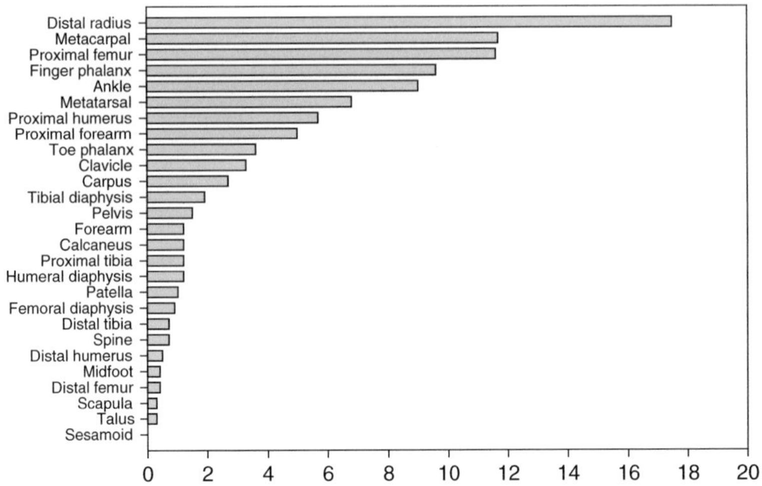

Fig. 1.1 Fractures arranged in order of decreasing frequency in % (Data from [3])

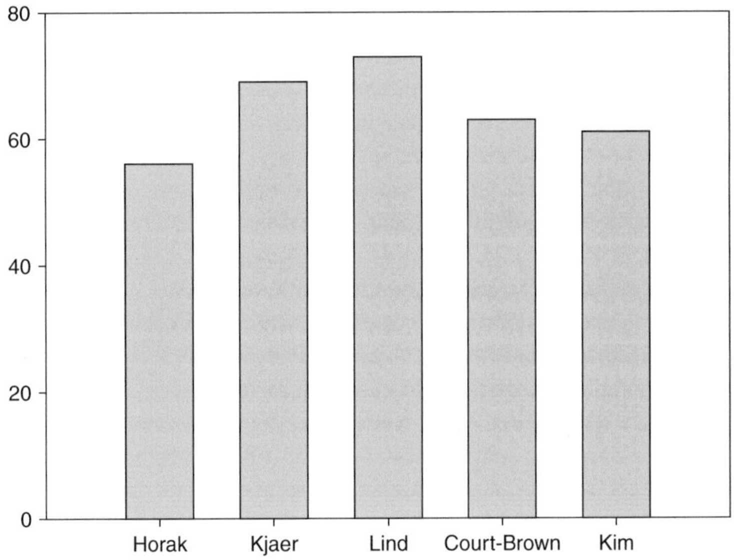

Fig. 1.2 Incidence rates of proximal humerus fractures (per 100,000 per year) (Data from [3, 9–12])

Incidence Rate

In general the incidence rate is defined as the number of new events occurring during a specified time period divided by the number of people at risk [8].

Dynamic variation of the incidence rate of proximal humerus fractures has been described by several authors between 1965 and 1989 [9] (see Fig. 1.2). Horak et al. showed an overall incidence rate of 56/100,000 [10], Kjær et al. described a rate of 69/100,000 [11] and Lind et al. reported an incidence rate of 73/100,000 per year. Current epidemiologic studies refute a further increase, presenting an incidence rate of 63/100,000 in 2006 [3] and 61/100,000 in 2008 [12]; this slight decrease might be due to improvements in prophylaxis on falling, progress in medical treatment of osteoporosis, more careful behavior of the elderly or even more active older patients.

Fracture Region

Humerus fractures are generally divided into three anatomic regions: proximal, mid-shaft and distal humerus fractures. In an epidemiologic study in the United States the proximal humerus was identified as the most common site of fracture accounting for approximately 50 % of humerus fractures [12] (Fig. 1.3). The distal humerus with approximately 35 % accounted for

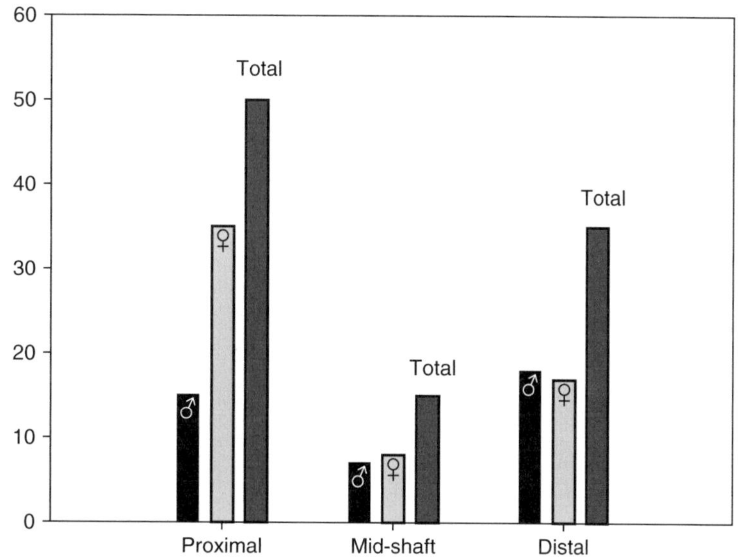

Fig. 1.3 Anatomic site of fracture in % (Data from [12])

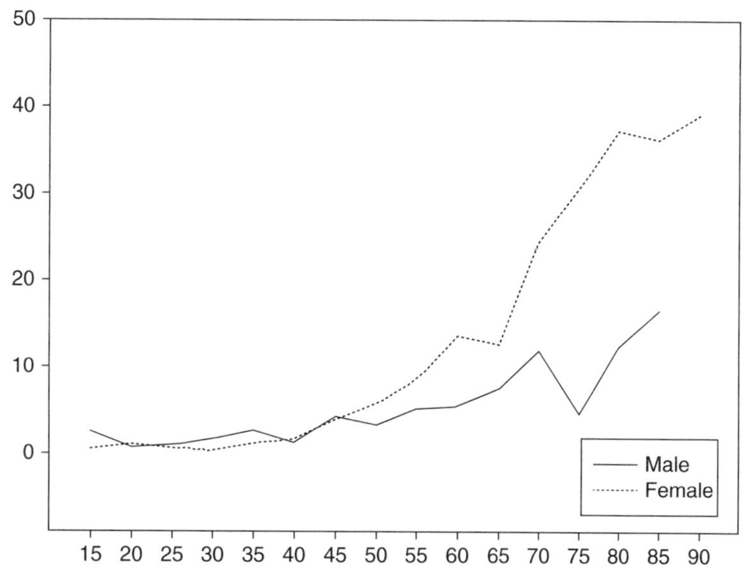

Fig. 1.4 Incidence of proximal humerus fracture dependent on age and gender (Data from [15])

the next most common site, whereas mid-shaft fractures occurred in only 15 %. A relevant impact of gender in terms of a female to male ratio was only found for the proximal region accounting for 2.3:1, whereas a ratio of 1.3:1 resulted for the humeral shaft, and of 0.9:1 for the distal humerus. In general the fracture location depends on the trauma mechanism and other patient-specific risk factors: in this context proximal humerus fractures are associated with an increased age, female gender and osteoporotic bone, compared to distal humerus fractures, which are associated with children's age.

Age and Gender

Fractures of the proximal humerus are seen most commonly in the elderly population [13, 14] with an average age accounting for approximately 65 years [3, 4, 9]. Incidence and severity of the fracture increase with the patient's age (Fig. 1.4) [4]. Especially in female patients the incidence increases exponentially at an age of 40 years and older. In contrast, male patients show an increased incidence in the youth, however, at an age of 50 years and older, women's incidence predominates [15, 16]. These gender differences might be

Table 1.1 Places of accident

	Under 60 years *n* (%)	Over 60 years *n* (%)
At home	60 (27.9)	280 (53.3)
Public areas	97 (45.1)	160 (31.1)
Place of work	10 (4.7)	1 (0.2)

Reprinted with permission from [9]

due to lower bone mineral density and a correspondingly higher prevalence of osteoporosis in women than in men [17].

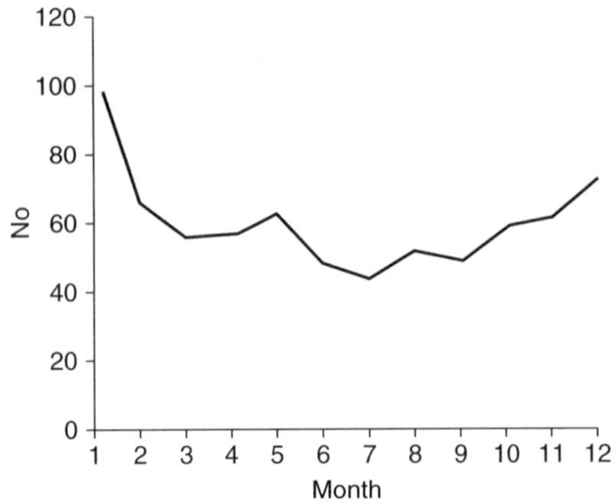

Fig. 1.5 Time of accident (months) (Reprinted with permission from [9])

Mechanism and Time of Accident

The chief cause of proximal humeral fractures is a simple fall onto the upper extremity with over 90 % happening in patients older than 60 years [4, 18], while only a few fractures are caused by traffic accidents or accidents at work [9]. In people younger 60 years of age most accidents happen in public, whereas in people older 60 years of age more than half of the accidents occur at home (see Table 1.1). Activity at the time of the accident is mainly walking straight ahead [18]. According to the patient's own judgment the main reason for the injury is tripping or slipping. In 76 % the main impact of the fall is directed straight to the shoulder or upper arm resulting in a concomitant subcutaneous hematoma at that particular site. Most of the patients report that they had fallen obliquely forward or to the side. Accumulation of accidents in the colder months (Fig. 1.5) [4, 9] is due to snow and ice on the streets as well as early darkness. The majority of accidents happens during the middle of the day, although a peak in incidence is recognizable before midnight (Fig. 1.6) [9].

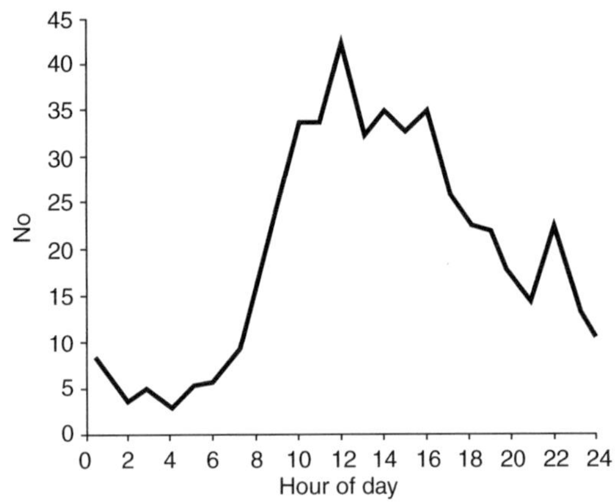

Fig. 1.6 Time of accident (hours of a day) (Reprinted with permission from [9])

What Brings the Future?

Improvements in medical treatment and social conditions have led to an increasingly aged population. Court-Brown et al. showed a quick change in the epidemiology of fractures [3]. In the current literature, a triplication of the incidence of osteoporotic proximal humerus fractures in Finnish people at an age of 60 years or older during the years 1970 and 1998 has been described [19]. Kim et al. expect nearly 275,000 emergency department visits due to proximal humerus fractures in the United States in the year 2030 as compared to 185,000 visits in the year 2008 [12]. Due to constant expansion of the population at risk, rigorous safety measures to reduce falls and preventive treatments of osteoporosis are needed in this specific age group.

Summary

Fractures of the proximal humerus account for approximately 10 % in the elderly population. Current epidemiologic studies show an incidence rate of 61/100,000 per year. Incidence rate and severity increase with patient's age, especially in female patients. The proximal humerus is the most common site of fractures of the humerus. A simple fall obliquely forward or to the side presents in over 90 % the cause of the fracture. In elderly people more than half of the accidents occur at home whereas in patients at an age younger 60 years accidents mostly happen in public. In our increasingly aged population we hypothesize that incidence rates of proximal humerus fracture will further increase and rigorous safety measures to reduce falls and preventive treatments of osteoporosis are inevitably necessary.

References

1. Kleinbaum D, Sullivan K, Barker N. A pocket-size introduction. In: A pocket guide to epidemiology. New York: Springer; 2007. p. 1.
2. Kristiansen B, Barfod G, Bredesen J, Erin-Madsen J, Grum B, Horsnaes MW, Aalberg JR. Epidemiology of proximal humeral fractures. Acta Orthop Scand. 1987;58(1):75–7.
3. Court-Brown CM, Caesar B. Epidemiology of adult fractures: a review. Injury. 2006;37(8):691–7.
4. Court-Brown CM, Garg A, McQueen MM. The epidemiology of proximal humeral fractures. Acta Orthop Scand. 2001;72(4):365–71.
5. Baron JA, Karagas M, Barrett J, Kniffin W, Malenka D, Mayor M, Keller RB. Basic epidemiology of fractures of the upper and lower limb among Americans over 65 years of age. Epidemiology. 1996;7(6):612–8.
6. Chu SP, Kelsey JL, Keegan TH, Sternfeld B, Prill M, Quesenberry CP, Sidney S. Risk factors for proximal humerus fracture. Am J Epidemiol. 2004;160(4): 360–7.
7. Jones G, Nguyen T, Sambrook PN, Kelly PJ, Gilbert C, Eisman JA. Symptomatic fracture incidence in elderly men and women: the Dubbo Osteoporosis Epidemiology Study (DOES). Osteoporos Int. 1994;4(5):277–82.
8. Greenland S, Rothman K-J. Measures of occurrence. In: Rothman K-J, Greenland S, Lash T-L, editors. Modern epidemiology, vol. 3. Philadelphia: Lippincott Williams & Wilkins; 2008. p. 34.
9. Lind T, Kroner K, Jensen J. The epidemiology of fractures of the proximal humerus. Arch Orthop Trauma Surg. 1989;108(5):285–7.
10. Horak J, Nilsson BE. Epidemiology of fracture of the upper end of the humerus. Clin Orthop Relat Res. 1975;112:250–3.
11. Kiaer T, Larsen CF, Blicher J. Proximal fractures of the humerus. An epidemiological and descriptive study of fractures. Ugeskr Laeger. 1986;148(30):1894–7.
12. Kim SH, Szabo RM, Marder RA. Epidemiology of humerus fractures in the United States: nationwide emergency department sample, 2008. Arthritis Care Res (Hoboken). 2012;64(3):407–14.
13. Jo MJ, Gardner MJ. Proximal humerus fractures. Curr Rev Musculoskelet Med. 2012;5(3):192–8.
14. Resch H. Fractures of the humeral head. Unfallchirurg. 2003;106(8):602–17.
15. Singer BR, McLauchlan GJ, Robinson CM, Christie J. Epidemiology of fractures in 15,000 adults. the influence of age and gender. J Bone Joint Surg Br. 1998;80(2):243–8.
16. Donaldson LJ, Cook A, Thomson RG. Incidence of fractures in a geographically defined population. J Epidemiol Community Health. 1990;44(3):241–5.
17. Cawthon PM. Gender differences in osteoporosis and fractures. Clin Orthop Relat Res. 2011;469(7):1900–5.
18. Palvanen M, Kannus P, Parkkari J, Pitkajarvi T, Pasanen M, Vuori I, Jarvinen M. The injury mechanisms of osteoporotic upper extremity fractures among older adults: a controlled study of 287 consecutive patients and their 108 controls. Osteoporos Int. 2000;11(10):822–31.
19. Kannus P, Palvanen M, Niemi S, Parkkari J, Jarvinen M, Vuori I. Osteoporotic fractures of the proximal humerus in elderly Finnish persons: sharp increase in 1970–1998 and alarming projections for the new millennium. Acta Orthop Scand. 2000;71(5):465–70.

Anatomy

2

Lukas K.L. Postl

Adequate reconstruction of fractures requires a profound knowledge of the respective anatomy. Whenever possible the treatment of fractures should aim for an anatomical reconstruction of the involved structures. This avoids problems arising from altered biomechanics after reconstruction. However, in case of complex injuries to the bone complete anatomical reconstruction may not be possible. If so, consideration should be given to the biomechanical situation after the anatomical reconstruction.

Basic Anatomy of the Shoulder Joint

In general four separate joints the gleno-humeral, the acromio-clavicular, the sterno-clavicular and the thoraco-scapular joint allow for movements of the arm. The proximal end of the humerus is part of the gleno-humeral joint. Therefore this joint is of great importance for the treatment of proximal humerus fractures. In the following relevant anatomical structures of the shoulder are described.

L.K.L. Postl
Department of Trauma Surgery,
Klinikum rechts der Isar, Technical University of Munich,
Munich, Germany
e-mail: lukasleo@gmx.at

Bony Elements

The gleno-humeral joint is formed by the hemispherical surface of the humeral head and the pear-shaped glenoid cavity. The shoulder's impressive range of motion is possible due to the disproportion between the size of the humeral head and the glenoid cavity. The disproportion is quantified by the gleno-humeral index, which is defined as normal when accounting for 0.86 in the sagittal and 0.58 in the axial axis [1, 2]. Besides the articular surface the greater tuberosity and the lesser tuberosity also have specific biomechanical functions. The greater tuberosity is the insertion site of the supraspinatus and the infraspinatus muscle's tendons. The subscapularis tendon inserts at the lesser tuberosity. Further bony structures of the shoulder joint that should be considered are the acromion and the coracoid process, which are both located cranial to the gleno-humeral joint [3, 4]. Two muscles, the coracobrachialis and the biceps brachii muscle, arise from the coracoid process. In addition, the pectoralis minor muscle inserts at the coracoid process. The coracoid process is located on the lateral edge of the antero-superior portion of the scapula. The acromion is also a bony process and together with the clavicle it forms the top of the shoulder. The acromio-clavicular joint is of importance for raising the arm above the shoulder level. [5]

P. Biberthaler et al. (eds.), *Fractures of the Proximal Humerus*, Strategies in Fracture Treatments,
DOI 10.1007/978-3-319-20300-3_2

Capsular and Ligamental Stabilizers

The circularly shaped glenoidal labrum enlarges the articular surface of the glenoid. The articular capsule arises from the medial glenoid surface and spherically encases the gleno-humeral joint [6, 7]. In neutral position and adduction of the arm the caudal parts of the capsule form the axillary recess. There are three gleno-humeral ligaments, the superior-, middle- and inferior gleno-humeral ligament,, which are all located ventral to the gleno-humeral joint to stabilize the articular capsule [8]. The subacromial space with the subacromial bursa is located between the articular capsule und the acromion. [5]

Muscles

The deltoid muscle determines the outer shape of the shoulder joint. It is involved in the movements of abduction, extension, flexion as well as in internal and external rotation. The biceps brachii muscle mainly provides flexion and supination movements in the elbow joint. Its long tendon arises from the supraglenoid tubercle as well as from the superior glenoid labrum. Forty percent to 60 % of the fibers arise from the supraglenoid tubercle. For the remaining fibers four different types of attachment to the glenoid labrum have been described. These types were defined depending on the distribution of the fiber attachment to the posterior and anterior labrum [9]. The long biceps tendon initially runs within the capsule and is encircled and supported by the biceps pulley. It continues into the bicipital groove [10, 11].

The four rotator cuff muscles, the supra- and infraspinatus muscle, the subscapularis and teres minor muscle are located between the deltoid muscle and the articular capsule. The rotator cuff is responsible for centering the humeral head in the glenoid cavity. In addition these muscles are very important for arm movements and provide stability of the shoulder joint. All four rotator cuff muscles arise from the scapula. The supraspinatus muscle initiates arm abduction. It lies ventro-cranially and inserts at the greater tuberosity. Both dorsal located muscles, the infraspinatus muscle and the teres minor muscle (dorso-caudal), are involved in adduction and external rotation. Both insert at the greater tuberosity. Internal rotation is provided by the subscapularis muscle, which is located on the ventral side and inserts at the lesser tuberosity [5].

Innervation

The supraspinatus muscle and the infraspinatus muscle are innervated by the suprascapular nerve (C5 and C6). The nerve arises from the upper trunk of the brachial plexus and reaches the supraspinous fossa from ventral through the suprascapular notch for the innervation of the suprascapularis muscle. The nerve runs under the supraspinatus muscle and supplies the articular capsule with some branches. After laterally curving around the scapula's spine, it reaches the infraspinatus muscle for innervation. The subscapularis muscle is innervated by the upper and lower subscapular nerves. Both arise from the posterior cord of the brachial plexus (C5–C6). The axillary nerve (C5, C6) also derives from the posterior cord of the plexus and supplies the teres minor muscle and the deltoideus muscle [5].

References

1. Gianotti SM, Marshall SW, Hume PA, Bunt L. Incidence of anterior cruciate ligament injury and other knee ligament injuries: a national population-based study. J Sci Med Sport. 2009;12(6):622–7.
2. McPherson EJ, Friedman RJ, An YH, Chokesi R, Dooley RL. Anthropometric study of normal gleno-humeral relationships. J Shoulder Elbow Surg. 1997;6(2):105–12.
3. Braunstein V, Korner M, Brunner U, Mutschler W, Biberthaler P, Wiedemann E. The fulcrum axis: a new method for determining glenoid version. J Shoulder Elbow Surg. 2008;17(5):819–24.
4. Bhatia DN, de Beer JF, du Toit DF. Coracoid process anatomy: implications in radiographic imaging and surgery. Clin Anat (New York, NY). 2007;20(7):774–84.
5. Thiel W. Photographischer Atlas der praktischen Anatomie. 2nd ed. Heidelberg: Springer Medizin Verlag; 2002.

6. Beltran J, Jbara M, Maimon R. Shoulder: labrum and bicipital tendon. Top Magn Reson Imaging. 2003;14(1):35–49.
7. Halder AM, Kuhl SG, Zobitz ME, Larson D, An KN. Effects of the glenoid labrum and glenohumeral abduction on stability of the shoulder joint through concavity-compression : an in vitro study. J Bone Joint Surg Am. 2001;83-A(7):1062–9.
8. Kirchhoff C, Imhoff AB. Posterosuperior and anterosuperior impingement of the shoulder in overhead athletes-evolving concepts. Int Orthop. 2010;34(7):1049–58.
9. Vangsness Jr CT, Jorgenson SS, Watson T, Johnson DL. The origin of the long head of the biceps from the scapula and glenoid labrum. An anatomical study of 100 shoulders. J Bone Joint Surg. 1994;76(6):951–4.
10. Gerber C, Sebesta A. Impingement of the deep surface of the subscapularis tendon and the reflection pulley on the anterosuperior glenoid rim: a preliminary report. J Shoulder Elbow Surg. 2000;9(6): 483–90.
11. Habermeyer P, Magosch P, Pritsch M, Scheibel MT, Lichtenberg S. Anterosuperior impingement of the shoulder as a result of pulley lesions: a prospective arthroscopic study. J Shoulder Elbow Surg. 2004; 13(1):5–12.

Risk Factors for Proximal Humerus Fractures

3

Moritz Crönlein

Introduction

Fractures of the proximal humerus belong to the second most common fractures of the upper extremity. Only fractures of the distal radius occur more often according to the current literature [1]. Through continuous improvement and development of different therapeutical options, the injured patients can be offered many different curative solutions nowadays.

However long term effects such as loss of motion or development of arthritis with corresponding negative impact on the outcome even after ideal conservative or surgical treatment still exist in the course of the healing.

Therefore it would be eligible to minimize the incidence of proximal humerus fractures, so that problems as just mentioned cannot arise or can be at least reduced to a minimum. For this purpose it is helpful to understand the risk factors for proximal humerus fractures to counteract them preemptively.

The following chapter provides an overview of the different risk factors for the development of proximal humerus fractures and the relevant prevention options shall be explained (Table 3.1).

Falls

More than 90 % of the proximal humerus fractures result from falls. The pathomechanism is in most cases the same, with the most common direction of the fall being forward to the fracture site, falling either on the outstretched arm, or directly onto the shoulder [2]. Correspondingly in patients who tend to suffer from frequent falls the risk of proximal humerus fractures is higher [1]. A history of at least one fall within the last 6 months increases the fracture risk of the patient in the future which becomes clear considering that 30 % of the patients of 65 years or older fall

Table 3.1 Risk for proximal humerus fractures [1]

Falls	Low bone mass/ Osteoporosis	Frailty
Diabetes mellitus	BMD	Control of falls
Epilepsy	Age	Physical activity
Handedness	Female gender	
Visual impairment	Nutrition	
Deafness	Glucocorticoids	
	BMI	
	Ethnical differences	

M. Crönlein
Department of Trauma Surgery, Klinikum rechts der Isar, Technical University of Munich, Munich, Germany
e-mail: moritz.croenlein@mri.tum.de

P. Biberthaler et al. (eds.), *Fractures of the Proximal Humerus*, Strategies in Fracture Treatments, DOI 10.1007/978-3-319-20300-3_3

at least once per year with 50 % of them suffering from recurrent falls. In this context it should be mentioned that people with recurrent falls tend to have general physical disabilities affecting their daily life also increasing their personal risk for a proximal humerus fracture [3, 4].

Besides the personal history of falling a history of maternal hip fracture also increases the personal fracture risk most likely being related to the predisposition of suffering from osteoporosis later [3].

Factors that go along with a higher fall risk are exemplarily listed below:

- Diabetes mellitus
- Epilepsy
- handedness
- visual impairment
- deafness

Diabetes Mellitus (DM)

Ivers et al. describe DM as risk factor to suffer from fractures, particularly in terms of fractures of the proximal humerus. Two different pathological explanations exist: on the one hand lower bone mineral density (BMD) scores are described in people with DM (especially type I DM) compared to healthy people. A low BMD results in higher fracture rates in patients with type I DM because of the higher bone fragility. On the other hand Ivers et al. showed different associations between the late-onset complications of DM, particularly in terms of diabetical retinopathy and neuropathy, and a higher risk for falls. Patients with diabetical retinopathy have a higher risk of falling as soon as DM affects their visual ability simply overlooking obstacles in daily life. This is similar to patients with diabetical neuropathy. An increasing loss of proprioception can lead to an impairment of balance resulting in falls. Hereby the possibility of suffering from a proximal humerus fracture is increased. The longer the patients suffer from DM and the worse the patients are adjusted to the diabetical medication, the higher is the probability of the occurrence of proximal humerus fractures. Preemptively attention should be paid to the guidelines of the "international diabetes federation" (http://www.idf.org/) [5, 6].

Epilepsy

About 50 million people worldwide suffer from epilepsy [7]. Most of them take antiepileptic drugs (AEDs) as prevention from seizures and to improve their quality of life.

A research group lead by Carbone tried to establish an association between the use of AEDs and the fracture risk. In a prospective study they were able to show that there is a significant correlation between taking AEDs and a higher risk to fall along with a higher fracture risk. There was no evidence of a correlation between changes in the bone mineral density though [7].

A combination of AEDs and antidepressants shows an increased fall risk and an increased fracture rate compared to a monotherapy with only AEDs [8].

However, not only the side effects of antiepileptic drugs lead to a higher fracture risk, but the acute seizure correlates with higher fracture rates as well. This might be due to falls in the beginning of the seizure and because of the enourmous forces affecting the patient during a generalized tonic clonic seizure (grand mal). The typical seizure induced fracture pattern is a bilateral locked posterior fracture dislocation of the shoulder [9, 10].

To minimize the fracture risk regular check-ups and an ideal adjustment to the antiepileptic medication is needed. Current guidelines can be found at the "American Epilepsy Society" (http://www.aesnet.org/).

Handedness

Left handed people have a higher fracture risk compared to right handed persons [11]. The reason for this phenomenon is not completely understood by now. It is supposed that left handed people do not get along well in a world created mostly for right handed people leading to a higher fall risk and thus a higher fracture risk [11, 12].

Visual Impairment/Deafness

Visual impairment is assumed as an indicator for a higher risk to fall since reduced vision leads to an possible overlooking of obstacles in the daily life on the one hand. On the other hand there are different comorbidities that go along with visual impairment e.g. DM going along with higher risk of falling. In the current literature a higher fracture risk is described for both explanations [13, 14].

Chu et al. describe a correlation between reduced hearing capability and risk of falling. Patients that suffer from hearing problems have a higher risk to fall. An explanation for this is the limited awareness of the environment that conciliates an insecurity in the daily routine. Above all presbyakusis, resulting of a degenerative process of the corti organ in the old age, is deemed to be a risk factor for recurrent falls [1].

Osteoporosis and Bone Mineral Density (BMD)

Osteoporosis is known as a systemic skeletal disease with corresponding higher fracture risk caused by microarchitectonical changes of the bone tissue [15]. A general greater average life expectancy explains the growing importance and relevance of osteoporosis in traumatology [16].

In the literature there are more than nine million fractures reported worldwide per year caused by osteoporosis [17] with fractures of the proximal humerus presenting the forth most common fracture entity [18].

The major risk factors for developing fractures due to osteoporosis are (see Table 3.2):

- BMD
- age
- female gender
- nutrition
- hormonal changes
- glucocorticoids
- BMI (body mass index)
- ethnic differences

BMD

The level of BMD is an indicator for fracture risk in osteoporosis. There is a negative correlation between BMD and fracture risk: the lower the BMD the higher the fracture risk being substantified by the EPIDOS study and a study of Keegan et al. [3, 19].

Age

Since over 70 % of the people suffering from a proximal humerus fracture are 60 years and older, a correlation of the age and fracture risk can be assumed [18]. This might be due to an age-depending distribution of the bone mass with a peak being reached in females at the age of thirty. From the beginning of the menopause the bone mass decreases continuously in most of the women [20]. Taking this into consideration the chances for proximal humerus fractures, even in low-energy injuries are increased whereas usually a high-energy injury is essential to cause such fractures in healthy bone [18].

Besides the risk of falling increases as well with increasing age leading especially in combination with low BMD to a higher fracture risk per se [15, 21].

Table 3.2 Risk factors for osteoporotic fractures [15]

Female sex	Low bone mineral density	Neuromuscular disorders
Premature menopause	Glucocorticoid therapy	Cigarette smoking
Age	High bone turnover	Excessive alcohol consumption
Primary or secondary amenorrhoea	Family history of hip fracture	Long-term immobilisation
Primary and secondary hypogonadism in man Asian or white ethnic origin	Poor visual acuity	Low dietary calcium intake
Previous fragility fracture	Low bodyweight	Vitamin D deficiency

Gender

As described above the chance to suffer from an osteoporosis related fracture is several times higher in women compared to men. On the one hand, the postmenopausal changes, on the other hand the overall lower bone mineral density are responsible for this fact. Due to the increasing age of the population the percentage of men developing osteoportic fractures increases as well since men lose about 1 % of their bone mass starting at the age of sixty with a raised conspicuously fracture risk [15, 22].

Nutrition

In general, nutrition plays an important role in the development of osteoporosis related fractures. The risk of suffering from a proximal humerus fracture is increased by low dietary calcium and vitamin D intake [1].

In accordance the literature provides evidence that an appropriate calcium intake combined with and without vitamin D significantly decreases the fracture risk among older patients [23, 24].

Following current guidelines of the "International Osteoporosis Foundation" an intake of 1000 mg calcium per day is recommended for women and men. For women at the beginning of the menopause and for men at the age of 65 the calcium intake should be increased to 1300 mg per day [24].

In this context it should be mentioned that alcohol consumption has an influence on BMD and fracture risk correspondingly. While alcohol abusus is known to inhibit bone formation and bone growth, moderate alcohol consumption seems to have a certain positive influence on BMD by metabolizing Aldosteron into Ostrogen which is needed to prevent osteoporosis related fractures [25].

Immoderate smoking has a negative impact on BMD. The higher rate of bone resorption in smokers is due to the lower circulation of estradiol in the blood. Lower levels of estradiol lead to an increase of FSH and LH production and thus increased bone resorption [26].

Hormonal Changes

When talking about hormonal changes influencing the fracture risk especially menopausal changes are considered. Ostrogens inhibit the apoptosis of osteoblastic cells and promote the apoptosis of osteoclastic cells at the same time. This has a positive impact on the bone formation. Because of the decrease of the oestrogen levels in the postmenopausal periode, the risk of developing osteoporosis and concomitant the risk of osteoporotic fractures is increased [27].

To minimize the fracture risk postmenopausal hormone therapy can be helpful. Keagen et al. showed that hormone replacement therapy (HRT) has a beneficial effect on the fracture risk. In contrast, the fracture risk among women who have not been treated with HRT in their postmenopausal period increases from year to year [19].

Glucocorticoids

An important factor for developing osteoporosis related fractures like proximal humerus fractures is the therapy with glucocorticoids. Glucocorticoid therapy is majorly used to treat allergies or systemic inflammatory and/or immunological diseases. There are several known side effects of a glucocorticoid therapy to name the most common muscular distrophy, glaucoma and immunosuppression as well as the induction of osteoporosis. Pathophysiologically glucocorticoids result in a reduced number of osteoblastic cells so that the bone production rate is lower than the bone resorption rate resulting in a higher fracture risk.

Body Mass Index/Body Weight

Another factor, which has an influence on the incidence of proximal humerus fractures is the body weight. The body mass index (BMI) helps to determine the ideal body constitution in relation to the patient's height.

Since there exists no adequate explanation for the correlation between body weight and proximal humerus fractures, yet, there are two different [28] possible approaches discussed in literature. In this context Holmberg et al. found out that a higher BMI is associated with a higher fracture risk in women, but a lower fracture risk in men [1, 29]. It is believed, that there is an increased risk of falling and clumsiness among people suffering from obesity leading to a higher fracture risk. A bad nutritional condition could be the reason for a bad bone quality with a higher fracture risk as well.

Hagino et al. propose that a low BMI is a significant risk factor for loss of bone mass which leads to a higher fracture risk, especially after falls [30]. However, there is no significant positive or negative correlation found between body weight and incidence of proximal humeral fractures.

Ethnical Differences

There are also ethnical differences having an impact on the fracture risk. In general black people have a minor fracture risk compared to white people. As an explanation for these findings, the bone conditions of Blacks and Caucasians had been analysed by several groups. It had been found that black people present with a higher BMD compared to white people lowering the fracture risk especially in low energy accidents [31–33].

Frailty

Frailty is another important risk factor to suffer from a proximal humerus fracture. There are two aspects in frail people. One is, that the risk of falling is higher than in people in a good health state. The other fact is, that if frail people fall, they can usually barely control the fall so that they can not avoid serious trauma. This leads to a higher fracture risk in general. Physical activity may have a positive effect on the bone mass, it also can be supposed, that physically inactive patients are in a bad medical health status which leads to a higher fall risk [1, 34].

Summary

To sum it up, proximal humerus fractures are severe fractures of the upper extremity that cause many problems for the injured patient. These fractures usually affect older people with altered bone structure. As mentioned above, the major risk factors for proximal humerus fractures are falls, osteoporosis and frailty. To reduce the number of these fractures it is necessary to treat the problems that lead to their development. Therefore an ideal medication status and regular check-ups are needed, when suffering from diseases such as diabetes, epilepsia or other chronic disorders. In addition the fracture risk especially in the osteoporotical bone can be reduced by ideal nutritional conditions and good physical activity of the patients.

References

1. Chu SP, et al. Risk factors for proximal humerus fracture. Am J Epidemiol. 2004;160(4):360–7.
2. Palvanen M, Kannus P, Parkkari J. The injury mechanisms of osteoporotic upper extremity fractures among older adults: a controlled study of 287 consecutive patients and their 108 controls. Osteoporos Int. 2000;11(10):822–31.
3. Lee SH, Dargent-Molina P. Risk factors for fractures of the proximal humerus: results from the EPIDOS prospective study. J Bone Miner Res. 2002;17(5):817–25.
4. Center JR, Bliuc D, Nguyen TV, Eisman JA. Risk of subsequent fractures. Am Med Assoc. 2007;297(4): 387–94.
5. Schwartz AV, Sellmeyer DE, Ensrud KE, Cauley JA. Older women with diabetes have an increased risk of fracture: a prospective study. J Clin Endocrinol Metab. 2001;86(1):32–8.
6. Ivers RQ, Cumming RG, Mitchell P, Peduto AJ. Diabetes and risk of fracture, the blue mountains eye study. Diabetes Care. 2001;24(7):1198–203.
7. Carbone LD, et al. Antiepileptic drug use, falls, fractures, and BMD in postmenopausal women: findings from the women's health initiative (WHI). J Bone Miner Res. 2010;25(4):873–81.
8. Shiek Ahmad B, et al. Falls and fractures in patients chronically treated with antiepileptic drugs. Neurology. 2012;79(2):145–51.
9. Engel T, Lill H, Korner J, Josten C. Die beidseitige verhakte hintere Schulterluxationsfraktur. Unfallchirurg. 1999;102(11):897–901.
10. Heckmann JG, Stangl R, Erbguth F, Rutherford H, Neundörfer B. Nontraumatic seizure- associated bilat-

eral fractures of the head of the humerus. Intensive Care Med. 1999;25(5):B548–9.
11. Luetters CM, et al. Left-handedness as a risk factor for fractures. Osteoporos Int. 2003;14(11):918–22.
12. Hemenway D, Azrael DR, Rimm EB. Risk factors for wrist fracture: effect of Age, cigarettes, alcohol, body height, relative weight, and handedness on the risk for distal forearm fractures in Men. Am J Epidemiol. 1994;140(4):361–7.
13. Klein BEK, et al. Associations of visual function with physical outcomes and limitations 5 years later in an older population. Ophthalmology. 2003;110(4):644–50.
14. Salonen L, Kivela SL. Eye diseases and impaired vision as possible risk factors for recurrent falls in the aged: a systematic review. Curr Gerontol Geriatr Res. 2012;2012:271481.
15. Kanis JA. Diagnosis of osteoporosis and assessment of fracture risk. Lancet. 2002;359(9321):1929–36.
16. Grifka J, Kuster M. Orthopädie und Unfallchirurgie. Berlin: Springer DE; 2011.
17. Borrelli J. Taking control: the osteoporosis epidemic. Injury. 2012;43(8):1235–6.
18. Lill H, et al. Osteoporotic fractures of the proximal humerus. Chirurg. 2012;83(10):858–65.
19. Keegan TH, et al. Hormone replacement therapy and risk for foot, distal forearm, proximal humerus, and pelvis fractures. Osteoporos Int. 2003;14(6):469–75.
20. Reeve J, Walton J, Russel LJ, Lunt R, Wolman R. Determinants of the first decade of bone loss after menopause at spine, hip and radius. Q J Med. 1999;92(5):261–73.
21. Ivers RQ, Cummings RG. Risk factors for fractures of the wrist, shoulder and ankle: the blue mountains eye study. Osteoporos Int. 2002;13(6):513–8.
22. Drake MT, Murad MH, Mauck KF. Risk factors for low bone mass-related fractures in men: a systematic review and meta-analysis. J Clin Endocrinol Metabol. 2012;97(6):1861–70.
23. Zhu K, Prince RL. Calcium and bone. Clin Biochem. 2012;45(12):936–42.
24. Baron JA, et al. Basic epidemiology of fractures of the upper and lower limb among Americans over 65 years of age. Epidemiology. 1996;7(6):612–8.
25. Eleftheriou KL, Rawal JS, James LE. Bone structure and geometry in young men: the influence of smoking, alcohol intake and physical activity. Bone. 2013;52(1):17–26.
26. Rapuri PB, Gallagher JC, Balhorn KE, Ryschon KL. Smoking and bone metabolism in elderly women. Bone. 2000;27(3):429–36.
27. Silbernagel S, Lang F. Taschenatlas Pathophysiologie. Stuttgart/New York: Georg Thieme Verlag; 2009.
28. Berry SD, Miller RR. Falls: epidemiology, pathophysiology, and relationship to fracture. Curr Osteoporos Rep. 2008;6(4):149–54.
29. Holmberg AH, et al. Risk factors for fragility fracture in middle age. A prospective population-based study of 33,000 men and women. Osteoporos Int. 2006; 17(7):1065–77.
30. Hagino H, et al. Case–control study of risk factors for fractures of the distal radius and proximal humerus among the Japanese population. Osteoporos Int. 2004;15(3):226–30.
31. Griffin MR, Ray WA. Black-white differences in fracture rates. Am J Epidemiol. 1992;136(11):1378–85.
32. Curtis JR, et al. Population-based fracture risk assessment and osteoporosis treatment disparities by race and gender. J Gen Intern Med. 2009;24(8): 956–62.
33. Cauley JA. Defining ethnic and racial differences in osteoporosis and fragility fractures. Clin Orthop Relat Res. 2011;469(7):1891–9.
34. Kelsey JL, Browner WS, Seeley DG, Nevitt MC, Cummings SR. Risk factors for fractures of the distal forearm and proximal humerus. Am J Epidemiol. 1992;135(5):477–89.

Biomechanics of the Shoulder

4

Philipp Ahrens

Introduction

The shoulder joint is the most flexible joint of the human body. The enormous range of motion is facilitated by the sequential connection of four bones. The balanced articulation of the glenohumeral joint is provided by the rotator cuff which inserts around the humeral head fulfilling the centering function aspect of the proximal humerus over the much smaller glenoid and provides adequate force distribution during shoulder motion. Besides these osseous and muscular parts, stabilizing effects are also contributed by ligaments and the capsule-ligamentous complex. If the fine composition of bones, muscles and surrounding soft tissue is affected by any kind of injury unbalanced motion or even instability may result. These changes may affect the biomechanics of the shoulder and alter the shoulder joint inducing loss of power and pain according to the underlaying pathology. This chapter concentrates on the physiological range of motion and the different stabilizing and anatomical aspects of the shoulder.

P. Ahrens
Department of Orthopedics and Sports Medicine, Klinikum rechts der Isar, Technical University of Munich, Munich, Germany
e-mail: ph.ahrens@gmail.com

Biomechanics of the Shoulder

The shoulder joint gains its range of motion from some groundbreaking anatomical developments. The high flexibility in shoulder motion is provided by the interaction of osseos structures, ligaments and the composition of muscles, covering the shoulder girdle. Four bones the clavicle, the scapula, the bony thoracic wall and the humerus, are composed to a sequential chain of four joints as follows: the sterno-clavicular, the acromioclavicular, the gleno-humeral and the scapulothoracic joint. In comparison to other joints especially of the lower extremity, the stability of the shoulder is mainly provided by the composition of static (osseous) and dynamic capsule, ligaments and muscles components so that any pathology may arise either from isolated or combined injuries of one or more of those structures.

During the evolution the glenoid had become a nearly pan shaped shallow bone, which is only in contact with the humeral head in a small predescribed area. This development comes along with an increased diameter of the humeral head which is centred onto the glenoid by a balanced force control concept of the four rotator cuff muscles, the Supraspinatus, Infraspinatus, Teres minor and Subscapularis muscle.

P. Biberthaler et al. (eds.), *Fractures of the Proximal Humerus*, Strategies in Fracture Treatments,
DOI 10.1007/978-3-319-20300-3_4

Kinematics of the Shoulder

The 3-dimensional movement of the shoulder is a complex process of different highly coordinated muscles. The wide range of motion (ROM) of the shoulder joint is strongly connected to the historical developments when the humans started walking on two instead of all four extremities. When the human changed his way of locomotion the arms became increasingly useful for manipulation. The ROM increased by different explicit developments as follows:

- Formation of sequentially ordered joints: the gleno-humeral, the sterno-clavicular, the acromio-clavicular joint.
- Downsizing of the osseous fitting between humeral head and glenoid,
- Development of a flexible joint edge (labrum glenoidale) and joint capsule,
- Growth of the muscle diameters and accordingly increase of the qualities of the deltoid, the infraspinatus and the subscapularis muscle.

Especially the reduction of the glenoid surface in relation to the circumference of the humeral head in the evolution enabled this expanded ROM on the account of form fitted stability.

This loss of stability needs to be compensated by the muscles of the rotator cuff. External rotation is limited by a slight retrotorsion of the humeral head in relation to the axis of the humerus [1, 2]. Comparing the gleno-humeral joint to the hip joint owning three degrees of freedom in motion, the gleno-humeral joint gains its flexibility in motion from additional anterior to posterior and cranial to caudal translation possibilities of the humeral head onto the shallow surface of the glenoid caused by the flexible glenoidal labrum. Thus, the shoulder joint reaches five degrees of freedom in motion and can be characterised as a "force stabilized" joint.

Even during normal shoulder motion the contact area between the humeral head and the glenoid varies and a roll- sliding mechanism supports the wide range of motion. Elevation of the arm de-centres the humeral head to a more posterior region of the glenoid, from a specific point the force vectors change their force approach and a sliding of the humeral head results [3, 4]. Nevertheless nearly the entire shoulder motion is a combination of motion of the shoulder girdle and the scapula-thoracic junction. During motion, only at the end of external rotation the scapula is approximated to the thoracic wall and removed from there at the end of internal rotation. In the sagittal plane anterior flexion is possible up to 170° and posterior flexion up to 50°. The rise of the arm sideways is divided into two phases, the abduction phase until 100° and the rise above 100° so-called elevation up to the end of approximately 170°. In the first phase the motion arises almost only from the gleno-humeral joint, all motion above this level is provided by a combination of the scapula, the gleno-humeral joint and the scapula-thoracic sliding.

Statics of the Shoulder

The muscle insertion at the scapula is a direct connector to the thoracic wall with its own basic tension. Already small changes of this sensibly balanced muscular construct affect the position of the scapula in relation to the posterior thoracic wall. This situation might be recognized when the Serratus anterior muscle is either destroyed or paralyzed known as Scapula alata syndrome. In this situation the scapula reacts with a protrusion of the patient's back in an abnormal position presenting a rare appearance with the potential to limit functional activity such as the ability to lift, pull, and push weight.

The synergistic work of the shoulder girdle allows for the broad range of motion since the glenoidal cavity is always put in a perfect position to allow increased motion. The trapezoid muscle and its minor supporters such as the levator scapulae muscle and sternocleidomastoideus muscle are stabilizing factors regarding cranial shoulder movement. The central forces, which are restraining anterior movement are distributed from the acromio-clavicular joint and the clavicle to the sterno-clavicular joint. The sliding suspension of the scapula-thoracic area is combined with the supporting sling of the superficial back muscles and the serratus muscle the only attachment to the thorax. Increasing abduction also increases the lever and in this combination also the forces applied to the scapula, thorax and clavicle. The multidirectional suspension of the scapula with its broad sliding freedom towards the thorax is nevertheless an isolated fixation concept and can thus be seen from a static point of view. It is unique that the shoulder joint is free of ligaments to provide an adequate fixation to the trunk.

The force transmission of the shoulder is provided by the surrounding muscles of the shoulder girdle. In the 0° -position in terms of a hanging arm, the forces to centre the humeral head on the glenoidal cavity are equivalent to the weight of the arm and the force vector aiming to the centre. The basic tension of the rotator cuff allows for a centering of the humeral head onto the glenoid. If the arm is abducted in the sagittal plane, this motion is majorly beard by the supraspinatus and deltoid muscles. In case of performing weight bearing the rotator cuff has to respond to this weight by developing immense forces to balance the humeral head in the right anatomical position. With increasing abduction the lever and its resulting forces are changing and the humeral head is ascending to the fornix humeri on the relatively flat glenoidal cavity. To hold against this ascending movement of the humeral head the adductor muscles have to re-center the humeral head.

Many statements exist regarding the disproportion of the humeral head's circumference and the much smaller glenoidal cavity being an aberrated development. But at a closer look, this development seems to be a perfect construction. The arrangement of the periarticular muscles shows that these muscles are able to centre the humeral head onto the glenoidal cavity according to the motion required with a fine adjustment of these mechanisms. Since the scapula is not rigidly fixed to the thorax, in the evolution process there was no need for increased bone or ligament fixation providing more stability. Instead the suspension of the shoulder is very flexible and allows for a combined sliding on the thoracic and rolling manoeuvres on the glenoidal cavity always being neuromuscularly stabilised by the rotator cuff. Only in cases when neurological or traumatic reasons are affecting the composition the risks of instability arises. Accordingly a misfunctional muscular balance leads to a rise of the humeral head against the fornix humeri or the roof of the shoulder. In this situation the fornix becomes an abutment to the humeral head with the clinically apparent typical impingement symptoms when in most cases the supraspinatus muscle tendon is compromised. In a normal physiologically working shoulder the greater tuberosity dives under the lateral edge of the acromion without pincing the supraspinatus tendon. Repeated squeezing of the supraspinatus tendon may harm it with, in the worst case, triggering a tendon tear.

Stability of the Shoulder Joint

To understand the stabilizing structures of the humeral head the differentiation into static and dynamic mechanisms is very useful. The dynamic or active stabilizers are the surrounding muscles of the shoulder girdle and corresponding tension whereas the passive stabilizers are the anatomical construct including the osseous and capsular structures.

Dynamic Mechanisms

The most important dynamic function is provided by the rotator cuff and its ability to balance the glenoid during all kinds of motion so that the resulting force vector runs through the centre of the glenoid. As long as this construct is stable, no further stabilizing forces are needed. But if the humeral head tends to move away from the centre, the risks of dislocation and rupture of the demarcating glenoidal labrum raise with the result of a massive loss of stability. Besides the osseous cavity of the glenoid, the labrum bordering the edge of the glenoid increases the construct of a pan or cavity by 50 % [5]. When the energy needed to keep the humeral head in the centre of the glenoidal cavity to avoid dislocation is measured, it is thereby possible to count the stability index (SI [%] = Shearforce/centre force) × 100 [6–8]. Due to the pear like shape of the glenoid the Stability Index is the lowest in anterior and posterior direction explaining the most common direction of shoulder dislocation.

Vacuum Effect

Inside the shoulder joint hypobaric conditions exist which may help to center the humeral head onto the glenoidal cavity. Since Habermeyer et al. [9] and Itoi [10] made an experimental approach to identify the stabilizing effects of the shoulder the low intraarticular pressure has been recognized to support the stability comparable to an O-ring in a motor's cylinder. In experiments they explored that a shifting of the humeral head produces a vacuum effect of approximately 7 kp [11] and that the venting of this pressure increases the instability, especially in the antero inferior direction [10].

Cohesion

Besides the described stabilizing mechanisms also the cohesion effect of form fitting surfaces has been known as shoulder joint stabilizer. Cohesion is the tendency of plane surfaces to stick together due to intermolecular forces. The two joint partners, the humerus and the glenoid, are seperated by a thin fluid layer of synovial fluid holding the two surfaces together through cohesion effects like two plane layers of glas with fluid in-between.

Static Mechanisms of Stability

The importance of the osseous configuration of the humeral head has often been overrated. The diameter of the humeral head is approximately 44 mm, the area of the glenoidal cavity is around 35 × 25 mm. To measure the proportion a vertical and transversal glenohumeral index was established [12, 13]. When the humeral head shifts in relation to the glenoid more than the normal range of motion, the capsule and the supporting gleno- humeral ligaments are participating to hinder dislocation and damage to the shoulder. Anatomically the fibres of the capsule are composed like a helix around the humeral head leading to a change in tension of the fibres according to the position [14]. Since the rotator cuff is directly connected to the capsule an active tensioning of the capsule is possible. In this meaning the capsule converts from a passive to an active stabilizer. In some exquisite positions, like elevation and rotation the active stabilizers are less effective with the capsule working like a hammock limiting the shift of the humeral head [15, 16]. The ligaments of the rotator cuff interval are shaped like a triangular space created by the intervention of the coracoid process between the subscapularis and supraspinatus muscles and tendons. The floor of the rotator cuff interval is the cartilage of the humeral head, and the roof is build by the rotator cuff and capsule, which links the subscapularis and supraspinatus tendons and is composed of two layers: the Coraco humeral ligament on the bursa side and the fasciculus obliquus on the articular side.

The rotator interval is an important stabilizer of the shoulder. During adduction the strongly developed coraco-humeral ligament and the superior gleno-humeral ligament limit the inferior translation and guarantee the posterior stability during abduction and anteversion [17, 18]. In the moderate position of abduction the middle gleno- humeral ligament limits the translation into anterior direction [14, 16, 17, 19]. From the biomechanical view the antero inferior part of the labrum is a functional part of the inferior gleno humeral ligament [14].

Active Stabilisators

The muscles of the rotator cuff are the main stabilizer of the shoulder joint. Their key function is the direct application of compression forces onto the humeral head, whereas the centering effect is also supported by the form fitting of the shallow glenoidal cavity and the surrounding labrum. The compression is not proportional to the applied pressure, since the glenoidal labrum is soft tissue and deforms with increasing pressure. The rotator cuff muscles also work as active depressors of the humeral head providing a neutralizing effect on the decentering shear forces, as result of the action of the deltoid muscle and an indirect creation of compressive forces at a decentering of the gleno-humeral joint. Each shift of the humeral head on the surface of the glenoid increases the pretension of the rotator cuff muscles and supports the recentering of the humeral head in relation to the glenoid. The rotator cuff is also connected to the joint capsule and therefore a tensioning of the capsule is possible when the muscles contract. The activity of the other muscles with insertion at the proximal humerus can create translational forces which may decentre the humeral head as well. Another destabilizing effect can be seen when the N. suprascapularis and its inervation to the M. infraspinatus and M. subscapularis is blocked or damaged. In this case the stability is heavily disturbed showing that these two muscles are very important active stabilizers [20]. The effect of a disturbed muscle balance appears in patients suffering from paralysis or other kinds of neurological pathologies which is very impressive when an asymmetrical failure of some branches of the deltoid muscle or the rotator cuff is present. In this case an antero-inferior or postero-inferior instability can result. In this context it is interesting to know that nearly 2/3 of patients after stroke suffer from pain due to a subluxation [15]. The mobility of the gleno-humeral joint is provided by a complex of 12 muscle unites with discriminable functional aspects. These unites are more categorized by their effects than by their anatomical properties.

The first group is labelled as the peripheral group and contains all muscles starting from the thorax inserting at the humerus. The superficial group mainly represented by the three parts of the arm elevating deltoid muscle. The group of the deep, controlling, muscles consist of the rotator cuff itself [16]. Inman and later Poppen et al. tried to calculate the forces having an effect on the GH joint. They calculated a maximum of 89 % of the body weight applied as a compression force against the glenoid surface in 90°. Assuming that the muscles diameter correlates proportionally to the strength a muscle can produce [17]. The most important shoulder muscles have a well known and described relation, in comparison to the M. supraspinatus (1) the cross section of the deltoid muscle is greater (anterior portion approx. by factor 1.2, middle approx. by 2.5 and rear area by approx. 1.5). This unfavorable relation is equalized by the other muscles of the rotator cuff (Infraspinatus/teres minor muscle approx. factor 2 and subscapularis muscle by factor 2.3). But all those experimental approaches did not provide realistic data. In reality the effect of the muscle is strongly connected to the physical moment and the orientation of the muscle fibres as well as the distance to the center of rotation; those facts have the highest influence on the power of each muscle. Van der Helm developed a dynamic Finite element Model of the shoulder, on basis of a 3 D analysis of all shoulder structures. It is actual the best approach to handle these problems, since with this setup every given position and direction can be computed and relatively exact results can be produced [21]. Kuechle et al. counted the torque of ten different muscles and showed that the pectoralis, latissimus dorsi and teres major muscles, are the most powerful depressors of the humeral head. They are more efficient as the entire rotator cuff [22, 23].

Not much is known about dynamic changes in connection to greater rotator cuff defects. Radiological examinations showed that symptomatic as well as asymptomatic shoulders with supraspinatus tendon lesions show a measurable cranialisation of the contact area of the humeral head.

A compensated biomechanical situation is reached while a force vector pair is working. The vector pair consists of the subscapularis muscle ventrally and infraspinatus/terres minor muscle dorsally. But also it is clear that a defect arthropathy cannot be explained by the biomechanical changes alone [24].

Nowadays possibilities with finite element computed models and adequate computer power will enhance further scientific work and may enlight a much more specific view onto the biomechanical workout and shoulder pathologies.

Summary

Considering the joints of the human body, the shoulder provides the most elaborate functional architecture. Anatomical developments like the reduction of the glenoid bearing in contrast to the enlarged diameter of the humeral head enabled an incomparable range of motion. The humeral head is centered like a golf ball on the T, on the glenoid, actively positioned by the muscles of the rotator cuff and passively secured off exorbitant motion by the ligaments and joint capsule as well as the anatomical bony structure. With the knowledge of these structures and their function, many pathologies of the shoulder stand on a rational basis and are approachable by different treatment options.

References

1. Gohlke F. Biomechanik der Schulter. Orthopade. 2000;10:835–44.
2. Clark J, Sidles JA, Matsen FA. The relationship of the glenohumeral joint capsule to the rotator cuff. Clin Orthop Relat Res. 1990;254:29–34.
3. Soslowsky LJ, Flatow EL, Bigliani LU, Mow VC. Articular geometry of the glenohumeral joint. Clin Orthop Relat Res. 1992;285:181–90.
4. Soslowsky LJ, Flatow EL, Bigliani LU, Pawluk RJ, Ateshian GA, Mow VC. Quantitation of in situ contact areas at the glenohumeral joint: a biomechanical study. J Orthop Res. 1992;10(4):524–34.
5. Howell SM, Galinat BJ. The glenoid-labral socket. A constrained articular surface. Clin Orthop Relat Res. 1989;243:122–5.
6. Lippitt S, Matsen F. Mechanisms of glenohumeral joint stability. Clin Orthop Relat Res. 1993;291: 20–8.
7. Matsen 3rd FA. The biomechanics of glenohumeral stability. J Bone Joint Surg Am. 2002;84-A(3): 495–6.
8. Matsen 3rd FA, Harryman 2nd DT, Sidles JA. Mechanics of glenohumeral instability. Clin Sports Med. 1991;10(4):783–8.
9. Habermeyer P, Schuller U, Wiedemann E. The intra-articular pressure of the shoulder: an experimental study on the role of the glenoid labrum in stabilizing the joint. Arthroscopy. 1992;8(2):166–72.
10. Itoi E, Motzkin NE, Browne AO, Hoffmeyer P, Morrey BF, An KN. Intraarticular pressure of the shoulder. Arthroscopy. 1993;9(4):406–13.
11. Hoffmeyer P. Biomechanics of the shoulder – kinematics and intra-articular vacuum. Orthopade. 1992;21(1):71–4.
12. Itoi E, Lee SB, Berglund LJ, Berge LL, An KN. The effect of a glenoid defect on anteroinferior stability of the shoulder after Bankart repair: a cadaveric study. J Bone Joint Surg Am. 2000;82(1):35–46.
13. Yamamoto N, Itoi E, Abe H, Kikuchi K, Seki N, Minagawa H, Tuoheti Y. Effect of an anterior glenoid defect on anterior shoulder stability: a cadaveric study. Am J Sports Med. 2009;37(5):949–54.
14. Warner JJ, Caborn DN, Berger R, Fu FH, Seel M. Dynamic capsuloligamentous anatomy of the glenohumeral joint. J Shoulder Elbow Surg. 1993;2(3):115–33.
15. O'Brien SJ, Neves MC, Arnoczky SP, Rozbruck SR, Dicarlo EF, Warren RF, Schwartz R, Wickiewicz TL. The anatomy and histology of the inferior glenohumeral ligament complex of the shoulder. Am J Sports Med. 1990;18(5):449–56.
16. Turkel SJ, Panio MW, Marshall JL, Girgis FG. Stabilizing mechanisms preventing anterior dislocation of the glenohumeral joint. J Bone Joint Surg Am. 1981;63(8):1208–17.
17. Harryman 2nd DT, Sidles JA, Clark JM, McQuade KJ, Gibb TD, Matsen 3rd FA. Translation of the humeral head on the glenoid with passive glenohumeral motion. J Bone Joint Surg Am. 1990;72(9):1334–43.
18. Harryman 2nd DT, Walker ED, Harris SL, Sidles JA, Jackins SE, Matsen 3rd FA. Residual motion and function after glenohumeral or scapulothoracic arthrodesis. J Shoulder Elbow Surg. 1993;2(6):275–85.
19. Harryman DT, Sidles JA, Harris SL, Lippitt SB, Matsen 3rd FA. The effect of articular conformity and the size of the humeral head component on laxity and motion after glenohumeral arthroplasty. A study in cadavera. J Bone Joint Surg Am. 1995;77(4):555–63.
20. Howell SM, Kraft TA. The role of the supraspinatus and infraspinatus muscles in glenohumeral kinematics of anterior should instability. Clin Orthop Relat Res. 1991;263:128–34.
21. van der Helm FC. A finite element musculoskeletal model of the shoulder mechanism. J Biomech. 1994;27(5):551–69.
22. Kuechle DK, Newman SR, Itoi E, Niebur GL, Morrey BF, An KN. The relevance of the moment arm of shoulder muscles with respect to axial rotation of the glenohumeral joint in four positions. Clin Biomech (Bristol, Avon). 2000;15(5):322–9.
23. Kuechle DK, Newman SR, Itoi E, Morrey BF, An KN. Shoulder muscle moment arms during horizontal flexion and elevation. J Shoulder Elbow Surg. 1997;6(5):429–39.
24. Thompson WO, Debski RE, Boardman 3rd ND, Taskiran E, Warner JJ, Fu FH, Woo SL. A biomechanical analysis of rotator cuff deficiency in a cadaveric model. Am J Sports Med. 1996;24(3):286–92.

5 Physical Examination

Ulrich Irlenbusch

In most cases proximal humerus fractures cause pain, pressure pain, swelling or local muscular defense representing an acute situation mostly caused by fall or traffic accidents. In this mostly acute situation in the emergency room or even on scene of the accident palpation of the bony contours is usually not possible. In case of a proximal humerus fracture during the inspection of the affected extremity a diffuse swelling associated with signs of a hematoma, which can extend in the course of the following 4–5 days onto the lower arm or the corresponding thorax side might be apparent. The presence of such hematomas might be an indicator for vascular damage secondary to the primary fracture incident [3], when diagnostics and therapy could only be initiated with delay

Is a dislocated fracture suspected often characteristic changes of the physiological shoulder contours might be present. Regarding an anterior dislocation fracture usually a prominent anterior portion of the humeral head along with a protruding acromion, an almost not palpable coracoid process and a flattening of the dorsal articular portion are apparent. Correspondingly contrary findings are visible in case of a rather rare occurring posterior dislocation of the shoulder.

In general the characteristic position of the arm in case of a dislocation fracture can be helpful in the diagnostics so that in case of an anterior dislocation the arm is positioned in slight abduction and external rotation along with a blocked internal rotation whereas in case of a posterior dislocation the arm is positioned in rather internal rotation along with a blocked external rotation.

In addition for the clinical examination the treating doctor should pay attention to external injury of the skin or soft tissue damage, which might influence the further treatment.

As it is common knowledge unnecessary manipulation of the fractured arm should be avoided if possible. The vascular and neurological state should be ascertained again after each manipulation/each reposition manoeuvre at the shoulder. At that it should be considered that the risk of vascular and neurological injuries increases because of adhesions after preceding surgeries [13].

Although the incidence of neuro-vascular lesions in case of non-dislocated fractures is rather low its exclusion is definitely necessary. However, in case of additional dislocation fractures the incidence of such neuro-vascular lesions significantly increases to up to 2–30 % [13].

A meticulous neurovascular examination is paramount, as the plexus brachialis – especially

U. Irlenbusch
Orthopaedic Clinic, Marienstift Arnstadt, Arnstadt, Germany

Sports Clinic Erfurt, Erfurt, Germany
e-mail: ulrich.irlenbusch@ms-arn.de

P. Biberthaler et al. (eds.), *Fractures of the Proximal Humerus*, Strategies in Fracture Treatments, DOI 10.1007/978-3-319-20300-3_5

the axillary nerve and the axillary artery might be endangered in case of a proximal humerus fracture [12]. Furthermore, secondary injury is possible [7, 8, 10]. Reliable diagnostics of the motoric qualities can often not be performed due to pain, but the presence of sensory deficits or paraesthesia should definitely be examined and documented. The examination of peripheral pulses is also obligatory [2]. An inferior subluxation of the humerus occurring immediately after the fracture incident can be a consequence of an atony of the deltoid muscle or the rotator cuff and has to be discerned from a paresis of the axillary nerve in the further course.

The thorax should also be included in the mentioned examinations, because concomitant thoracic injuries such as a pneumothorax or even intrathoracic penetration of the humerus head can occur [1, 3–6, 9, 11].

References

1. Abellan JF, Melendreras E, Gimenez DJ, Carrillo FJ, Ruano L, Rivkin J. Intrathoracic fracture-dislocation of the humeral head: a case report. Orthop Surg. 2010;18(2):254–7.
2. Barvencik F, Gebauer M, Janssen A, Ismail M, Rupprecht M, Rueger JM, Briem D. Prolonged vascular complications with subsequent finger necrosis after humeral head luxation fracture in the elderly. Unfallchirurg. 2007;110(1):78–85. [German].
3. Bigliani LU, Flatow EL, Pollock RG. Fractures of the proximal humerus. In: Rockwood AC, Matsen A, editors. The shoulder, vol. I. 2nd ed. Philadelphia: W.B. Saunders; 1998. p. 337–89.
4. Daffner SD, Cipolle MD, Phillips TG. Fracture of the humeral neck with intrathoracic dislocation of the humeral head. J Emerg Med. 2010;38(4):439–43.
5. Galois L, Siat J, Reibel N, Valentin S, Gasnier J, Mainard D. Intra-thoracic fracture-dislocation of the humeral head: a case report and review of the literature. Rev Chir Orthop Reparatrice Appar Mot. 2007;93(8):854–58.
6. Griffin NC, Temes RT, Gill IS, Rice TW. Intrathoracic displacement of a fractured humeral head. Ann Thorac Surg. 2007;84(4):1400.
7. Mouzopoulos G, Lassanianos N, Mouzopoulos D, Tzurbakis M, Georgilas I. Axillary artery injury associated with proximal humerus fractures. Vasa. 2008;37(3):274–7. doi:10.1024/0301-1526.37.3.274.
8. Mouzopoulos G, Lasanianos N, Mouzopoulos D, Batanis G, Tzurbakis M, Georgilas I. Acute renal failure due to rhabdomyolysis after proximal humerus fracture associated with axillary artery rupture. Int Urol Nephrol. 2008;40(3):855–8.
9. Salhiyyah K, Potter D, Sarkar PK. Fracture-dislocation of humeral head with intrathoracic displacement. Asian Cardiovasc Thorac Ann. 2012;20(2):196–8.
10. Somville FJ. Plexus injury after reduction of anterior caudal dislocation of the shoulder. Acta Chir Belg. 2008;108(3):362–4.
11. Tan GJ, Tan AG, Peh WC. Wandering humeral head mimicking a breast mass. Med J Malaysia. 2008;63(2):164–5.
12. Traxler H, Surd R, Laminger KA, Windisch A, Sora MC, Firbas W. The treatment of subcapital humerus fracture with dynamic helix wire and the risk of concommitant lesion of the axillary nerve. Clin Anat. 2001;14(6):418–23.
13. Zuckermann JD, Checroun AJ. Fractures of the proximal humerus: Diagnosis and management. In: Ianotti JP, Williams GR, editors. Disorders of the shoulder. Philadelphia: Lippincott; 1999. p. 639–85.

Plain Imaging

6

Sonja M. Kirchhoff

Introduction

After detailed clinical examination including check up of perfusion, motor function and sensitivity in case of a proximal humeral fracture attention should be paid to possible concomitant injuries especially in the area of the shoulder girdle and the thorax.

Radiographic Diagnostics

However if from the clinical side a proximal humeral fracture is suspected x-rays of the shoulder joint are the first step in the diagnostical cascade. Despite the increasingly available high tech imaging diagnostics such as computed tomography (CT) radiographs of the shoulder joint still own a significant value regarding the exact analysis of the form and localisation of osseous injuries respectively fractures of the proximal humerus if they are responsibly performed. After the initial physical examination plain X-rays are essential for the diagnostic evaluation of proximal humeral fractures. High-quality radiological diagnostics are based on correct x-ray exposure, presentation of the shoulder joint in two views perpendicular to each other with minimal overlap of the fractured region by surrounding osseous structures and soft tissue [1]. Only if these requirements are met, an adequate evaluation of the individual topography, severity and direction of displacement of the fracture fragments is possible, and the fracture can reliably be classified. A review of literature showed that the "normal" a-p view as well as the scapular y-view along with the axial view are most often used but more important most helpful in daily clinical routine [2–6].

In the following in case of suspected proximal humeral fracture the most important x-ray projections of the proximal humerus and shoulder joint respectively are explained.

True a-p View (Glenoidal-Tangential View)

Typical indications for this projection are suspected fractures or dislocation of the shoulder joint, but also more generally speaking suspected inflammatory, degenerative or tumorous diseases. For this a-p view the patient is positioned with the back towards the stand, the healthy side is lifted by 45° whereas the affected side bears on with a slight abduction and the hand in a supined position and the upper arm hanging down in a

S.M. Kirchhoff
Department of Clinical Radiology,
Munich University Hospital,
Downtown Campus, Ludwig Maximilian University
of Munich, Munich, Germany
e-mail: sonja.kirchhoff@me.com

P. Biberthaler et al. (eds.), *Fractures of the Proximal Humerus*, Strategies in Fracture Treatments,
DOI 10.1007/978-3-319-20300-3_6

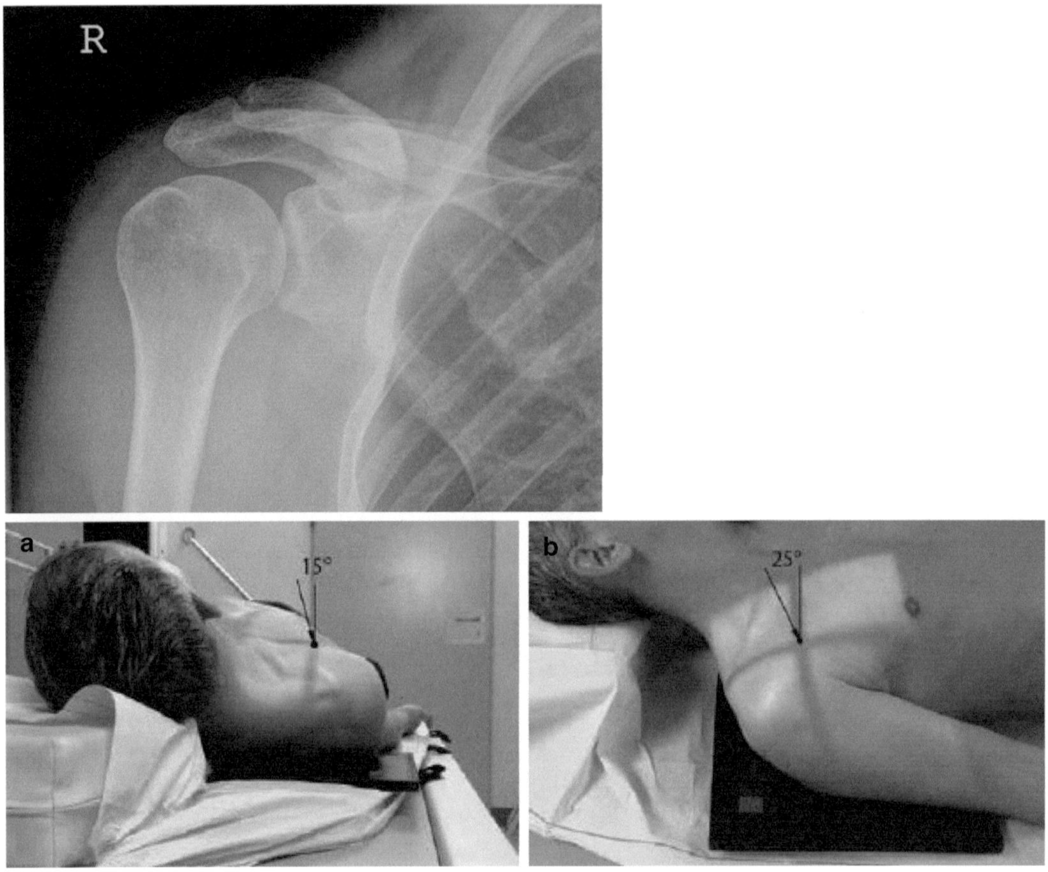

Fig. 6.1 True-ap view of a right shoulder joint. Normal findings (Reprinted with permission from *Lehrbuch der röntgendiagnostischen Einstelltechnik*, 6th edition, 2008)

neutral position. The central ray directs from anterior to posterior direction with approximately 25° cranio-caudal and 15° medio-lateral tilt. Crucial for the so called "true" a-p view is the x-ray tube being tilted in cranio-caudal direction approximately 12 to maximal 15° to get a better insight into the gleno-humeral joint. However, for acute diagnostics one should be content with an x-ray overview including the acromio-clavicular joint as well as the lateral clavicle without tilting the x-ray tube.

Criteria for a well-performed radiograph are the overprojection of the anterior and posterior rim of the cavitas glenoidalis as **one** contour. The bearing area of the scapula should be pictured streak like, the humeral head should not be overlaid and correspondingly the subacromial space as well as the gleno-humeral articular space should be greatly visible (see Fig. 6.1).

Axial View

Usually the axial view is performed with the patient laying onto the x-ray table with his body axis in parallel to the table, but may also be performed with the patient sitting next to the table. The affected side is abducted to an angle between 60° and 90° and stuffed so that the shoulder joint is positioned in the center of the x-ray film (see Fig. 6.2). The x-ray tube is in a 90° position with cranio-caudal central ray being focused on to the humeral head almost parallel to the body axis (see Fig. 6.3). This view allows for an undistorted

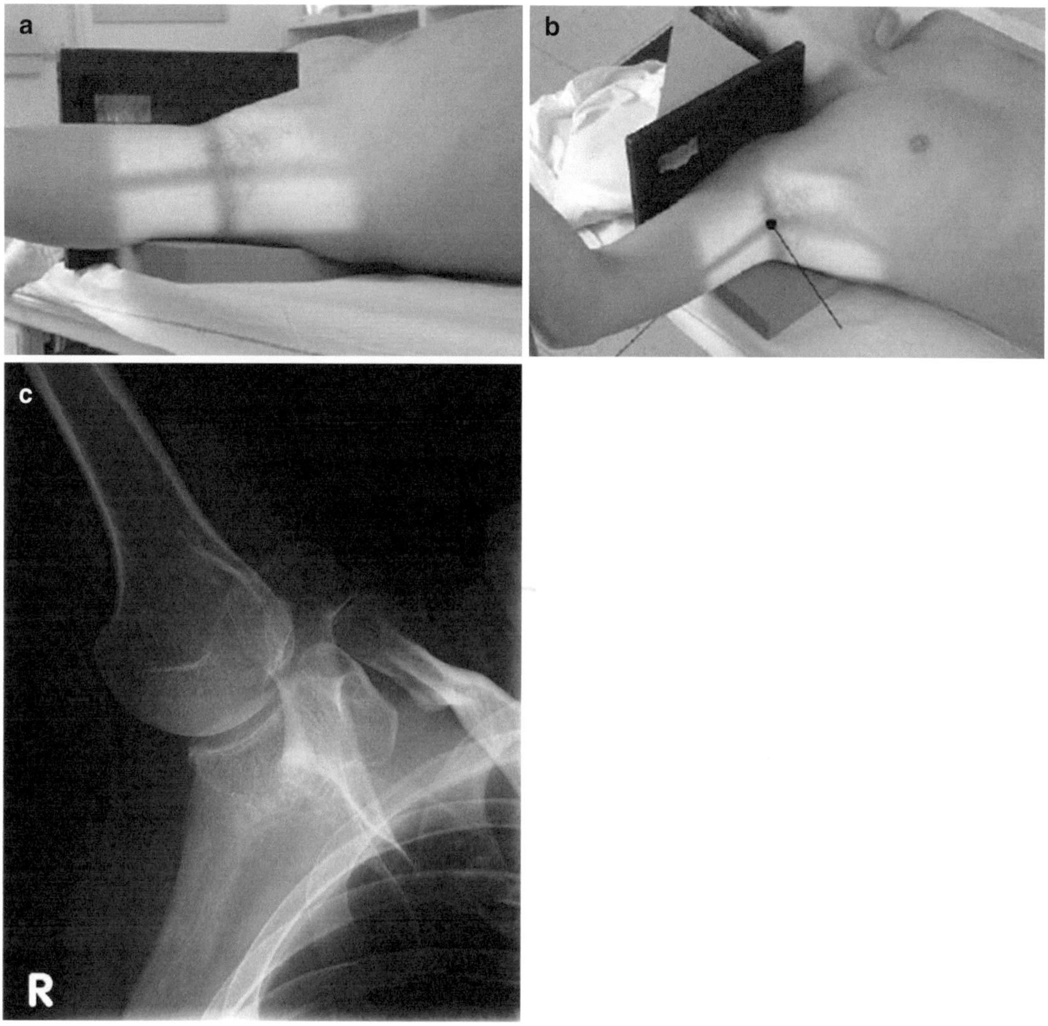

Fig. 6.2 Axial view of a right shoulder joint. Normal findings (Reprinted with permission from *Lehrbuch der röntgendiagnostischen Einstelltechnik*, 6th edition, 2008)

view of the coracoid process and the acromioclavicular joint being projected onto the upper arm. A well adjusted radiograph shows the humeral head and glenoid clearly arranged and without any severe overlap. The shoulder joint region is virtually seen bottom-up like.

Alternative: Velpeau View

As alternative to the axial view the technique according to Velpeau should be mentioned. This technique offers in comparison to the axial view the advantage that the affected side does not necessarily need to be taken out of the sling [7]. For this x-ray technique the patient is sitting with his back opposite to the x-ray table leaning backwards for approximately 30°. The central ray hits the center of the shoulder joint running perpendicular to the x-ray film. This radiographic view presents the gleno-humeral joint in an augmented way with the humeral shaft appearing shortened and thus the relation between the humeral head and the glenoid is well evaluatable. However, several bony overprojections might be present so that in general the axial view should preferably be performed.

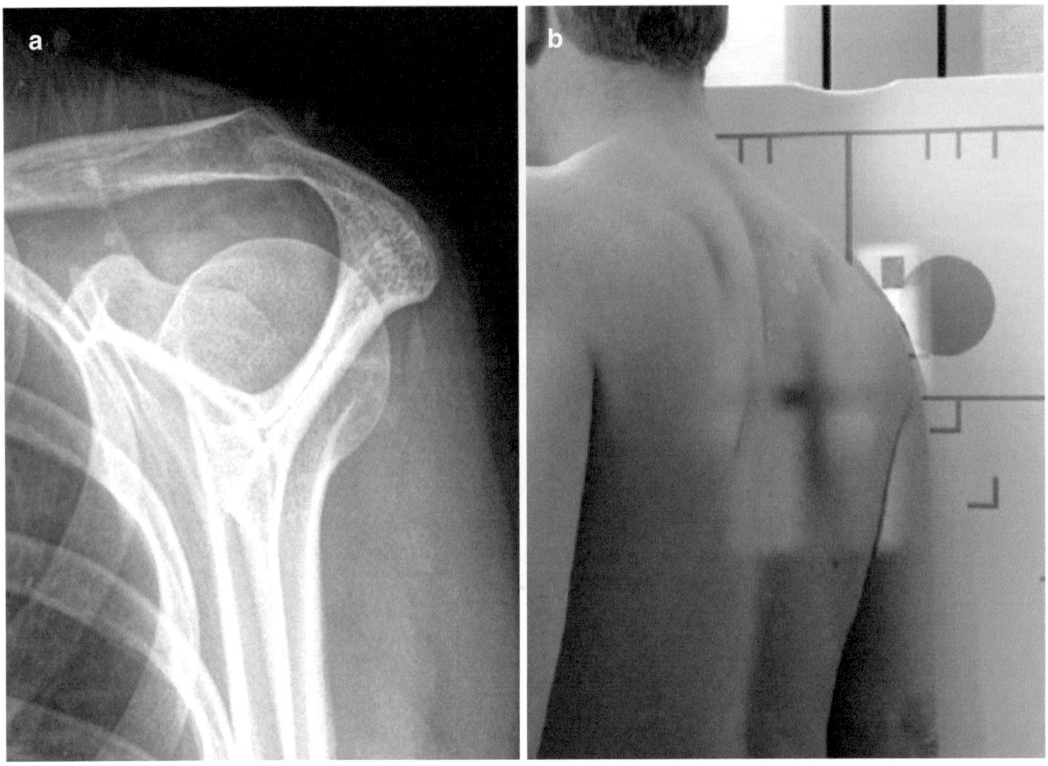

Fig. 6.3 Scapular y-view of a right sighted shoulder joint. Normal findings (Reprinted with permission from *Lehrbuch der röntgendiagnostischen Einstelltechnik*, 6th edition, 2008)

Lateral View (y-View, Transscapular View)

The patient is standing sideways to the stand with the affected side bearing on with both arms hanging down. The healthy side is tilted ventrally for approximately 45° so that the plain scapular bone is positioned perpendicular to the x-ray film (see Fig. 6.3). The x-ray beam is focussed vertically running latero-medial through the scapula.

In case of a dislocated shoulder joint this radiograph can be performed additionally to the (true) a-p view without any problems since the axial projection is often not possible due to pain. The scapula is pictured as the long bracket of a "y" whereas the short bracket on the ventral side is the coracoid process and on the dorsal side the spina scapulae without overprojection of the ribs. The humeral head is projected onto the glenoid. In case of a dislocation the joint socket looks "empty".

Trauma Series (True a-p, y-View, Axial-View)

In case a fracture of the proximal humerus is clinically suspected the so-called trauma series consisting of three radiographs as follows:

(a) (true) a-p view
(b) y-view
(c) axial view [8] should be performed (Table 6.1).

Discussion

The plain X-rays are still the most important tool for initial fracture diagnostics. In the commonly used trauma series the gold standard for initial evaluation is an AP view in the plane of the scapula, a scapular Y- and the axial view. According to Neer, for the initial evaluation of proximal

Table 6.1 Overview of indications for radiographical examinations of the shoulder joint and proximal humerus respectively

Indication	Choice of x-ray projection
Basic Trauma diagnostics	Shoulder joint in 2 planes:
	1. a-p view in neutral position (standard view)
	2. Axial view
Subcapital humeral fracture	1. a-p view in neutral position (standard view)
	2. Transcapular view
Anterior/posterior dislocation	1. a-p view in neutral position (standard view)
Control after repositioning	2. Transscapular view
Fracture of greater tuberosity	1. a-p view in neutral position (standard view)
Often associated with subcapital humeral fracture	2. a-p view in internal rotation
or dislocation of the shoulder	3. a-p view in external rotation
Minor tuberosity fracture	1. a-p view in neutral position (standard view)
	2. Axial view

humeral fractures an AP-view and a scapular Y-view are recommended. If the exact classification of the fracture remains unclear, an axial view needs additionally be performed [9]. Bahrs et al. [10] demonstrated in their study the superiority of the axial view regarding overlap and assessment of the relevant osseous structures, when compared to the scapular Y-view. Similar to their study, other authors also strictly recommend the axial view as standard view in combination with the AP view [6, 11–13].

Sidor et al. [14] classified 50 cases of proximal humeral fractures using the trauma series (AP, axial, scapular Y-view). The trauma series was evaluated for information regarding fracture classification. The authors showed that a correct fracture classification was possible in 99 % of the cases by combining the AP with the axial view. However, a combination of AP and scapular Y-view resulted only in 79 % of the cases in a correct fracture classification with the conclusion that an axial view delivers significantly more information regarding fracture classification than the scapular Y-view.

In general the performance of the AP view is not associated with technical difficulties. This view provides a visualization almost overlap free of the proximal humerus so that an adequate assessment of osseous structures such as the greater tuberosity, the glenoid and the subacromial space is possible in most cases. However, problems arise, if for the AP radiograph the arm is positioned in internal rotation and/ or the x-ray beam is inclined so that the joint gap is only inadequately seen. This might lead to a misdiagnosis especially in cases of a posterior dislocation of the shoulder due to an overlap of the humeral head and the glenoid (Fig. 6.4) [12, 15, 16].

The scapular y-view allows for an evaluation of the position of the joint and the relationship between the humeral shaft and head. Bahrs et al. found in their study [10] a decent osseous overlap of the proximal humerus and the shoulder joint in about 70 % with a considerably limited evaluation of especially the glenoid, the humeral head and the minor tuberosity as well.

Concomitant injuries such as fractures of the greater tuberosity, fractures of the glenoid rim, Hill-Sachs-lesion but also bony Bankart lesions can be clearly diagnosed. However especially for the diagnosis of a posterior dislocation of the shoulder this view is essential. About 60 % of the cases of a posterior dislocation are primarily overlooked in other x-ray projections since a posterior dislocation in contrast to an anterior dislocation might pretend normal articular conditions in AP view.

Regarding the axial view it can possibly deliver valuable additional information regarding bony concomitant injuries to fractures and luxations, although this technique is quite demanding. In case of a posterior luxation the focus is set on the proof and size of the often present reversed Hill Sachs lesion. Also fractures of the minor

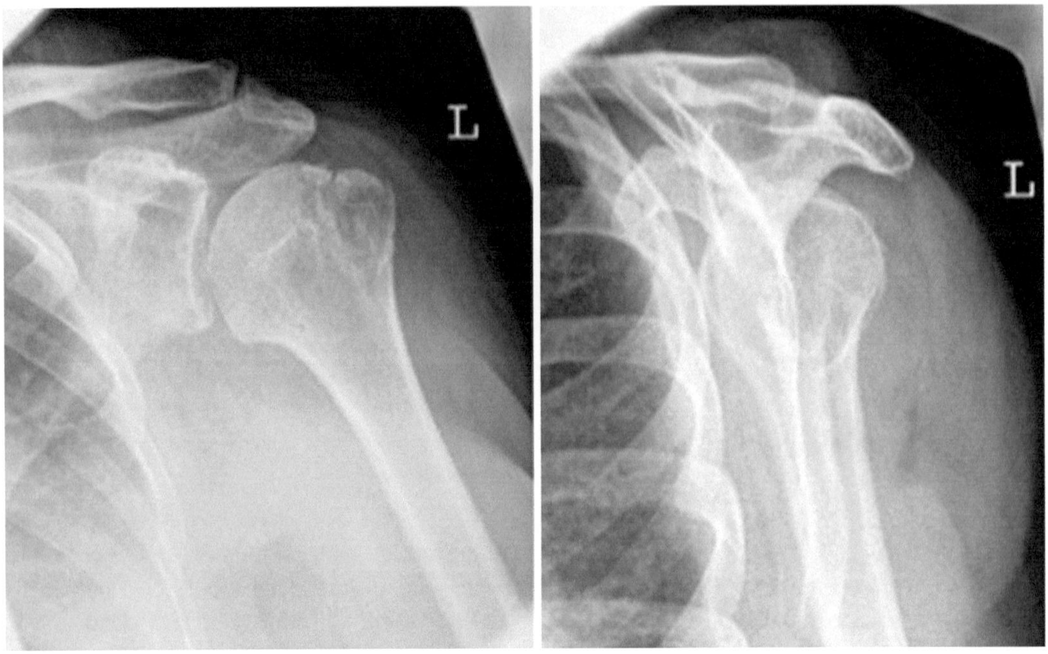

Fig. 6.4 Non-dislocated fracture of the greater tuberosity

tuberosity and the glenoid can more adequately be displayed compared to other x-ray projections.

Due to the mostly severe pain associated with relieving posture of the affected extremity the requested active excursion of the arm necessary for this x-ray projection is usually not possible. However, if the treating doctor performs a passive abduction of the affected arm and also explains the need of this special x-ray view in detail to the patient in most cases the performance of the axial view is still possible.

In summary although the performance of the axial view is in most cases stressful for patients with acute humeral head fractures the traumatologist should not resign from it since this is the only x-ray view with a good depiction of the humeral head – humeral shaft axis in sagittal plane delivering sufficient information about the minor tuberosity (Fig. 6.5).

Summary

Plain radiographs including ap-view and high-quality axillary view are useful for primary diagnostics of proximal humeral fractures and often but not always show a clear presentation of the relevant bony structures such as both tuberosities, the glenoid and the humeral head. It is common knowledge that not in all cases of injury to the proximal humerus all described x-ray views need to be performed. However, in general a documentation in two different orthogonal planes should be carried out.

If image quality impairs fracture visualization or if osseous overlap prevents from a visualization of the fractured structures, conventional radiography is not sufficient. In such situations computed tomography (CT) should be performed if the proximal humerus and the shoulder joint are not sufficiently presented on x-rays to be able to establish an optimal treatment plan.

The knowledge on x-ray techniques and application of the presented x-ray setting possibilities are major prerequisites for an adequate classification according to the commonly used classification systems. The imaging modality has partly considerable influence onto the way of treatment and at the end onto the prognosis. In this context a good, complementable interdisciplinary teamwork among radiologists and trauma surgeons has a major impact.

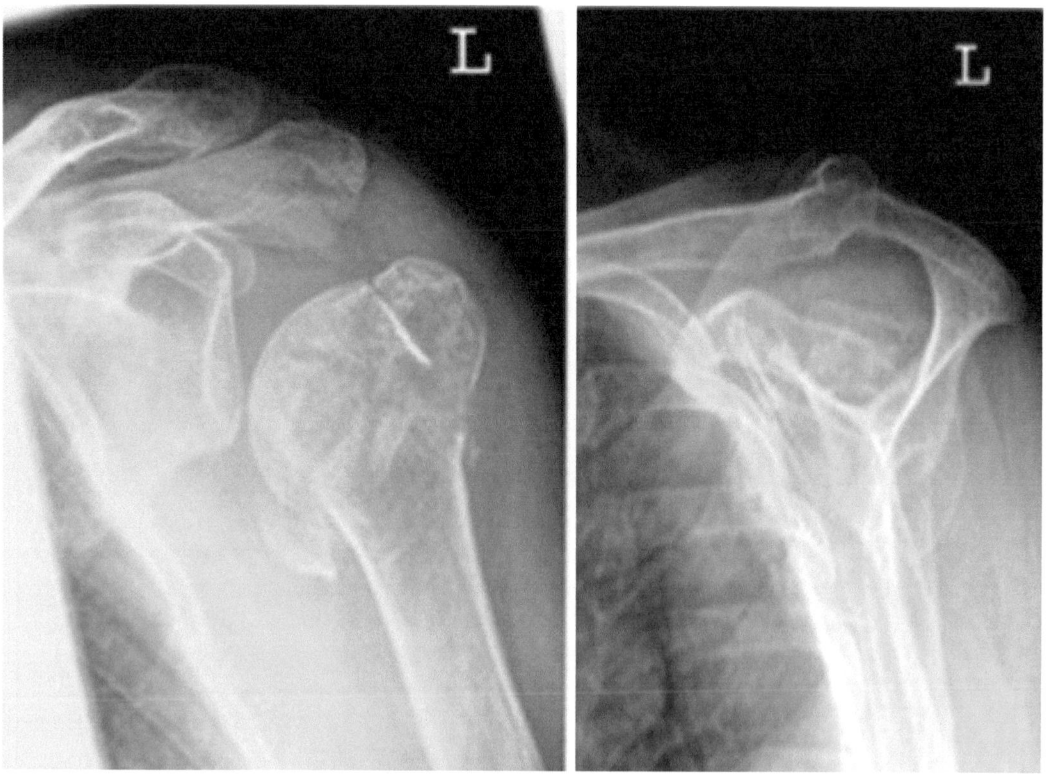

Fig. 6.5 Multi-fragment fracture of the humeral head

References

1. Nicholson DA, Lang I, Hughes P, Driscoll PA. ABC of emergency radiology. The shoulder. BMJ. 1993;307:1129–34.
2. Iannotti JP, Ramsey ML, Williams Jr GR, Warner JJ. Nonprosthetic management of proximal humeral fractures. Instr Course Lect. 2004;53:403–16.
3. Neer 2nd CS. Four-segment classification of proximal humeral fractures: purpose and reliable use. J Shoulder Elbow Surg. 2002;II(4):389–400.
4. Lill H, Josten C. Proximal and distal humerus fractures in advanced age. Orthopade. 2000;29:327–41.
5. Szyszkowitz R, Schippinger G. Fractures of the proximal humerus. Unfallchirurg. 1999;102:422–8.
6. Resch H. Fractures of the humeral head. Unfallchirurg. 2003;106:602–17.
7. Bloom MH, Obata W. Diagnosis of posterior dislocation of the shoulder with use of Velpeau axillary and angle up roentgenographic views. J Bone Joint Surg. 1967;49(A):943–9.
8. Bigliani LU. Fractures of the shoulder. Part I: fractures of the proximal humerus. In: Rockwood CA, Green DP, Buchholz RW, editors. Fracture in adults. 3rd ed. Philadelphia: JB Lippincott; 1991. p. 871–927.
9. Neer 2nd CS. Displaced proximal humeral fractures part I. Classification and evaluation 1970. Clin Orthop Relat Res. 2006;442:77–82.
10. Bahrs C, Rolauffs B, Südkamp NP, Schmal H, et al. Indications for computed tomography (CT) diagnostics in proximal humeral fractures: a comparative study of plain radiography and computed tomography. BMC Muskuloskelet Dis. 2009;10:33. doi:10.1186/1471-2474-10-33.
11. Schnabel M, Bahrs C, Walthers E, Gotzen L. Marburg shoulder radiography splint for standardized and high quality plain film radiography in fractures of the proximal humerus. Unfallchirurg. 2004;107:1099–102.
12. Clough TM, Bale RS. Bilateral posterior shoulder dislocation: the importance of the axillary radiographic view. Eur J Emerg Med. 2001;8:161–3.
13. Heyer D. Imaging methods in traumatology of the shoulder and elbow joint. Aktuelle Radiol. 1996;6:225–31.
14. Sidor ML, Zuckerman JD, Lyon T, Koval K, Schoenberg N. Classification of proximal humeral fractures: the contribution of the scapular lateral and axillary radiographs. J Shoulder Elbow Surg. 1994;3:24–7.
15. Hatzis N, Kaar TK, Wirth MA, Rockwood Jr CA. The often overlooked posterior dislocation of the shoulder. Tex Med. 2001;97:62–7.
16. Perron AD, Jones RL. Posterior shoulder dislocation: avoiding a missed diagnosis. Am J Emerg Med. 2000;18:189–91.

7 Special Imaging

Sonja M. Kirchhoff

Introduction

Fractures of the proximal humerus present the third most common fracture type of the elderly population following proximal femur and distal radial fractures. In the diagnostic cascade the intensive initial clinical exam of the affected extremity should be followed by conventional radiographs in at least two planes which had and still has an essential and dominant role in acute trauma care.

Imaging Modalities

Computed Tomography (CT)

Due to the nature of radiographs it is often not possible to definitely rule out a proximal humerus fracture especially when the x-rays are not adequately performed mostly due to patient's discomfort. Also in cases of complex proximal humerus fractures further imaging examinations in terms of computed tomography (CT) should be performed to get further information of the bony situation [1].

S.M. Kirchhoff
Department of Clinical Radiology, Munich University Hospital, Downtown Campus, Ludwig Maximilian University of Munich, Munich, Germany
e-mail: sonja.kirchhoff@me.com

Because of recent technical breakthroughs multidetector CT (MDCT) of the latest generation allows for performing two-dimensional reformats (multiplanar reconstruction MPR) as well as three dimensional (3D) surface rendering of excellent quality in very little amount of time because of fast image processing.

Compared to helical CT, MDCT presents a faster imaging modality with lesser artifacts, reduced partial volume effects along with decreased image noise and the possibility of assessing high quality MPRs. These qualities increase the diagnostic power of MDCT resulting in a definite benefit for trauma patients. High quality MPRs are especially useful when it comes to complex fractures of the shoulder joint and therefore coronal as well as sagittal oblique reformats should be acquired in the daily clinical routine when scanning a patient with proximal humerus fracture.

In general but also regarding proximal humerus fractures the radiation exposure of MDCT should always be concerned. It is usually higher compared to conventional radiography, but CT of the bones can be regarded as rather low dose examination especially providing important information for the treating surgeon to decide for the optimal therapy.

By CT it is possible to better demonstrate the displacement, rotation and integrity of the articular surface of the humeral head [2, 3] (see Fig. 7.1). Nowadays the performance of CT after

P. Biberthaler et al. (eds.), *Fractures of the Proximal Humerus*, Strategies in Fracture Treatments,
DOI 10.1007/978-3-319-20300-3_7

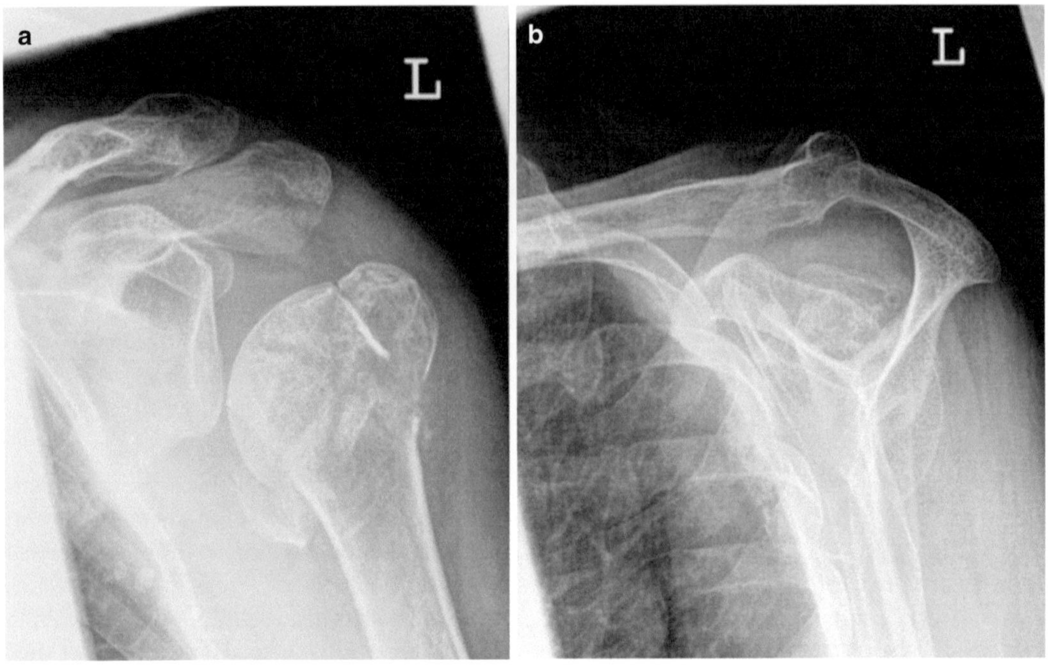

Fig. 7.1 Radiographs in a-p (**a**) and lateral (**b**) view of a 74 year old patient who fell onto his left shoulder showing a multi-part fracture of the proximal humerus

proximal humerus fracture is indispensable for the preoperative planning. In case of a head split fracture, impression fractures of the humeral head as well as suspected bony concomitant lesions e.g. of the glenoid or the scapula CT helps to detect otherwise often not recognized bony lesions (Fig. 7.2).

In general CT is a commonly used imaging modality when it comes to the assessment of traumatic injuries of the shoulder. In comparison to conventional radiography already axial CT images help to increase the accuracy of classifying the fracture adequately as well as help to correctly plan the surgical procedure and to decide for the optimal therapy regimen.

It is known that especially displaced three- or even four-part fractures of the proximal humerus are associated with a high incidence of humeral head avascular necrosis. Thus, these fractures have to be treated adequately depending on the number and dislocation of the fragments [4, 5] so that the extent of the fracture itself as well as number and localisation of the fragments need to be correctly identified. Although the diagnostic cascade after proximal humerus fracture starts with conventional radiography of the affected extremity it is sometimes quite difficult for several reasons (see Chap. 6) to adequately assess fracture fragments and their exact location especially if the lesser tuberosity is affected on plain radiography. Not only in exactly describing the fracture and its extent itself but also in detecting concomitant bony lesions such as fractures of the coracoid process x-rays provide only poor sensitivity. However, for the identification of bony Bankart lesions on conventional x-rays Haapamaki et al. reported a rather good sensitivity [6] which is of great importance since fractures of the glenoid with large fragments might cause an anterior instability of the shoulder joint [7]. Also in this context CT provides superior image quality compared to conventional radiography [8] as described by Haapamaki et al. [6] as well (Figs. 7.3 and 7.4).

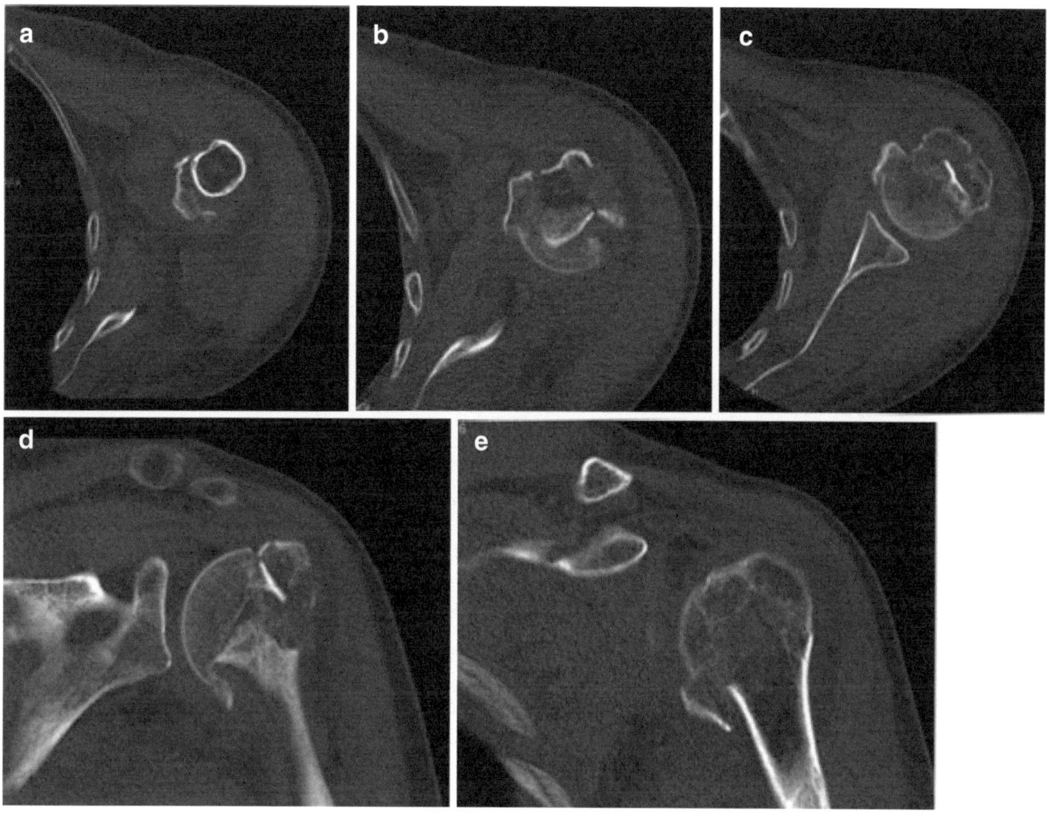

Fig. 7.2 Although the radiographs (Fig. 7.1) showed the presence of multi-part fracture of the proximal humerus of the left side a MDCT exam of the patient's left shoulder was performed to get information on the exact number of fragments, the fracture lines as well as whether the humeral head calotte is affected or not. (**a**–**c**) show CT-images in axial orientation with (**d**) and (**e**) presenting coronal reformats exactly presenting a four-part fracture of the proximal humerus without affecting the humeral head calotte

To summarize it is recommended to perform CT of the shoulder including multiplanar reformats and a 3D reconstruction on a routine basis in case of especially complex proximal humerus fractures to be able to adequately evaluate fracture morphology and to assess prognostic factors. So that in general on the basis of the CT images it should be evaluated whether there is valgus or varus position of the calvarium along with a flexion/extension position and/or rotational malposition, if there is an impaction or distraction present, determine the number of fragments as well as the length of the posteromedial calcar and the dislocation at the medial hinge to be able to choose for the optimal treatment.

Magnetic Resonance Imaging (MRI)

In general MRI is known for its superb soft tissue contrast and missing radiation exposure as compared to x-rays and CT so that MR-examinations own a high significance when it comes to musculoskeletal imaging especially as imaging modality for evaluating joints and traumatic joint injuries [9].

The typical disadvantages of MRI especially compared to CT are known as follows: first of all its availability, its cost and the compared to CT significantly prolonged examination times which makes MRI rather useless for acute trauma care.

Performing MRI it is possible to show that a proximal humerus fracture is not just an injury to

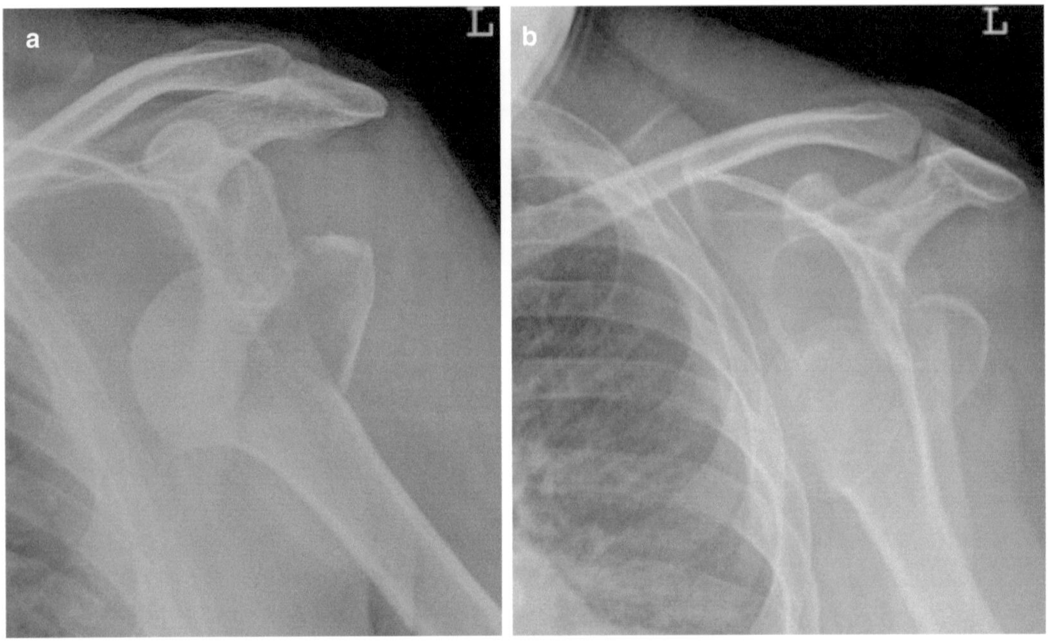

Fig. 7.3 The radiographs in a-p (**a**) and lateral (**b**) view under suboptimal conditions show an anterior-inferior dislocation of the left shoulder of a 65 year old patient after a fall. The greater tuberosity seems fractured and slightly displaced with a non-axial alignment within the gleno-humeral joint

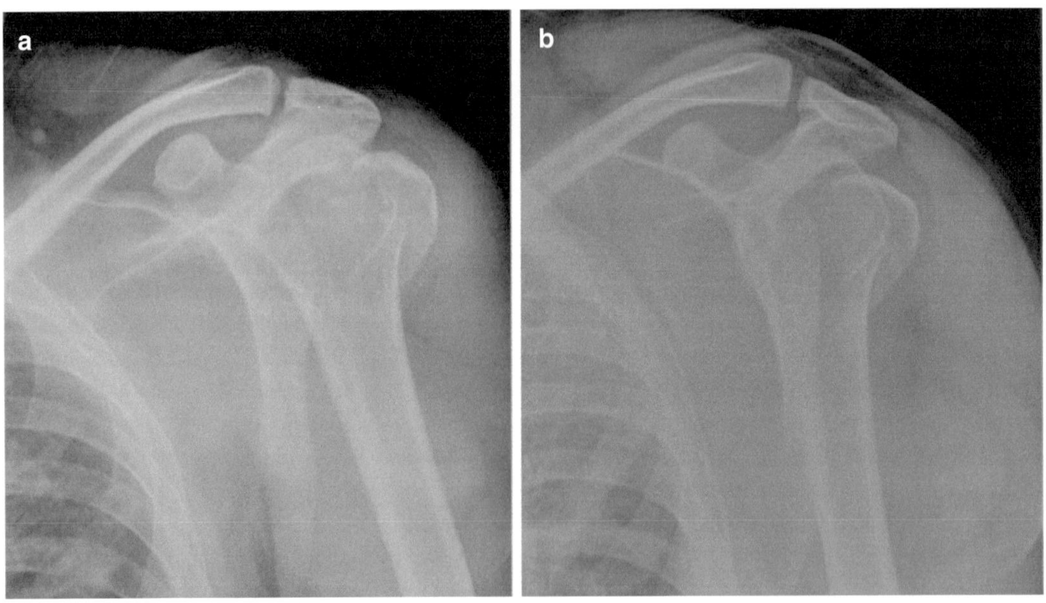

Fig. 7.4 These radiographs (**a**) a-p view, (**b**) lateral view show the status after closed reduction of the left shoulder of a 65 year old patient. A good axial alignment is reached. However the fracture of the greater tuberosity is still visible but seems not as much displaced as in the previous radiographs (Fig. 7.3)

the bone but is usually associated with injuries to the surrounding tissues such as the rotator cuff (RC) and others.

In the current literature a positive correlation between the severity of proximal humerus fractures and RC lesions had been described by several authors [10, 11]. However, the definite role of the RC injury to the functional outcome after proximal humerus fractures is yet not completely understood, however recent studies in the literature state that RC injuries along with a proximal humerus fracture do not result in significantly worsened functional outcome of the shoulder joint [10, 12].

The domain of CT is the depiction of the osseous changes whereas MRI's domain lays within the demonstration of soft tissue and its pathological changes. Since due to the increasing patients' age and activity more and more older people do suffer from proximal humerus fractures possibly presenting with degenerative changes of the RC. Concludingly, in singular cases depending on the clinical evaluation a preoperative MRI might be useful to rule out pathologies e.g. of the RC or to define the extent of soft tissue injury for the exact planning of the surgical intervention [13]. However, 50 % of the patients older than 60 years show signal abnormalities in the RC being consistent with signs of tears [14]. Therefore regarding a screening tool for patients suffering from proximal humerus fractures MRI has not been proven to be a cost-effective economic tool and neither has arthroscopy.

In this context the work of Wilmanns et al. [11] should be mentioned describing a correlation between RC injuries and the proximal humerus fracture type according to the AO classification. Their findings are supported by the results of Fjalestad et al. [15] suggesting that additional RC tears are not caused by degeneration but are rather part of the injury leading primarily to the proximal humerus fracture.

However, reading an MR-exam after proximal humerus fractures with injured soft tissues and of course an abnormal anatomy, does raise some difficulties especially regarding the exact detection of partial and full thickness tears respectively of the RC tendons. In this context Potter et al. [16] described in their study a high detection rate of 98 % for full thickness tears whereas for partial thickness tears only 70 % of the cases were recognized which is equal to results known from ultrasound [13].

Another factor deteriorating MR images is blood in the articular cavity of the shoulder joint especially when it is located in the subacromial-subdeltoid bursa since it may derive from a full thickness tear of the RC, but may also be of secondary character due to posttraumatic bursitis.

In addition in case of proximal humerus fractures MRI should be performed to be able to clarify whether the quality of the RC allows for the implantation of a fracture prosthesis which is considered due to severe soft tissue – as well as bony injuries.

If in the posttraumatic or even post-operative phase when an avascular necrosis (AVN) of the humeral head is clinically or radiographically suspected MRI presents the imaging method of choice to confirm or exclude the diagnosis of an AVN. On MR-images it is possible to assess vitality of the humeral head and the exact extent of the AVN. In case of diagnosis of an AVN also MRI-follow-up exams should be considered to evaluate progressive or stable conditions of the humeral head to be able to adequately react in every case with the optimal treatment (Fig. 7.5).

If posttraumatically a lesion of the plexus brachialis is suspected MR-images are definitely helpful to demonstrate first of all the continuity of the plexus which is of great prognostic value, but also to rule out significant injury to soft tissue of the shoulder joint such as hematomas especially along the anatomic course of the plexus brachialis. In this context it should be mentioned that plexus brachialis lesions are of rather rare incidence in "normal" proximal humerus fractures but might occur in cases of motor cycle accidents (Fig. 7.6).

In summary MRI has no significance in the acute diagnostic work up following proximal humerus fractures. However, for the evaluation of

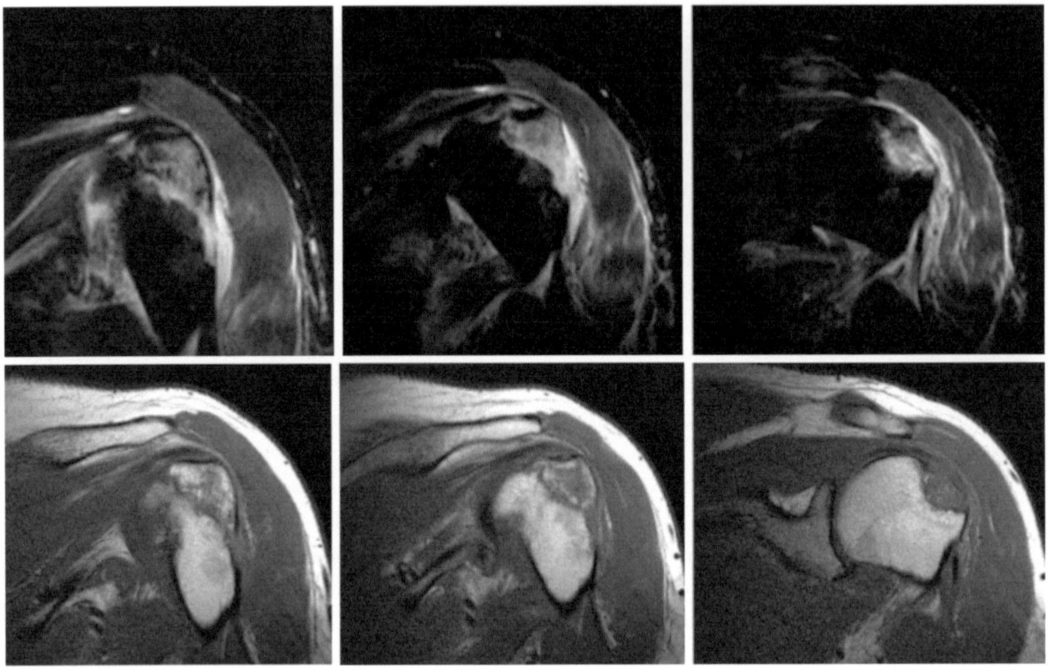

Fig. 7.5 Since the radiographs pointed out that the greater tuberosity was fractured a lesion to the rotator cuff was suspected so that the decision was made to perform a MR-examination of the shoulder. The *upper row* of images presents T2-weighted STIR images in coronal orientation with corresponding T1-weighted coronal images in the *lower row*. On the STIR-sequence a bone marrow edema of the fractured but not displaced greater tuberosity is visible along with effusion in the bursa subdeltoidea and subacromialis as well as a slight hyperintensity of the insertion of the supraspinatus tendon with corresponding hypointensity on T1-w images suspicious for traumatic lesion of the rotator cuff

a clinically suspected RC lesion MRI might be performed although these lesions can basically be determined by US as well depending on the examiner's experience. In the posttraumatic course however MRI is of great importance regarding the determination of a posttraumatic avascular necrosis (AVN) of the humeral head since on MR images it is possible to assess the vitality of the head fragments and of course to perform follow-up exam to rule out and confirm a progress of AVN respectively.

However, up to date there exists no consensus regarding the performance of MRI for imaging of the RC in context with the presence of a proximal humerus fracture. Since proximal humerus fractures provide a high incidence and there is a possible contribution to an unpredictable outcome, the tendons of the RC warrant a significant diagnostic work-up and corresponding treatment especially in case of three- and four-part fractures and all two-part fractures with dislocation of the greater tuberosity >5 mm. For these type of fractures the RC tendons should either be visualized directly during the fracture fixation or in case of conservative treatment MRI or US should be performed if the patient is however a candidate for surgery. In this context we agree with the diagnostic work-up algorithm as suggested by Gallo et al. [17]. The authors suggest that no initial MRI is necessary in case of any one-part or two-part fractures with only minimal displacement of the greater tuberosity (GT) since the incidence for RC tears is low. For more displaced GT in case of two-part or three- or more part fractures with a high incidence of RC lesions and inconsistent functional results advanced imaging or even direct visualisation of the RC is recommended.

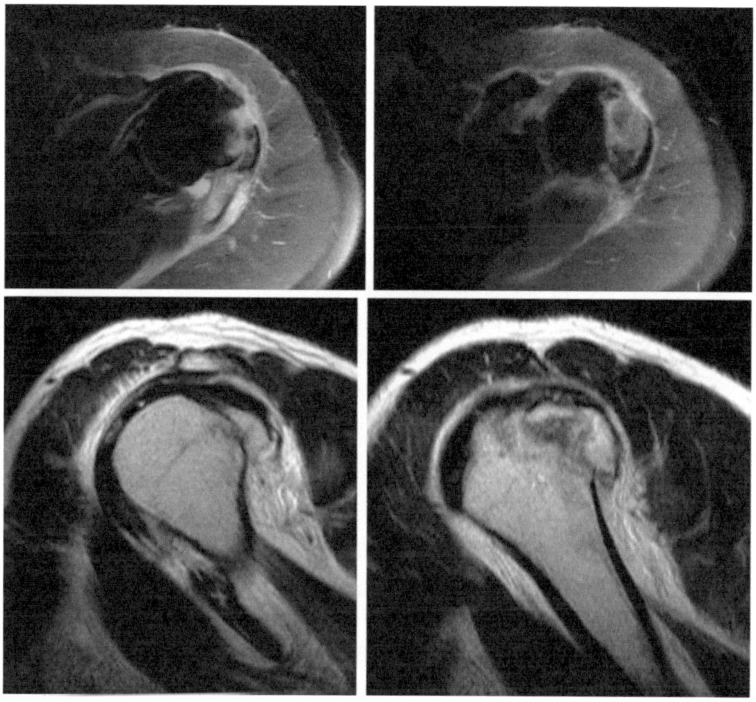

Fig. 7.6 The *upper* 2 MR-images show a proton density fat saturated axial view onto the left shoulder (see Figs. 7.3, 7.4 and 7.5). On these axial MR-images effusion is recognizable but here in the posterior part of the shoulder joint along the capsule as well as in the bursa subcoracoidea. As far as possibly evaluated no greater lesion of the glenoid is visible. The *lower row* presents T2-weighted sagittal images of the shoulder showing the fractured slightly displaced greater tuberosity along with the slight distraction of the supraspinatus tendon and surrounding fluid

Ultrasound (US)

A well-known cost-efficient alternative imaging modality to MRI for the evaluation of the soft tissue situation of the shoulder joint or of the musculoskeletal system in general is ultrasound (US) being performed using a linear usually 7.5 MHz transducer [18]. Performing ultrasound of the shoulder joint it is possible to evaluate the conditions of the RC especially regarding the presence of partial or full thickness tears, the extent of hematoma, fragments and possible soft tissue interposition.

The well known, most important advantage of US in comparison to the other described imaging modalities is the fact that US can also be performed dynamically as well as in comparison to the other side.

In addition, possible lesions of the long head of the biceps tendon as well as its dislocation out of the sulcus intertubercularis or its rupture can be proven.

The most important disadvantage of US is the fact that this examination is examiner-dependent as compared to CT and MRI and is thus restricted to centers with radiologists or orthopedic surgeons experienced with this technique. Another disadvantage lays in the lower sensitivity and importance in the diagnostics of proximal humerus fracture itself. However detection and correct classification of proximal humerus fractures [19] and the differentiation from RC tears is very important since therapy differs [20]. Rutten et al. [21] as well as Zanetti and coworkers [22] reported in their publications that often in patients suffering from a trauma to the upper extremity proximal humerus fractures are missed on conventional radiographs but can reliably be detected by MRI [22], CT and/ or US. Furthermore, US may be too painful for the patients with proximal humerus fractures to tolerate.

It is reported in the literature that Hill-Sachs lesions are frequently missed on x-rays [23] where they can reliably be detected using US [24]. However in this context it needs to be mentioned that these studies are rather old and that the currently required trauma series or at least x-rays in 2 orthogonal planes usually allow for a distinct detection of Hill-Sachs-lesions if performed adequately. Another reason is the fact that MRI as well as US are not commonly performed in the initial work-up of patients with traumatized shoulders.

In summary US as well as MRI do not pertain to the initial diagnostic work up of patients with proximal humerus fractures.

However, US of the shoulder after proximal humerus fracture is recommended in case the examiner is experienced to assess the status of the RC and potential tears despite possible limits of the exam due to swelling, hematoma etc.

Angiography

Vascular complications along with a traumatized shoulder joint are relatively rare but if so most of them resulted from an anterior dislocation of the gleno-humeral joint [25] whereas an injury to the axillary artery after proximal humerus fracture were also reported in the literature [26, 27]. Injury to the axillary artery after proximal humerus fracture are mostly due to a laceration of the circumflex arteries or subscapularis artery by the effect of abduction of the distal fragment. However, Neer et al. [19] did not describe a single case of axillary artery injury in their series on 117 patients with proximal humerus fractures. But in the few cases of a with a proximal humerus fracture associated vascular injury the results were either acute ischemia of the affected extremity or neuronal damage and the diagnosis was obvious [28, 29]. Even of more rare incidence is the presence of late vascular injury which happen to be more serious than the common vascular complications. However, every sign of vascular injury following shoulder trauma should carefully be evaluated and considered as emergency whereas the treating physician should not hesitate to perform angiography and consult surgery.

If there is no angiography setting available the treating physician should consider performing a CT-angiography applying intravenous iodinated contrast media to rule out and/or detect respectively eventual vascular lesions of the upper thorax aperture or the shoulder area.

In summary, trauma to the shoulder joint may end in fatal axillary artery injury. To prevent from iatrogen vascular lesions one should perform maneuvers of fracture reduction or of reposition in case of dislocation gentle and should avoid excessive forces. However, if the peripheral pulse is reduced or progressive signs of ischemia of the affected extremity are present an emergency situation has occurred and accordingly emergent angiography should be performed or alternatively a non-invasive CT-angiography to get an overview of the vascular situation and plan the further proceeding.

Summary

In patients with complex proximal humerus fractures if the extent and morphology of the fracture itself and the exact position and origin of dislocated fragments respectively is not quite clear on conventional x-rays the performance of MDCT including reformats in sagittal and coronal orientation is recommended as complimentary examination. This imaging modality usually increases the accuracy of classifying the fracture correctly and may detect on radiography occult fractures of the shoulder joint.

MRI does not represent an imaging modality of the initial diagnostic work-up after proximal humerus fracture. However, the performance of MRI should be considered to assess the status of the RC especially in elderly patients to differentiate potential traumatic tears of the RC tendons from degenerative changes but also to evaluate the injury to the surrounding soft tissue in terms of hematoma, status of the long head of the biceps tendon etc as well as of the bone in terms of bone bruise or detection of occult fractures. Another typical indication for MRI following proximal humerus fracture is suspicion for AVN and to determine its extent and the vitality of the bone. However, MRI presents with the known disadvantages such as its availability, cost and also duration of the examination itself as compared to CT.

US as well as MRI do not pertain to the initial diagnostic work up of patients with proximal humerus fractures. However, US of the shoulder joint after proximal humerus fracture is recommended in case the examiner is experienced to assess the status of the RC when clinically RC tears are suspected and to diagnose the extent of soft tissue injury. US presents with the commonly known disadvantages such as examiner dependant, often limited evaluation due to swelling, hematoma etc but in comparison to MRI US is cost-effective, highly available and offers the possibility to perform dynamic exams also compared to the healthy side.

Trauma to the shoulder joint may end in fatal axillary artery injury. To prevent from iatrogen vascular lesions one should perform maneuvers of fracture reduction or of reposition in case of dislocation gentle and should avoid excessive forces. However, if the peripheral pulse is reduced or progressive signs of ischemia of the affected extremity are present an emergency situation has occurred and accordingly emergent angiography should be performed or alternatively a non-invasive CT-angiography to get an overview of the vascular situation and plan the further proceeding.

References

1. Forurla AM, de Gracia MM, Larson DR, et al. The pattern of the fracture and displacement of the fragments predict the outcome in proximal humeral fractures. J Bone Joint Surg Br. 2011;93:378–86.
2. Castagno AA, Shuman WP, Kilcoyne RF, Haynor DR, Morris ME, Matsen FA. Complex fractures of the proximal humerus: role of CT in treatment. Radiology. 1987;165:759–62.
3. Kilcoyne RF, Shuman WP, Matsen III FA, Morris M, Rockwood CA. The Neer classification of displaced proximal humeral fractures: spectrum of findings on plain radiographs and CT scans. AJR Am J Roentgenol. 1990;154:1029–33.
4. Tanner MW, Cofield RH. Prosthetic arthroplasty for fractures and fracture-dislocations of the proximal humerus. Clin Orthop. 1983;179:116–28.
5. Resch H, Povacz P, Frohlich R, Wambacher M. Percutaneous fixation of three- and four part fractures of the proximal humerus. J Bone Joint Surg Br. 1997;79:295–300.
6. Haapamaki VV, Kiuru MJ, Koskinen SK. Multidetector CT in shoulder fractures. Emerg Radiol. 2004;11:89–94.
7. Aston JW, Gregory CF. Dislocation of the shoulder with significant fracture of the glenoid. J Bone Joint Surg Am. 1973;55:1531–3.
8. Itoi E, Lee SB, Amrami KK, Wenger DE, An KN. Quantitative assessment of classic anteroinferior bony Bankart lesions by radiography and computed tomography. Am J Sports Med. 2003;31: 112–8.
9. Bohndorf K, Kilcoyne RF. Traumatic injuries: imaging of peripheral musculoskeletal injuries. Eur Radiol. 2002;12:1605–16.
10. Gallo RA, Sciulli R, Daffner RH, et al. Defining the relationship between rotator cuff injury and proximal humerus fractures. Clin Orthop. 2007;44: 131–8.
11. Wilmanns C, Bonnaire F. Rotator cuff alterations resulting from humeral head fractures. Injury. 2002;33:781–9.
12. Nanda R, Goodschild L, Gamble A, Campbell R, Rangan A. Does the presence of a full thickness rotator cuff tear influence outcome after proximal humerus fracture? J Trauma. 2007;62:1436–9.
13. Teefy SA, Rubin DA, Middleton WD, et al. Detection and quantification of rotator cuff tears: comparison of ultrasonographic, magnetic resonance imaging and arthroscopic findings in seventy one consecutive cases. J Bone Joint Surg Am. 2004;86:708–16.
14. Sher JS, Uribe JW, Posada A, et al. Abnormal findings on magnetic resonance images of asymptomatic shoulders. J Bone Joint Surg Am. 1995;77:10–5.
15. Fjalestad T, Hole M, Blücher J, et al. Rotator cuff tears in proximal humerus fractures: an MRI cohort study in 76 patients. Arch Orthop Trauma Surg. 2010;130:575–81.
16. Potter HG, Birchansky SB. Magnetic Resonance Imaging of the shoulder: a tailored approach. Tech Shoulder Elbow Surg. 2005;6:43–56.
17. Gallo RA, Altman DT, Altman GT. Assessment of rotator cuff tendons after proximal humerus fractures: is preoperative imaging necessary? J Trauma. 2009;66:951–3.
18. Kaplan PA, Matamaros AJ, Anderson JC. Sonography of the musculoskeletal system. AJR Am J Roentgenol. 1990;155:237–45.
19. Neer CS. Displaced proximal humeral fractures. 1. Classification and evaluation. J Bone Joint Surg Am. 1970;52A:1077–89.
20. Bassett RW, Cofield RH. Acute tears of the rotator cuff. The timing of surgical repair. Clin Orthop. 1983;175:18–24.
21. Rutten MJ, Jager GJ, et al. Double line sign: a helpful sonographic sign to detect occult fractures of the proximal humerus. Eur Radiol. 2007;17:762–7.
22. Zanetti M, Weishaupt D, Jost B, Gerber C, Hodler J. MR imaging for traumatic tears of the rotator cuff: high prevalence of greater tuberosity fractures and subscapularis tear. AJR Am J Roentgenol. 1999;172: 463–7.
23. Workman TL, Burkhard TK, Resnick D, et al. Hill-Sachs lesion: comparison of detection with MR

imaging, radiography and arthroscopy. Radiology. 1992;185:847–52.
24. Cicak N, Bilic R, Delimar D. Hill-Sachs lesions in recurrent shoulder dislocation: sonographic detection. J Ultrasound Med. 1998;17:557–60.
25. Jardon OM, Hood LT, Lynch RD. Complete avulsion of the axillary artery as a complication of the shoulder dislocation. J Bone Joint Surg Am. 1973;55A:189–92.
26. Byrd RG, Byrd Jr RP, Roy TM. Axillary artery injuries after proximal fracture of the humerus. Am J Emerg Med. 1998;16:154–6.
27. McLaughlin JA, Light R, Lustrin I. Axillary artery injury as a complication of proximal humerus fractures. J Shoulder Elbow Surg. 1998;7:292–4.
28. Leborgne J, LeNeel J, Mitard D, et al. Les lesions de l' artere axillaire et de ses branches consecutives a un traumatisme ferme de L' epaule. Ann Chir. 1973;27: 587–9.
29. Theodorides T, de Keizer G. Injuries of the axillary artery caused by fractures of the neck of the humerus. Injury. 1976;8:120–3.

Part II

Fracture Morphology and Injury Pattern

8 Classifications

Arne J. Venjakob

Proximal humeral fractures portray 5 % of all fractures in adults and represent the third most common fracture in adults over 65 years old [1]. Despite that there is no definite consensus in literature regarding the classification system so far.

In the following the most common classification systems will be presented:

Neer Classification

The Neer classification was established by Charles Neer II in 1970 [2]. This classification represents a modification of the Codman classification and implies the four-segment theory. This classification is based on the occurrence of displacement of one or more of the four major segments in terms of humeral shaft, humeral head, greater and lesser tuberosity. Six different fracture type groups have been introduced based on a patient collective of 300 patients with undislocated and dislocated proximal humeral fractures treated in the New York Orthopaedic Hospital between 1953 and 1967.

The Neer classification may represent the most commonly used classification for proximal humeral fractures although several authors determined a low intraobserver reproducibility and interobserver reliability [3–7]. The Neer classification presents a descriptive classification without any recommendation of therapy for the different fracture types. In general for the Neer classification a segment is considered as displaced when a dislocation >1 cm or an angle >45° is present.

Group I consists of all undislocated fractures regardless of the number of fracture lines (see Fig. 8.1). Neer stated that the treatment of this group would be identical and in most cases of conservative character.

Group II includes a displacement of the articular-segment at the anatomical neck without separation of one or both tuberosities (see Fig. 8.1). Although being rare this fracture configuration needs to be identified by strict anteroposterior radiographs of the shoulder in order to prevent malunion and vascular necrosis.

Group III characterizes fractures at the level of the surgical neck being displaced more than 1 cm or angulated more than 45°. Three variations of this fracture have been described in terms of an (A) impacted and angulated surgical neck fracture, (B) separated surgical neck fracture and (C) comminuted surgical neck fracture. In 1970

A.J. Venjakob
Sports Orthopaedics Department, Marienkrankenhaus Kaiserswerth, Duesseldorf, Germany

Department of Trauma Surgery, Klinikum rechts der Isar, Technical University of Munich, Munich, Germany
e-mail: Arne.Venjakob@lrz.tu-muenchen.de

P. Biberthaler et al. (eds.), *Fractures of the Proximal Humerus*, Strategies in Fracture Treatments,
DOI 10.1007/978-3-319-20300-3_8

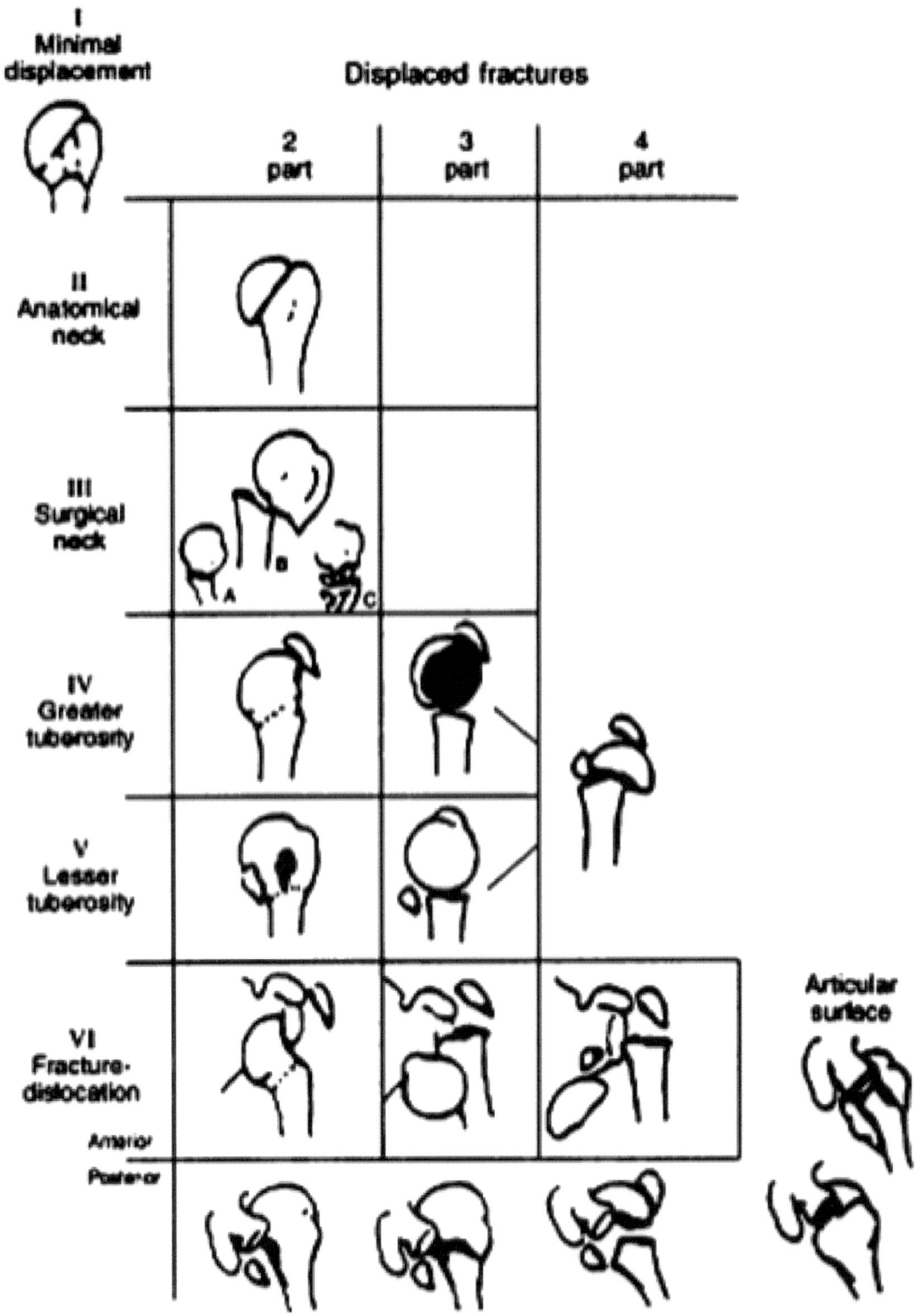

Fig. 8.1 Neer classification (Reprinted with permission from Neer [2])

conservative treatment options have been described by Charles Neer for group III fractures, whereas today displaced surgical neck fractures mainly are treated operatively.

In summary Group II and III fractures are classified as two-part fractures (see Fig. 8.1).

Group IV includes fractures of the greater tuberosity and may occur as two-, three- and four-part fractures (see Fig. 8.1). Two-part fractures reveal an articular segment which remains in normal position to the humeral shaft. A minimally displaced fracture of the surgical neck may be present as well. Three-part fractures are characterized by an additional fracture of the surgical neck often appearing due to an application of force by the subscapularis tendon resulting in internal rotation position. In four-part fractures a further detachment of the humeral head is present (see Fig. 8.1). Closed reduction of group IV fractures led to high rates of unsuccessful results mainly due to malunion [8].

In group V fractures a displacement of the lesser tuberosity is present. The two-part fracture of this group is characterized by a displacement of the lesser tuberosity, in some cases associated with an undisplaced fracture of the surgical neck. In three part fractures the surgical neck appears dislocated leading to abduction and external rotation position of the articular segment due to the attachment of the supraspinatus and infraspinatus tendon. The four-part fracture additionally reveals retraction of both tuberosities (see Fig. 8.1). Again closed reduction of group V fractures resulted in a high incidence of unsuccessful outcome.

In group VI fractures caused by a dislocation of the proximal humerus are summed up. Antero-inferior and posterior dislocation may occur in two-, three- and four-part fractures (see Fig. 8.1). It has been stated that a posterior displacement in combination with damage of more than 20 % of articular cartilage predisposes for recurrent shoulder instability and may require a so-called McLaughlin procedure in terms of a transplantation of the subscapularis tendon [9]. Defects greater than 50 % of the articular cartilage may even require prosthetic treatment.

Hertel Classification

The Hertel classification is predicated on the article "Fractures of the proximal humerus in osteoporotic bone" published by Ralph Hertel in the *Journal of Osteoporosis International* in 2005. In this article the author reviewed effective treatment options for proximal humeral fractures in patients suffering from severe osteoporosis [10]. In this context based on the original drawings [11] of Codman et al. a descriptive fracture classification was introduced by Hertel (see Fig. 8.2). In contrast to Neer's classification [2] based on the four segment theory, this classification is based on five fracture planes.

In this context five questions have been released to identify the basic fracture planes:

1. Is there a fracture between the greater tuberosity and the humeral head?
2. Is there a fracture between the greater tuberosity and the humeral shaft?
3. Is there a fracture between the lesser tuberosity and the humeral head?
4. Is there a fracture between the lesser tuberosity and the humeral shaft?
5. Is there a fracture between the lesser and the greater tuberosity?

Consequently these fracture planes lie between the greater tuberosity and the humeral head, the greater tuberosity and the humeral shaft, the lesser tuberosity and the humeral head, the lesser tuberosity and the humeral shaft and the lesser and greater tuberosity. The combination of these fracture planes results in 12 possible fracture patterns as illustrated in Fig. 8.2. Hertel pointed out that several additional aspects need to be considered regarding an appropriate fracture classification: subsequently the length of the postero-medial metaphyseal head extension and the integrity of the medial hinge present the most important criteria (see Fig. 8.3). Furthermore the displacement of the tuberosities, the amount of angular displacement of the humeral head, the occurrence of glenohumeral dislocation, an impression fracture of the humeral head, a headsplit component and the

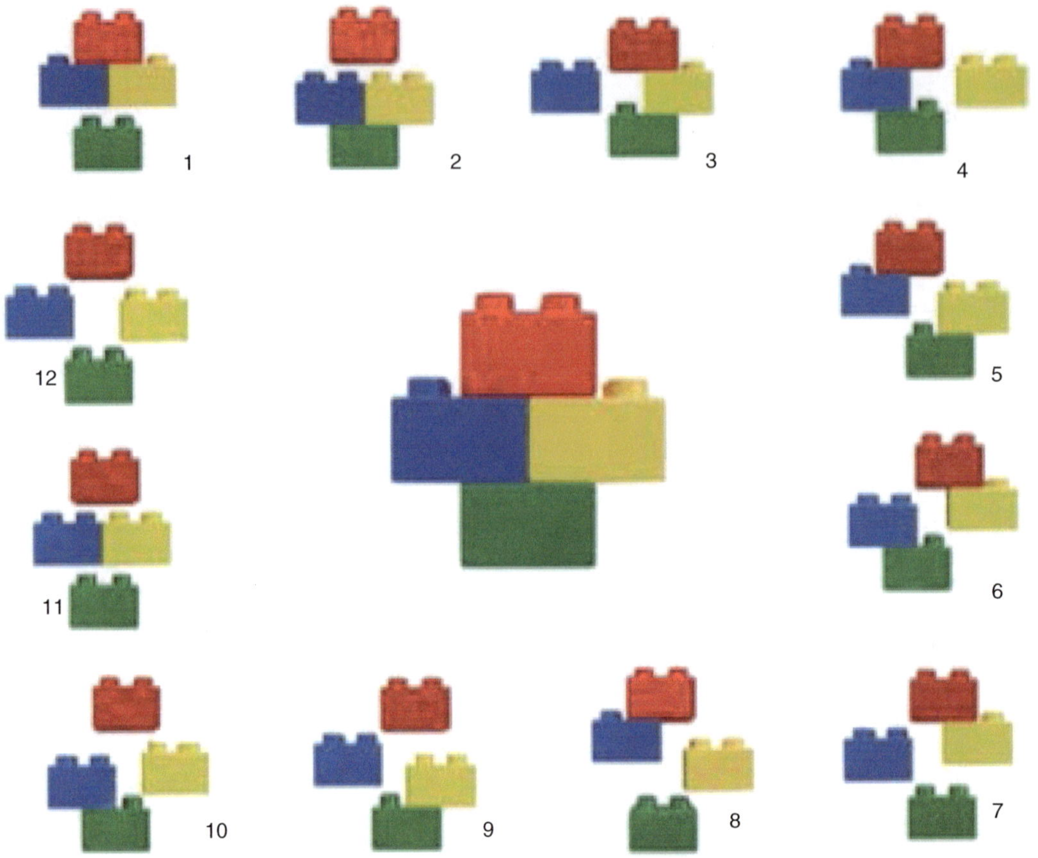

Fig. 8.2 Binary or "LEGO" descriptory system. The image illustrates the five basic fracture planes, resulting in 12 possible basic fractures: Six possible fractures devide the humerus into two fragments (figs. 1–6), five possible fractures devide the humerus into three fragments (figs. 7–11) and one single fracture devides the humerus into four fragments (fig. 12) (Reprinted with permission from Hertel [10])

mechanical quality of the bone are of utmost importance. All criteria are considered as predictors for the perfusion of the humeral head. Accordingly 100 consecutive fractures were prospectively analysed by Hertel et al. [11] in respect of humeral head ischemia, revealing the length of the metaphyseal head extension and the integrity of the medial hinge as good predictors for ischemia (see Fig. 8.3).

AO (Association for Osteosynthesis)/OTA (American Orthopaedic Trauma Association) Classification of Fractures and Dislocations

The AO classification (Association for Osteosynthesis, AO Foundation, Davos, Switzerland) for fractures of long bones was established in 1990 by Müller et al. [12]. Later this initial classification was further developed by surgeons and researchers of the AO and the American Orthopaedic Trauma Association (OTA) and is now officially named the AO/OTA Classification of Fractures and Dislocations.

This classification may contain the most accurate fracture-morphology compared to all other classification systems, being more comprehensive than the most commonly used Neer classification [13].

The first number of this classification represents the long bone (1 = humerus, 2 = radius/ulna, 3 = femur and 4 = tibia/fibula), the following defining the bone segment (1 = proximal, 2 = middle, 3 = distal and 4 = malleolar).

Proximal humeral fractures are therefore classified as 1.1-fractures and have been divided into extra-articular unifocal fractures (A), extra-

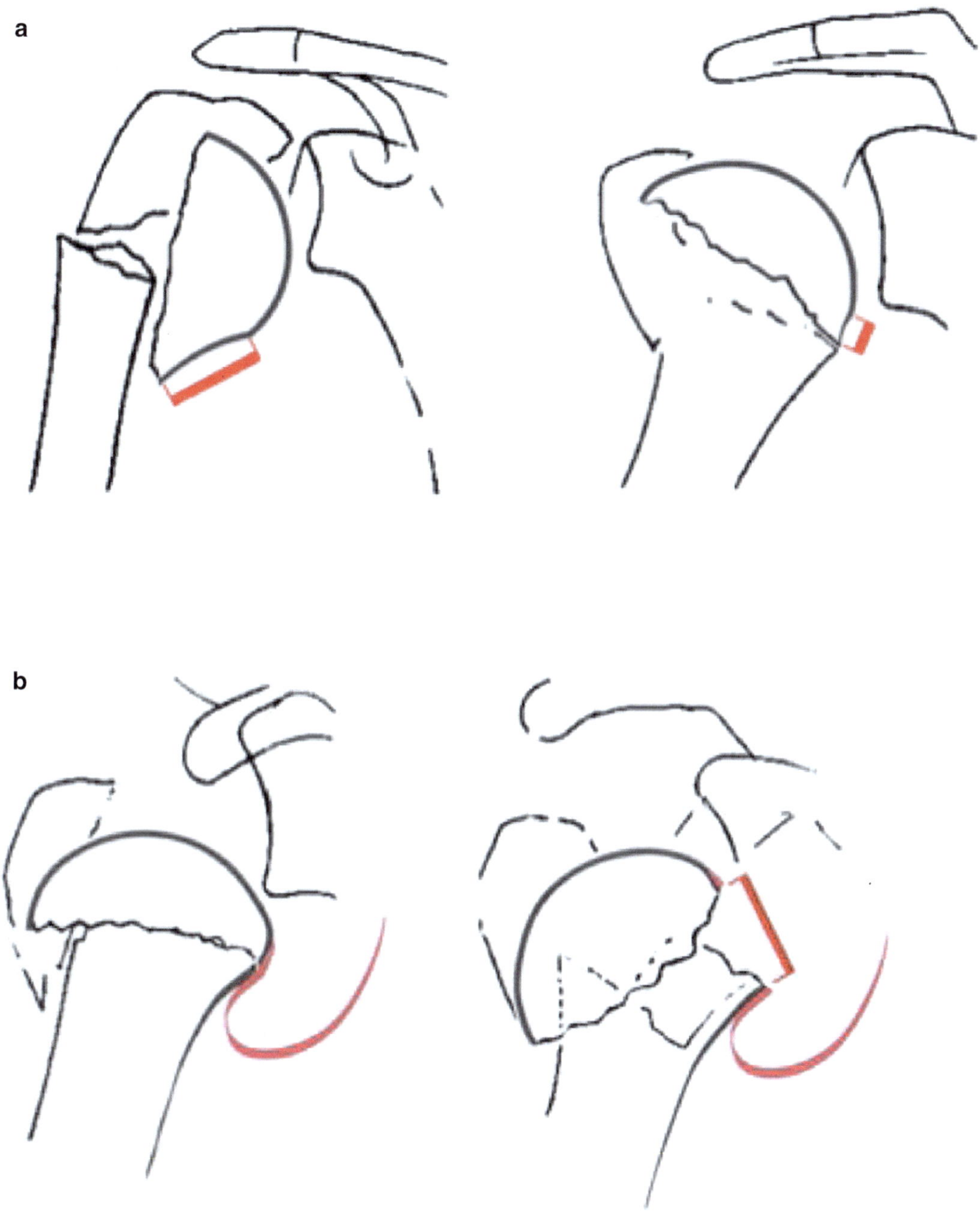

Fig. 8.3 Additional criteria as predictor for humeral head ischemia: (**a**) length of the medial metaphyseal head extension, (**b**) integrity of the medial hinge (Reprinted with permission from Hertel [10])

articular bifocal fractures (B) and articular fractures (C) (Fig. 8.4).

Type A fractures comprise non-articular, definite fractures which are rarely associated with the development of humeral head necrosis.

Type B fractures summarize bifocal fractures and type C fractures include severe, articular fractures which are associated with a higher risk of osteonecrosis of the humeral head [12].

All groups (proximal/diaphysal/distal) have been divided into 9 additional subgroups resulting in 27 fracture types of the humerus.

Due to its high number of fracture types the AO/OTA Classification of Fractures and

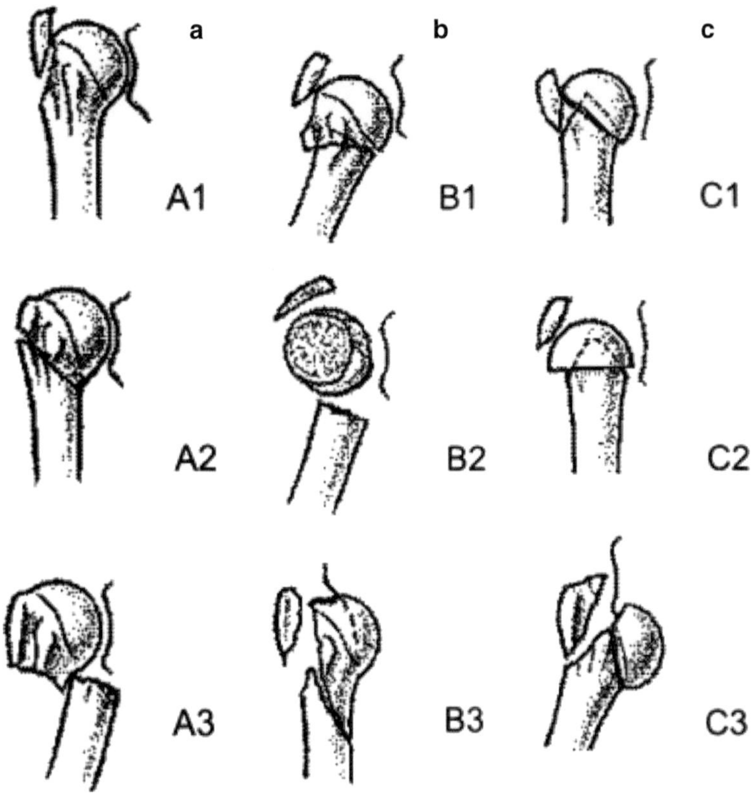

Fig. 8.4 Depiction of the AO classification system showing an extra-articular fracture of the tuberosity (A1), an impacted metaphyseal fracture (A2) and a non impacted metaphyseal fracture (A3). Extra-articular bifocal fracture patterns include fractures with metaphyseal impaction (B1), without metaphyseal impaction (B2) and with glenohumeral dislocation (B3). Articular fractures are classified with slight displacement (C1), impacted with marked displacement (C2) and dislocated (C3) (Reprinted with permission from Muller et al. [12])

Dislocations is not as commonly used as the Neer classification. Furthermore a low reproducibility and reliability has been assessed in the literature with the AO/OTA Classification of Fractures and Dislocations [4, 14].

References

1. Baron JA, Barrett JA, Karagas MR. The epidemiology of peripheral fractures. Bone. 1996;18:209S–13.
2. Neer 2nd CS. Displaced proximal humeral fractures. I. Classification and evaluation. J Bone Joint Surg Am. 1970;52:1077–89.
3. Kristiansen B, Andersen UL, Olsen CA, Varmarken JE. The Neer classification of fractures of the proximal humerus. An assessment of interobserver variation. Skeletal Radiol. 1988;17:420–2.
4. Gumina S, Giannicola PA, Passaretti D, Cinotti G, Postacchini F. Comparison between two classifications of humeral head fractures: Neer and AO-ASIF. Acta Orthop Belg. 2011;77:751–7.
5. Sidor ML, et al. The Neer classification system for proximal humeral fractures. An assessment of interobserver reliability and intraobserver reproducibility. J Bone Joint Surg Am. 1993;75:1745–50.
6. Petit CJ, et al. Management of proximal humeral fractures: surgeons don't agree. J Shoulder Elbow Surg. 2010;19:446–51.
7. Shrader MW, Sanchez-Sotelo J, Sperling JW, Rowland CM, Cofield RH. Understanding proximal humerus fractures: image analysis, classification, and treatment. J Shoulder Elbow Surg. 2005;14:497–505.
8. Neer 2nd CS. Displaced proximal humeral fractures. II. Treatment of three-part and four-part displacement. J Bone Joint Surg Am. 1970;52:1090–103.
9. Mc LH. Posterior dislocation of the shoulder. J Bone Joint Surg Am. 1952;24-A-3:584–90.
10. Hertel R. Fractures of the proximal humerus in osteoporotic bone. Osteoporos Int. 2005;16 Suppl 2:65–72.
11. Hertel R, Hempfing A, Stiehler M, Leunig M. Predictors of humeral head ischemia after intracapsular fracture of the proximal humerus. J Shoulder Elbow Surg. 2004;13:427–33.
12. Müller ME, et al. The comprehensive classification of fractures of long bones. Berlin, Heidelberg, New York: Springer Verlag, 1990.
13. Court-Brown CM, Garg A, McQueen MM. The epidemiology of proximal humeral fractures. Acta Orthop Scand. 2001;72:365–71.
14. Sallay PI, et al. Reliability and reproducibility of radiographic interpretation of proximal humeral fracture pathoanatomy. J Shoulder Elbow Surg. 1997;6: 60–9.

Fracture Dislocation of the Humeral Head

9

Florian B. Imhoff and Chlodwig Kirchhoff

Introduction

As already mentioned in Chap. 1 fractures of the proximal humerus account for approximately 5 % of all fractures of the human body [1] and present the seventh most common fracture following fractures of the distal radius, metacarpal fractures, femur, phalanx, ankle and metatarsal fractures. Incidence and severity increase with patient age especially in the female population [2]. In general the proximal parts are the most common site of fractures of the humerus.

However, the combination of fractures of the humeral head and luxation of the glenohumeral joint is often associated with poor long-term outcome [3, 4]. Acute fracture dislocation requires fast therapeutic action mostly in terms of surgery in terms of open reduction and internal fixation (ORIF) in order to allow for primary fracture healing. Multiple fragments as well as concomitant nerval and vascular injuries increase the intricacy of surgical therapy [5].

F.B. Imhoff (✉) • C. Kirchhoff
Department of Trauma Surgery,
Klinikum rechts der Isar, Technical University of Munich, Munich, Germany
e-mail: florian-imhoff@gmx.de; dr.kirchhoff@mac.com

Classification

Since the previous chapter focusses on the classification of proximal humeral fractures only a short summary of the most commonly used classification systems will be provided here. In 1970 Neer et al. established a classification of fractures of the humeral head as a modification of the Codman classification with the basic principle being the displacement of one or more of the four defined segments. Overall six fracture types were described by Neer whereas Neer type 6 stands for a dislocation of the glenohumeral joint in combination with any type of fracture of the humeral head [6] (see Fig. 9.1).

An also commonly used classification system was established by the Association of Osteosynthesis (AO) in 1990 by Müller et al. [7, 8].

Regarding fracture dislocation of the proximal humerus the definition of a particular classification system was not found to be necessary even though it presents a special type of proximal humeral fracture. However, for the general understanding of fracture dislocation two pathophysiological entities have to be considered [9, 10]:

1. Anterior dislocation of the shoulder associated with fractures of the greater or minor tuberosity
2. Dislocation of the humeral head associated with a subcapital fracture or multi part fracture of the humeral head.

P. Biberthaler et al. (eds.), *Fractures of the Proximal Humerus*, Strategies in Fracture Treatments,
DOI 10.1007/978-3-319-20300-3_9

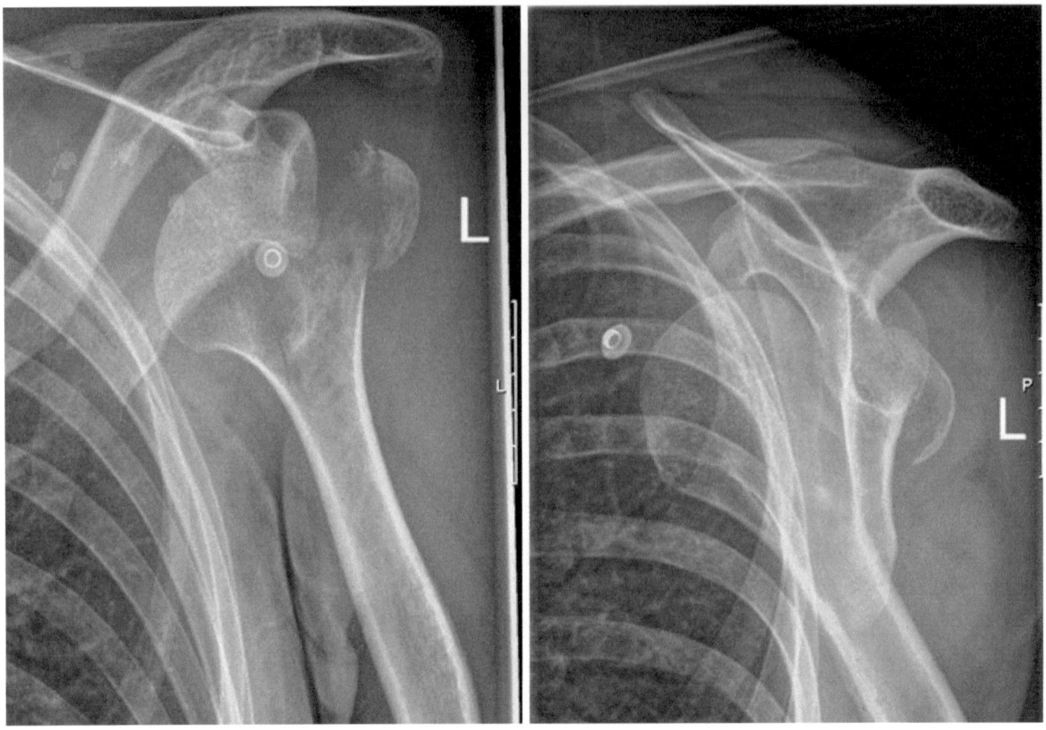

Fig. 9.1 True-ap view and y-view of a left shoulder joint showing an anterior dislocation of the humeral head along with an at least 2-part fracture of the humeral head

Trauma Mechanisms

In most cases simple falling onto the extended arm results in a fracture of the humeral head associated with rupturing of the anterior or posterior shoulder joint capsule depending on the direction of dislocation. As already described in Chap. 1 over 90 % of proximal humeral fractures occur in patients with age >60 years.

Especially in this elderly population even low impact trauma can result in multi part fractures along with fracture dislocation due to general disorders such as osteoporosis, diabetes mellitus, or neoplasia compromising bone mineral density and quality respectively. Another factor considered as predisposition of multi part and even fracture dislocation are degenerative changes of the rotator cuff tendons as well as atrophy of the shoulder girdle muscles.

Fracture dislocation of the proximal humerus can also evolve from epileptic seizures, in up to 60 % following posterior luxation of the shoulder joint presenting a characteristic impression among the humeral bearing area and the minor tuberosity, which can be fractured or dislocated [11].

Diagnostics and Therapy

After initial clinical examination of the patient including an exact documentation of nerval and pulse status, radiographs in at least two planes (true a-p, axillary view) should be performed. In case of clinically suspected vascular lesions a CT scan including CT angiography administering iv iodinated contrast agent of the shoulder should be performed to detect bony as well as vascular pathologies. If furthermore nerval lesions are suspected even additional imaging in terms of e.g. magnetic resonance imaging might be considered. In any case of suspected nerval injury an electrophysiologic exam is to be performed to assess nerval lesions accurately.

The incidence of collateral nerve lesions reaches from 30 to 40 % in fracture dislocation of the humeral head [9]. In particular, most commonly the axillary nerve is affected, in rather rare cases the suprascapularis nerve, the musculocutaneus nerve and the radial nerve as well.

Depending on the two different pathophysiological types of fracture dislocation, the position and displacement of the humeral head in refer to the humeral stem is of particular importance regarding prognosis and outcome.

In general any dislocation of the shoulder joint should immediately be reduced. In case of a gleno-humeral dislocation also if associated with a fracture of the greater tuberosity closed reduction presents usually the adequate type of initial treatment followed by X-ray or CT in order to verify the reduction's result as well as to complete the diagnostics regarding adequate fracture classification. Dislocated fractures of the greater tuberosity present shearing fractures of the supraspinatus as well as of the infraspinatus muscle tendon and displace corresponding to the traction direction of the inserting muscle in cranial and dorsal direction resulting in an abduction and external rotation blockade. In patients older than 60 years about 30 % of all traumatic shoulder dislocations are associated with fractures or infraction of the greater tuberosity [10]. Regarding treatment already shearing fractures of the supraspinatus muscle tendon with a dislocation of less than 5 mm should be treated surgically since the fragments lying on the top of the cartilage of the humeral calotte will not consolidate and thus can result in a loss of function of the supraspinatus muscle [12]. However, in case of younger patients already a dislocation distance of 3 mm should be considered as indication for surgical refixation. In conclusion typical indications for surgery are greater tuberosity fractures with a dislocation >3 mm as well as shearing fractures of the supra- and infraspinatus muscle tendons. Most commonly these fractures are treated by osteosynthesis using 2 screws with the option of additionally using cerclages in case of osteoporotic bone in older patients and presence of several fragments. According to Resch percutaneous transfixation using two cannulated small fragment screws can be performed as well after reduction of the fragments.

In dislocation fractures associated with subcapital fractures and isolated fragments of the calotte close reduction is not possible. In these cases the so-called "head-fragment" needs to be repositioned out of an anterior luxation pouch by surgery in term of open reduction.

Internal fixation using osteosynthesis presents the adequate treatment option for the subcapital fracture in order to reduce the risk of developing necrosis of the humeral head and also concomitant nerval lesions. Especially in these cases a preoperative CT-scan and an exact documentation of the neuro-vascular status is recommended. From the surgery technical point of view achieving sufficient medial support of the calotte in a correct position is often difficult. However, endoprothetic treatment is also challenging in this context since due to the tendency of dislocation in an anterior direction often only insufficient ventral stability is achieved (see Figs. 9.2 and 9.3). To overcome this problem additionally the subscapularis muscle should be gathered along with the anterior capsule.

As mentioned before dorsal fracture dislocation of the proximal humerus can also evolve from epileptic seizures, in up to 60 % following posterior luxation of the shoulder joint presenting a characteristic impression ("reversed Hill-Sachs-lesion") among the humeral bearing area and the minor tuberosity, which can be fractured or dislocated [11]. In case the reverse Hill-Sachs-lesion comprises only 20 % immediate closed reduction presents the adequate treatment with consecutive short-term immobilisation of the shoulder. If irreversible greater lesions are present immediate lift of the impressed bone and performance of screw fixation or alternatively the so-called Mc Laughlin technique and its modification following Neer in terms of transfer of the minor tuberosity into the impression defect respectively are recommended.

Implantation of endoprosthesis is indicated in case of an impression defect>40 % or persisting dislocation for more than 6 months. In patients younger than 60 years of age and dorsal locked dislocation an augmentation of the humeral head using iliac crest bone should be performed to achieve congruency of the joint surface (Figs. 9.4 and 9.5).

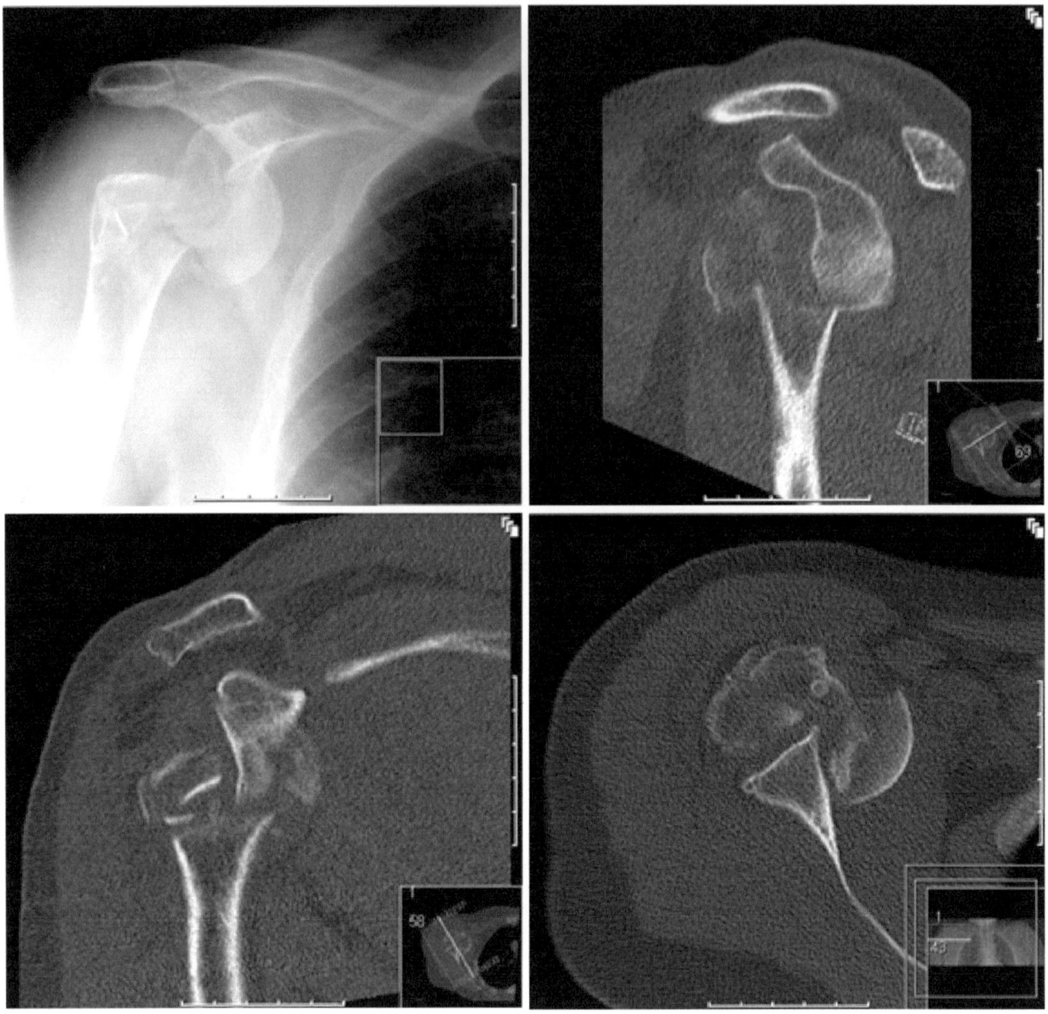

Fig. 9.2 The *left upper* image presents an a-p view of a right shoulder with corresponding native CT-images in coronal (*upper right* and *lower left* image) and axial orientation (*lower right* image) showing a dislocated shoulder in anterior-inferior direction along with multi-part fracture of the humeral head whereas CT provides a more detailed overview on the number and location of the fragments compared to conventional radiography

Fig. 9.4 The *upper row* presents true a-p and y-view of a right shoulder demonstrating a multi-part fracture of the humeral head with suspected posterior dislocation. The *lower row* presents the corresponding CT images in axial (*left*) and coronal (*right*) orientation confirming the suspected posterior dislocation along with fracture dislocation

Fig. 9.3 True a-p and y-view of the same right shoulder as shown in Fig. 9.2 following surgical treatment by implantation of an endoprosthesis

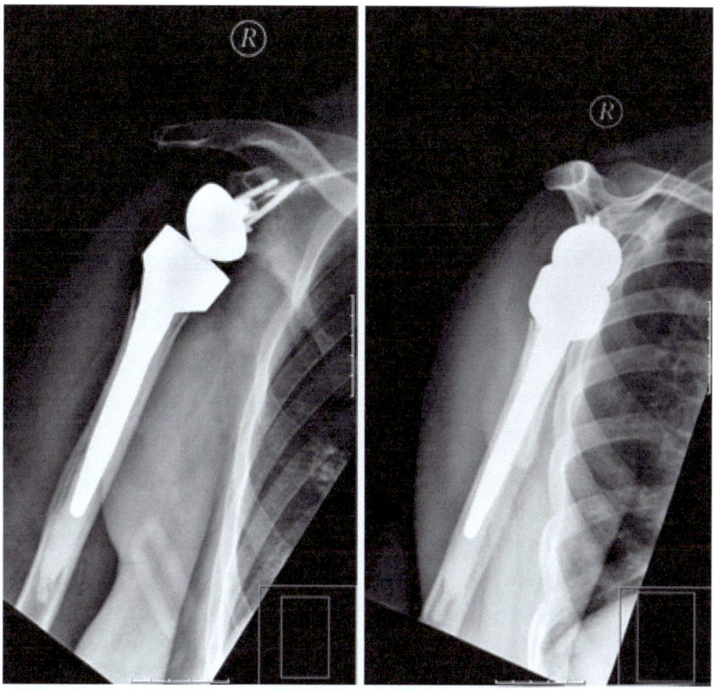

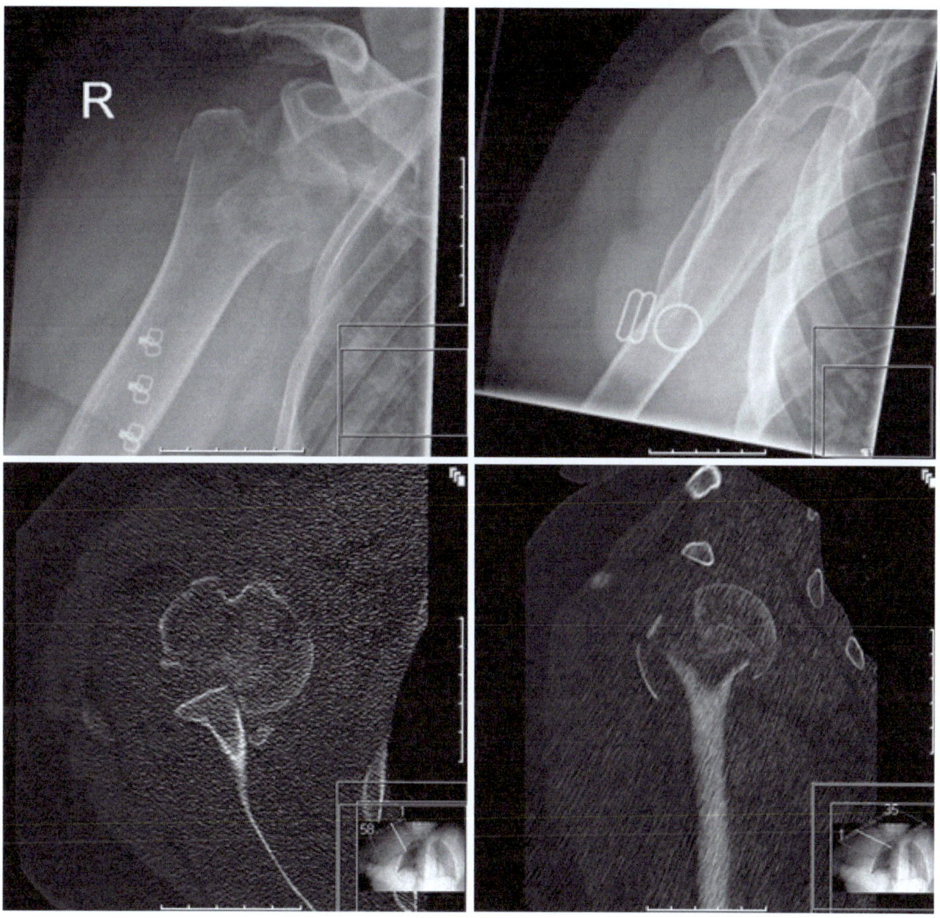

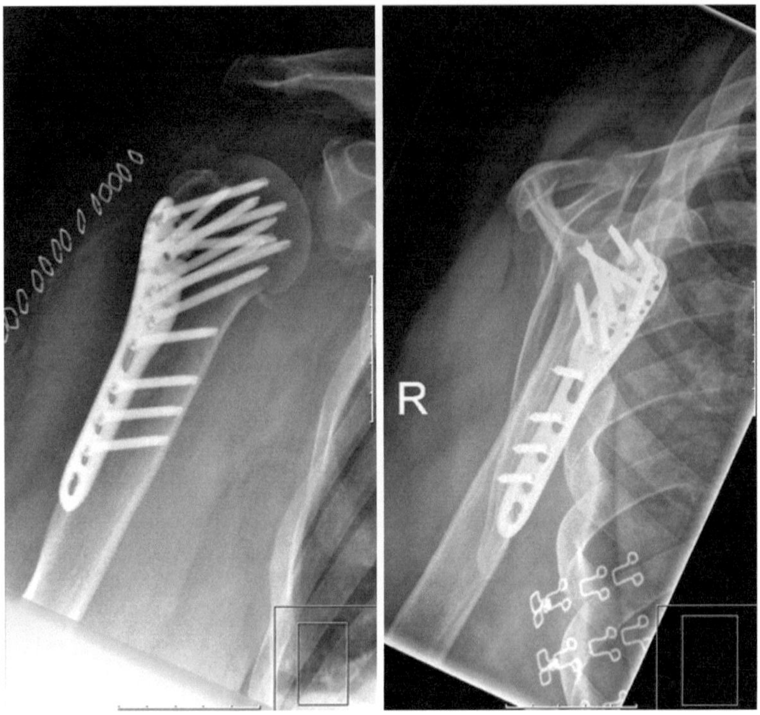

Fig. 9.5 True a-p and y-view of the same right shoulder as shown in Fig. 9.4. but this following reduction and treatment by locking plate osteosynthesis

Summary

Regarding the shoulder joint and the proximal humerus respectively the combination of fractures of the humeral head and luxation of the glenohumeral joint is often associated with poor long-term outcome. Acute fracture dislocation requires fast therapeutic action mostly in terms of closed or open reduction depending on the degree of impressed joint surface. The presence of multiple fragments as well as of concomitant nerval and vascular injuries increase the intricacy of surgical therapy. In case of fracture dislocation along with fractures of the greater tuberosity typical indications for surgery are dislocation >3 mm as well as shearing fractures of the supra- and infraspinatus muscle tendon. Most commonly these fractures are treated by screw osteosynthesis, with the option additionally using cerclages in case of osteoporotic bone in older patients and presence of several fragments.

Regarding the second pathophysiological entity in terms of fracture dislocation of the proximal humerus along with subcapital fractures or multiple fragments close reduction is not possible. Open reduction needs to be performed with consecutive internal fixation using osteosynthesis of the subcapital fracture in order to reduce the risk of developing necrosis of the humeral head and also concomitant nerval lesions. In this context endoprothetic treatment is also challenging since due to the tendency of dislocation in an anterior direction often only insufficient ventral stability is achieved.

In case of posterior fracture dislocation special attention should be paid to the so-called "reversed Hill-Sachs-lesion" since the adequate treatment relies on it. If the reversed Hill-Sachs-lesion is <20 % also conservative treatment including closed reduction is possible. However if the impressed area reaches 40 % and more especially patients >60 years should be treated with primary endoprosthesis and in younger patient bony augmentation and ventral reconstruction of the capsulo-ligamentous complex is recommended.

References

1. Court-Brown CM, Caesar B. Epidemiology of adult fractures: a review. Injury. 2006;37(8):691–7.
2. Court-Brown CM, Garg A, McQueen MM. The epidemiology of proximal humeral fractures. Acta Orthop Scand. 2001;72(4):365–71.
3. Blom S, Dahlbäck LO. Nerve injuries in dislocations of the shoulder joint and fractures of the neck of the humerus. Acta Chir Scand. 1970;136:461–6.
4. de Laat EAT, Visser CPJ, Coene LNJ, Pahlpatz PVM, Tavy DLJ. Nerve lesions in primary shoulder dislocations and humeral neck fractures. J Bone Joint Surg [Br]. 1994;76:381–3.
5. Michael Robinson C, Akhtar A, Mitchell M, Beavis C. Complex posterior fracture-dislocation of the shoulder: epidemiology, injury patterns, and results of operative treatment. J Bone Joint Surg Am. 2007;89(7):1454–66.
6. Neer CS. Displaced proximal humeral fractures. I: classification and evaluation. J Bone Joint Surg Am. 1970;52-A:1077–89.
7. Müller ME, Allgöwer M, Schneider R, Willenberger H. Manual der Osteosynthese. Berlin/Heidelberg/New York: Springer; 1992.
8. Mueller ME, Nazarian S, Koch P. The comprehensive classification of fractures oft he long bones. Berlin: Springer; 1990.
9. Laat EA, et al. Nerve lesions in primary shoulder dislocations and humeral neck fractures. J Bone Joint Surg. 1994;76(3):381–3.
10. Loew M, Thomsen M, Rickert M, Simank HG. Verletzungsmuster bei der chulterluxation des älteren Patienten. Unfallchirurg. 2001;104:115–8.
11. Neer CS. Displaced proximal humeral fractures. II: treatment of three-part and four-part displacement. J Bone Joint Surg Am. 1970;52(6):1090–103.
12. Brunner UH. Humeruskopffraktur. In: Habermeyer P (Hrsg) Schulterchirurgie. München: Urban & Fischer; 2002. p. 403–436.

Multiple Injury

10

Stefan Huber-Wagner, Elaine Schubert, Rolf Lefering, and Peter Biberthaler

Introduction

Proximal humeral fractures account for 4–9 % of all fractures [1–3], most commonly associated with age over 60 years, osteoporosis and female gender [4–8]. An overall increase of proximal humeral fractures has been reported [4, 6, 7, 9]. The most common mode of injury was found to be simple falls from a standing position [6] or low energy moderate trauma [4, 5, 8, 10].

Numerous studies or reviews exist about the incidence, therapy and outcome [3, 11–15] of proximal humeral fractures including complications [7, 16]. The initial patterns of humeral fractures [16] and fragment displacement on the outcome have also been studied. Little is known yet about concomitant injuries [17]. Clement et al. investigated multiple fractures in the elderly, where proximal humeral fractures, distal radial and pelvic fractures were associated with an increased risk of sustaining associated fractures. Proximal humeral fractures amount to 9.9 % of single fractures and 35.3 % of multiple fractures, being among the six most common fractures overall. The largest percentage of multiple fractures occurred after road traffic accidents. In fall-related double fractures, those of the proximal femur, distal radius, proximal humerus and pelvis occurred most often. The most common combination of injuries were proximal femur and proximal humeral fractures with an incidence of 34 %. Overall, proximal humeral fractures were involved in 38 % of fracture combinations. The mortality rates of proximal humeral fractures were 2 % in isolated fractures and 5 % in multiple fractures of all evaluated age groups. A combination of proximal humeral and femoral fractures was associated with the highest mortality risk. Patients who were frailer were most likely to develop proximal limb fractures such as proximal humeral and femoral fractures [10].

In a longitudinal analysis over 6 years including 815 proximal humeral fractures, only 15 (1.8 %, with ISS $\geq$ 16) polytrauma patients were identified [4]. A greater incidence of polytrauma occurred in the younger group with proximal humeral fractures of patients in a study by Jones et al. determining treatment and outcome [12].

S. Huber-Wagner, MD (✉) • P. Biberthaler
Department for Trauma Surgery, Klinikum rechts der Isar, Technical University Munich, Ismaninger Straße 22, 81675 Munich, Germany
e-mail: huber-wagner@mri.tum.de; Peter.Biberthaler@mri.tum.de
http://www.unfallchirurgie.mri.tum.de

E. Schubert
Institute for Diagnostic and Interventional Radiology, Klinikum rechts der Isar, Technical University Munich, Ismaninger Straße 22, 81675 Munich, Germany

R. Lefering
Institute for Research in Operative Medicine (IFOM), University Witten/Herdecke, Ostmerheimer Str. 200, 51109 Cologne, Germany

P. Biberthaler et al. (eds.), *Fractures of the Proximal Humerus*, Strategies in Fracture Treatments, DOI 10.1007/978-3-319-20300-3_10

Severe trauma was a more frequent cause of proximal humeral fractures in the group with an age below 40 years in an analysis of Kristiansen et al. [8].

The patient outcome was worse in polytrauma than in isolated fractures. With older age, isolated injuries and less complex injury patterns, an improved functional outcome was reported [12].

Up to this date, there is not much data available on fractures of the proximal humerus following multiple injuries, as it only accounts for a very small percentage of patient cases of the overall number of such fractures.

On the other hand, more than half of 24,885 major trauma patients presented with a significant extremity injury in an analysis of Banerjee et al. [18]. Fractures of the femur (16.5 %), the tibia (12.6 %) and clavicle (10.4 %) were the most common types. Injuries of the upper extremity (21.9 %) amounted to the largest number of injuries overall, followed by lower extremity injury (19.0 %). Both upper and lower extremity injuries were found in 17.7 % of cases. Fractures of the humerus were reported in 7.4 % of all patients. Overall, patients without significant extremity injury showed a different posttraumatic course and outcome, although they had a comparable injury severity to those with significant extremity injury. Patients with extremity injury presented a higher rate of severe chest trauma, a larger number of blood transfusions, more operative procedures and a longer hospital length of stay. These groups therefore may be regarded as two different populations in posttraumatic course and survival [18].

In a study by Bell et al. with 38 patients who showed fractures of the humeral shaft, 26 patients had additional head injuries, 26 showed chest injury and 7 abdominal injuries. Of 52 additional fractures among the collective of patients with humeral fractures, femur fractures were most common with 15 occurrences, followed by pelvis fractures in 13 cases [19].

The impact of fractures of the upper extremities on mortality is marginal which may lead to a lower priority in the course of treatment. However, this should be individually questioned [20]. Regel et al. report that 86 % of all patients with multiple injuries showed fractures of the extremities. Most of these were located in the lower extremities [21].

The therapy of humeral head fractures has generally changed in the last 20 years from an exclusively conservative to a more frequently applied operative treatment [1]. The therapy and operational procedure is discussed controversially, especially regarding osteoporotic patients [3, 22]. Patients with multiple injuries require a special treatment strategy, as fractures cannot be treated isolatedly but have to be seen in the whole context of injury patterns.

Bell et al. first analyzed the treatment of humeral shaft fractures with plate fixation particularly in patients with multiple injuries in 1985 [19]. Blum et al. later analyzed the timing and treatment strategy of upper limb fractures especially in polytraumatized patients. They found the quality of available data on this topic to be low. On grounds of the available publications they concluded that if vessels are injured additionally, they require fast diagnosis and operative reconstruction in cardiopulmonarily stable patients. Furthermore, open fractures that are combined with vessel or nerve lesions should have a higher therapeutic priority. The occurrence of compartment syndrome is seldom in fractures of the upper extremity long bones, but requires quick operative decompression. Amputations are only indicated in rare cases of upper extremity injuries in polytraumatized patients [20].

As far as surgical treatment goes for proximal humeral fractures in polytrauma patients, external fixation should be reserved for those patients [3]. A case series of polytrauma patients with proximal humeral fractures reported a satisfactory outcome by applying an Ilizarov external fixator [23].

We intended to analyze the incidence and injury pattern of severely injured patients with fractures of the humerus in the TraumaRegister DGU® (TR-DGU).

Methods

Since 1993, the TraumaRegister DGU® (TR-DGU) collects data from severely injured patients for the purpose of external quality control. Until 2009, data of 51,425 trauma patients were collected. The data collected cover the pre-hospital phase, the early in-hospital treatment in the emergency room, the following phase of intensive care, and the final outcome including a complete list of diagnoses. Data are collected via a web-based password-protected documentation system. The registry is managed, owned and hosted by the Academy for Trauma Surgery (AUC – Akademie der Unfallchirurgie GmbH), a company affiliated to the German Trauma Society (DGU, Deutsche Gesellschaft für Unfallchirurgie). The scientific leadership is provided by the Committee on Emergency Medicine, Intensive Care and Trauma Management (Sektion NIS – Sektion Notfall-, Intensivmedizin und Schwerverletztenversorgung) of the German Trauma Society. The participating hospitals are expected to include patients admitted alive to the emergency room with subsequent ICU treatment, including those patients who die before reaching the ICU.

The present retrospective analysis included only patients with an Injury Severity Score (ISS) of 16 points or more, which left a total of 34,049 individuals. Among these patients, we analysed the subgroup of patients with a humeral fracture. Specifically, fracture incidence, morphology and pattern of injury were analysed. Continuous and categorical data are presented as mean with standard deviation (SD), or as percentages, respectively.

Results

Table 10.1 shows the main characteristics of the investigated patients. 2,709 (8.0 %) out of 34,049 patients had a humeral fracture. Of 2,709 patients with humeral fractures, the mean ISS was 31.4. The age of patients with humeral fractures was between 0 and 101, with a mean of 41.6 years, 66 % were male. Furthermore, 95.7 % of patients presented with blunt trauma. The mortality was 21.7 %.

Table 10.1 Data description, n=2,709 (8 %) patients with humeral fractures out of 34,049 patients of the TR-DGU

Characteristic	Mean value or %
ISS	31.4±12.4
Age	41.7±20.5
Male	66.0
Blunt trauma	95.7
Mortality	21.7

Table 10.2 Location of fractures, overall collective with 34,049 patients TR-DGU

Location of fracture	Percentage all patients (%)
Shoulder	22.9
Clavicle	10.6
Humerus	8.0
Scapula	7.3

Table 10.3 Humeral fracture and concomitant fractures, n=2,709 (8 %) cases with humeral fractures

Location of fracture	Percentage of concomitant injuries of the upper extremity (%)
Radius	18.3
Ulna	13.8
Clavicle	11.9
Scapula	10.8
Hand	5.3

Table 10.2 presents the percentage of specific locations of fractures reported in the total of 34,049 patients with an ISS of more than 16. Most fractures occurred in the shoulder in 22.9 % of the cases, followed by 10.6 % fractures of the clavicle, 8 % of the humerus and 7.3 % of the scapula.

The percentage of concomitant fracture locations of 2,709 patients with a humeral fracture are shown in Table 10.3. The most common type of fracture were fractures of the radius in 18.3 % of cases, followed by fractures of the ulna in 13.8 % of patients, 11.9 % of clavicular fractures, 10.8 % of scapula fractures and 5.3 % fractures of the hand.

Table 10.4 Injury pattern, overall collective 34,049 patients TR-DGU

Location of injury	%
Head AIS ≥3	50.1
Chest AIS ≥3	67.7
Abdominal AIS ≥3	25.6
Extremities AIS ≥3	32.8

AIS Abbreviated Injury Scale

Table 10.5 Basic therapeutic data, n = 2,709 patients with humeral fractures

Treatment	%
Open fracture	15.4
Operative treatment	69.2
External fixators	17.0
Number of necessary humeral operations on average	1.6

Table 10.4 summarizes the injury patterns of all patients with humeral fractures. Most common were injuries of the chest in 67.7 % of cases. Injuries of the extremities were reported in 62.8 % of cases, 50.1 % head injuries and 25.6 % of abdominal injuries (only AIS ≥3 injuries, AIS = Abbreviated Injury Scale).

Table 10.5 shows that 15.4 % of humeral fractures were open fractures, 69.2 % were treated surgically and 17.0 % were treated with external fixators. Overall, 1.6 surgical interventions were necessary in the treatment of humeral fractures.

Discussion

We present epidemiological data in a polytrauma collective with humeral fractures. Compared to other recorded trauma populations, where the mean age was 37.5 years with a majority of men (67.5 %) and mean ISS of 34.3 [24], our data showed very similar findings with a mean age of 41.7 years, mean ISS of 31.4 as well as mainly male patients (66.0 %).

As known from several studies, the mean age for proximal humeral fractures generally is higher and related to low energy trauma in elderly women, whereas the age relatively decreases in multiple trauma patients which are also mainly male.

In our analysis, humeral fractures were recorded in 8 % of all patients with severe trauma and ISS greater than 16 which is a similar percentage as found by Banerjee et al. According to their data, humeral fractures occurred in 7.4 % of all major trauma patients [18].

In our analysis, the most common additional fracture in patients with humeral fractures is the radius fracture, followed by fractures of the ulna. Chest injuries were the most frequently observed injured body region, similar to findings by Banerjee et al., where patients with extremity injury often showed severe chest trauma [18]. Bell et al. report about femur fractures being the most commonly associated fracture in patients with humeral fractures [19].

Regel et al reported that 86 % of multiple injured showed extremity injuries [21], compared to 62.8 % injuries of extremities in our collective.

We observed a general mortality of 21.7 % compared to 5.0 % reported by Clement et al. in patients with humeral fractures that showed multiple fractures [10].

The diagnostic and therapeutic effort in patients with multiple injuries is especially demanding. The average number of necessary operations for humeral fractures in our collective was 1.6.

Multiply injured patients should be diagnosed according to the local trauma protocols such as ATLS® [25]. Whole body-computed tomography should be performed if possible [26, 27]. After analysis of the whole injury pattern, targeted and priority-orientated therapy must be started.

Limitations

All humeral fractures were included in our data collection and not only the proximal ones. Like all analyses coming from large registries, data completeness and data quality usually have a lower level than in prospective clinical studies. This remains true although we have implemented multiple plausibility checks and cross-validations in our data collection tool.

Summary

The incidence of humeral fractures was 8 % in multiply injured patients. This means that every 13th patient was affected. Data on humeral fractures in the young, mainly male collective of patients with multiple injuries, has not been studied much in the past. Our analysis presents a group of 34,049 patients with an ISS ≥ 16 in which the incidence of fractures was analyzed. In addition, we show data of humeral fractures and concomitant fractures as well as overall injury patterns. We also recorded basic therapeutic data in our relatively large sample of patients that can be of interest. To the best of our knowledge, most of the data we collected has not been analyzed with the main emphasis on humeral fractures in multiply injured before. Therefore, it was only possible to compare certain small partial aspects with existing data in the literature.

References

1. Seidel H. Proximal humeral fractures. In: Leung K-S et al., editors. Practice of intramedullary locked nails. Berlin/Heidelberg: Springer; 2006. p. 159–67.
2. Court-Brown CM, Garg A, McQueen MM. The epidemiology of proximal humeral fractures. Acta Orthop. 2001;72(4):365–71.
3. Karataglis D, Stavridis SI, Petsatodis G, et al. New trends in fixation of proximal humeral fractures: a review. Injury. 2011;42(4):330–8.
4. Bahrs C, Tanja S, Gunnar B, et al. Trends in epidemiology and patho-anatomical pattern of proximal humeral fractures. Int Orthop. 2014;38(8):1697–704.
5. Bahrs C, Bauer M, Blumenstock G, et al. The complexity of proximal humeral fractures is age and gender specific. J Orthop Sci. 2013;18(3):465–70.
6. Clement ND, Duckworth AD, McQueen MM, et al. The outcome of proximal humeral fractures in the elderly: predictors of mortality and function. Bone Joint J. 2014;96-B(7):970–7.
7. Tepass A, Rolauffs B, Weise K, et al. Complication rates and outcomes stratified by treatment modalities in proximal humeral fractures: a systematic literature review from 1970–2009. Patient Saf Surg. 2013;7(1):34.
8. Kristiansen B, Barfod G, Bredesen J, et al. Epidemiology of proximal humeral fractures. Acta Orthop Scand. 1987;58(1):75–7.
9. Dimai H, Svedbom A, Fahrleitner-Pammer A, et al. Epidemiology of proximal humeral fractures in Austria between 1989 and 2008. Osteoporos Int. 2013;24(9):2413–21.
10. Clement ND, Aitken S, Duckworth AD, et al. Multiple fractures in the elderly. J Bone Joint Surg Br. 2012;94(2):231–6.
11. Liu J, Li SH, Cai ZD, et al. Outcomes, and factors affecting outcomes, following shoulder hemiarthroplasty for proximal humeral fracture repair. J Orthop Sci. 2011;16(5):565–72.
12. Jones CB, Sietsema DL, Williams DK. Locked plating of proximal humeral fractures: is function affected by age, time, and fracture patterns? Clin Orthop Relat Res. 2011;469(12):3307–16.
13. Kettler M, Biberthaler P, Braunstein V, et al. Treatment of proximal humeral fractures with the PHILOS angular stable plate. Presentation of 225 cases of dislocated fractures. Unfallchirurg. 2006;109(12):1032–40.
14. Robinson CM, Bell KM, Court-Brown CM, et al. Locked nailing of humeral shaft fractures. Experience in Edinburgh over a two-year period. J Bone Joint Surg Br. 1992;74(4):558–62.
15. Kuner E, Siebler G. Luxationsfrakturen des proximalen Humerus. Unfallchirurgie. 1987;13(2):64–71.
16. Robinson CM, Stone OD, Murray IR. Proximal humeral fractures due to blunt trauma producing skin compromise. J Bone Joint Surg Br. 2011;93(12):1632–7.
17. Marquaß B, Schiffner E, Theopold J, et al. Ipsilaterale Begleitverletzungen an der oberen Extremität und des Schultergürtels nach proximalen Humerusfrakturen. Obere Extremität. 2012;7(3):150–7.
18. Banerjee M, Bouillon B, Shafizadeh S, et al. Epidemiology of extremity injuries in multiple trauma patients. Injury. 2013;44(8):1015–21.
19. Bell MJ, Beauchamp CG, Kellam JK, et al. The results of plating humeral shaft fractures in patients with multiple injuries. The Sunnybrook experience. J Bone Joint Surg Br. 1985;67(2):293–6.
20. Blum J, Gercek E, Hansen M, et al. Operative strategies in the treatment of upper limb fractures in polytraumatized patients. Unfallchirurg. 2005;108(10):843–4, 846–9.
21. Regel G, Lobenhoffer P, Lehmann U, et al. Ergebnisse in der Behandlung Polytraumatisierter. Eine vergleichende Analyse von 3406 Fällen zwischen 1972 und 1991. Unfallchirurg. 1993;96(7):350–62.
22. Solberg BD, Moon CN, Franco DP, et al. Surgical treatment of three and four-part proximal humeral fractures. J Bone Joint Surg Am. 2009;91(7):1689–97.
23. Dhar SA, Butt MF, Mir MR, et al. Use of the Ilizarov apparatus to improve alignment in proximal humeral fractures treated initially by a unilateral external fixator. Strategies Trauma Limb Reconstr. 2008;3(3):119–22.
24. Aldrian S, Koenig F, Weninger P, et al. Characteristics of polytrauma patients between 1992 and 2002: what is changing? Injury. 2007;38(9):1059–64.

25. Kreimeier U, Reith M, Huber-Wagner S, et al. Interdisciplinary trauma room treatment. Notfall Rettungsmedizin. 2008;11(6):399–406.
26. Huber-Wagner S, Lefering R, Qvick L-M, et al. Effect of whole-body CT during trauma resuscitation on survival: a retrospective, multicentre study. Lancet. 2009;373(9673):1455–61.
27. Huber-Wagner S, Biberthaler P, Häberle S, et al. Whole-body CT in haemodynamically unstable severely injured patients – a retrospective, multicentre study. PLoS One. 2013;8(7), e68880.

Part III

Preoperative Considerations

Cuff Disorders

11

Stefan Buchmann

Introduction

Bony anatomy and rotator cuff (RC) integrity are fundamental for a proper shoulder function, which is often impaired after humeral head fracture. In the last decades functional outcome after proximal humeral fractures was mainly brought in line with restoration of the bony anatomy. Little attention was paid to already preoperative existing or due to trauma developed rotator cuff lesion. As current studies on conservative and surgical treatment show a significant correlation between rotator cuff tears (RCTs) and poor clinical outcome, these pathologies should be considered carefully before final treatment decision regarding proximal humerus fractures [1–3]. Furthermore the option of anatomic or reverse arthroplasty for complex fractures of the proximal humerus in the elderly patients requires detailed information about the status of the RC [4, 5]. The following chapter accordingly focuses on preoperative diagnostics and considerations regarding pre-existing and concomitant RCTs in case of proximal humeral fractures to allow for an individual treatment decision for satisfying clinical results:

S. Buchmann
Department of Orthopedic Sports Medicine, Klinikum rechts der Isar, Munich, Germany
e-mail: s_buchmann17@hotmail.com

Etiology of Concomitant RCTs

The prevalence of asymptomatic RCTs increases with age so that in patients younger than 50 years less than 5 % of RCTs were found whereas patients older than 80 years show an asymptomatic RCT in up to 80 % [6]. Accordingly in the elderly patients a preexisting RCT is supposed to be more frequent (Fig. 11.1). But also trauma associated lesions of the rotator cuff are described in case of proximal humeral fractures [1, 7, 8]. In the era of open surgery a tear of the rotator interval (longitudinal or complex shape) has been described as the most common traumatic tear pattern besides bony avulsions [2]. However, arthros-

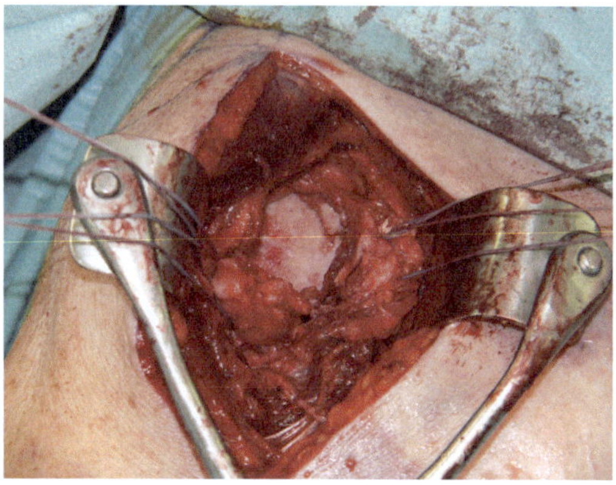

Fig. 11.1 Intraoperative situs of a chronic massive RCT in a humeral head fracture (Courtesy of Dr. V. Braunstein, Munich)

P. Biberthaler et al. (eds.), *Fractures of the Proximal Humerus*, Strategies in Fracture Treatments,
DOI 10.1007/978-3-319-20300-3_11

copy revealed a higher incidence of intraarticular lesions which have not been diagnosed in open surgery due to the limited exposure from the bursal side [9, 10]. A progression of the preexisting tear size or combined injuries are also described in proximal humeral fractures so that in some cases uncommon tear patterns may result.

Preoperative Diagnostics

A detailed acquisition of history of shoulder complaints (pain, weakness, active deficit in range of motion (ROM), instability, previous surgery) may provide a first hint to pre-existing rotator cuff pathologies. But in the elderly patient a proper evaluation of pre-traumatic shoulder function might be difficult due to reduced practice of the arm and altered pain perception. According to the increasing prevalence of RCTs with age the patient's age gives an idea of the overall tear probability [6, 11].

Clinical examination of the acute injured patient is mainly limited due to pain. But a careful inspection of the periscapular muscle status may already reveal an atrophy of the fossa supraspinata and/or infraspinata as a sign of a large chronic RCT (see Fig. 11.2). Significant haematoma or soft tissue swelling complicate this assessment. Traumatic lesions of the suprascapular nerve often combined with high velocity trauma and fractures of the scapula are also difficult to examine clinically. If due to the trauma mechanism a nerve injury is suspected additional neurologic diagnostics are indicated.

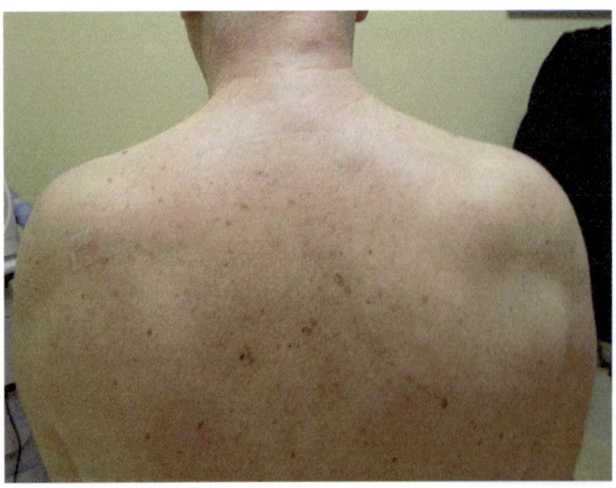

Fig. 11.2 Clinical sign of a chronic postero-superior RCT: Atrophy Fossa supra-/infraspinata right shoulder

Imaging

Plain radiographs of the shoulder are accepted as basic diagnostics for suspected proximal humeral fractures. For a standardized evaluation at minimum two planes ("true ap" and axial view/Velpeau) are required, an additional "outlet view" gives further information. Due to the inability to be visualized directly on plain radiographs, soft tissue structures have been neglected during initial evaluation of proximal humeral fractures. Nevertheless there are secondary signs of chronic rotator cuff insufficiency that are displayed on plain radiographs. The most obvious changes are seen in advanced cuff arthropathy with changes of the shape of the glenoid and acromion (acetabularisation) [12]. In early stages subchondral sclerosis of the acromion and cystic changes in the footprint of the rotator cuff might be evitable (see Fig. 11.3). An advanced osteoarthritic deformation of the head (fragments) or a posterior osteoarthritic glenoid bone loss gives no evidence of rotator cuff insufficiency.

The validity of the combination fracture pattern/dislocation and rotator cuff tear is discussed controversially. Biomechanically a typical fracture dislocation (greater tuberosity – postero-superior, lesser tuberosity – antero-inferior)

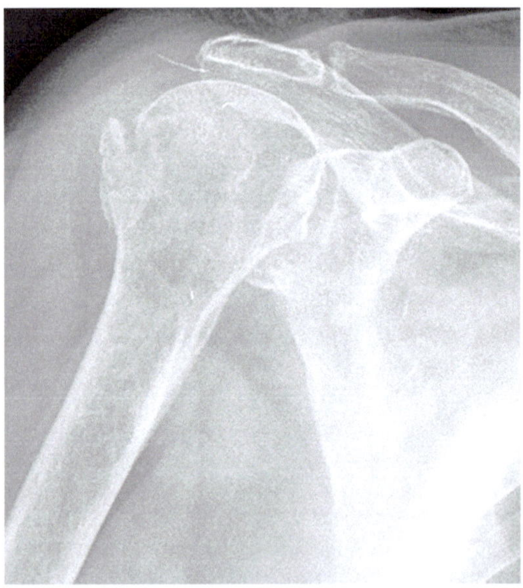

Fig. 11.3 Preexisting early cuff arthropathy (Hamada II) with reduced acromio-humeral distance, subchondral sclerosis of the acromion and cystic changes of the greater tuberosity [12]

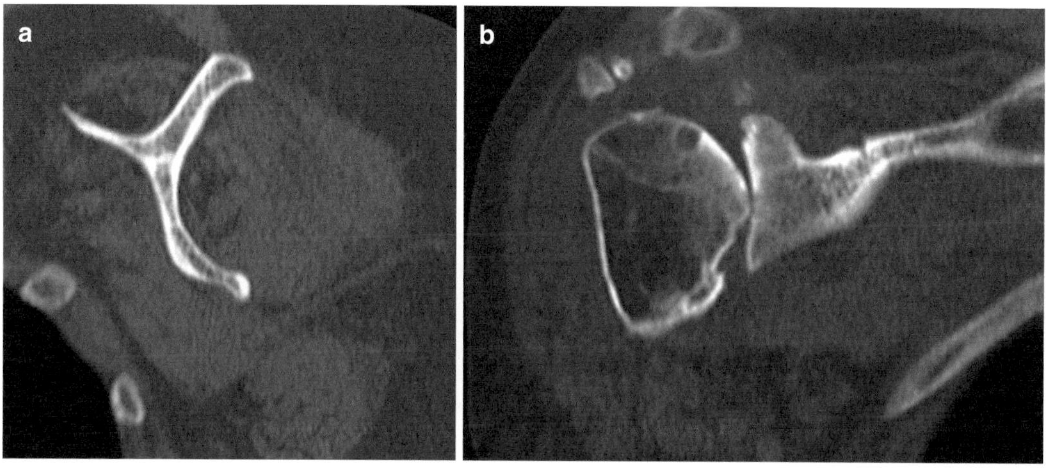

Fig. 11.4 CT-Scan (**a**) parasagittal reconstruction with a Grade III/IV fatty infiltration of SSP/ISP according to Goutallier et al. [14] (**b**) coronary reconstruction with significant fatty infiltration of the SSP muscle belly and cranialisation of the humeral head

concludes intact tension vectors (RC) and might be seen as a sign for functional integrity of the rotator cuff. But smaller rotator cuff tears may not be evident for changes in tension vectors. On the other hand two current studies show a positive correlation between severity/displacement of the fracture and prevalence of RCTs [1, 7]. But these differences might be due to different fracture mechanisms and age of the patients. In massive RCTs especially fracture patterns with compression fractures between acromion and humeral head are described.

In complex fractures a computed tomography (CT) scan enhances the consistency in understanding these fractures [13]. Additionally the fatty infiltration of the rotator cuff muscles can be evaluated in the parasagittal reconstruction according to Goutallier et al. [14]. In the elderly patient a generalized mild fatty infiltration in all parts of the RC is a common finding due to muscle inactivity whereas a localized fatty infiltration degree III/IV according to Goutallier is a certain sign for a biomechanically relevant chronic RCT (see Fig. 11.4a, b).

Besides the muscle structure also the muscle volume especially of the supraspinatus muscle can be estimated in CT according to the Thomazeau MRI classification in the parasagittal reconstruction, but changes in the cross-sectional area due to retraction of the musculo-tendinous junction have to be considered [15].

Additional ultrasonographic examination can give further information about the status of the rotator cuff. In traumatic or degenerative RCTs ultrasonography showed a sensitivity and specificity of 85–91 % regarding a detection of RCTs when compared to MR-arthrograms of the shoulder or arthroscopic findings of the shoulder at time of surgery [16]. But this accuracy is strongly dependent on the experience of the investigator. In fracture cases the examination accuracy is additionally limited due to haematoma and fracture dislocation of the RC insertion so that it cannot be recommended as standard diagnostic tool in dislocated multifragmentary fractures. Besides regarding the evaluation of the continuity of the RC some studies show the possibility of evaluating fatty infiltration but haematoma and investigator's experience may limit this technique [17, 18].

In daily clinical practice Magnetic resonance Imaging (MRI) diagnostics are performed only in few cases of proximal humeral fracture due to its availability and often misinterpretation of bony defect areas (bone bruise). But non- or minimally-displaced humeral head fractures are often not recognized until MRI reveals the fracture. In current radiological studies MRI showed information on fracture morphology comparable to CT but due to the above mentioned reasons it has not found the way to regular clinical practice yet. But in cases of persisting pain after conservative treatment MRI is accepted as standard diagnostic tool besides x-ray.

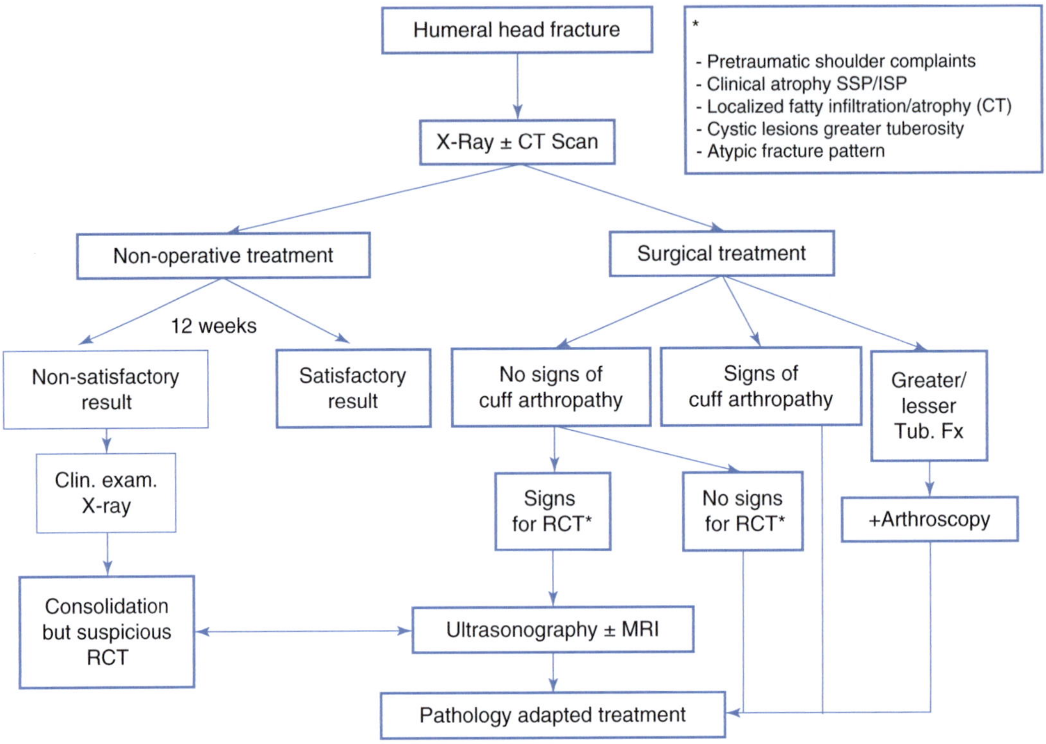

Fig. 11.5 Algorithm for imaging rotator cuff tendons in the setting of proximal humerus fractures

Arthroscopy

Diagnostic arthroscopy may reveal especially intraarticular lesions of the RCT and pathologies of the long head of the biceps tendon. But arthroscopy ahead of open refixation is technically limited to 2-Part fractures or minor dislocated fracture patterns. In comminuted or massive dislocated fractures the joint capsule continuity is completely destroyed so that an intraarticular visualisation cannot be achieved [9, 10]. As disadvantage prolonged arthroscopic diagnostics or treatment can cause massive periarticular swelling due to joint capsule interruption and complicate the open surgery itself. So the extent of arthroscopic diagnostics and treatment should be planned carefully.

Algorithm for Diagnostics

Already in 2009 Gallo et al. presented a simple algorithm based on the number of fragments and displacement of the greater tuberosity for additional diagnostics in proximal humeral fractures [19]. However the data about the relevance of fracture displacement remains unclear and especially preexisting lesions are not considered in the published algorithm. In fact the indication for additional diagnostics remains an individual decision. The following algorithm should provide a guideline for clinical practice (see Fig. 11.5).

Clinical Data and Treatment Considerations

The aforementioned additional diagnostic tools support the surgeon in his preoperative and also intraoperative considerations [20].

Preoperative considerations are mainly focussed on treatment modality (surgical vs. conservative treatment) and surgical technique. In most of the cases the indication of treatment modality (surgical vs. conservative) is not influenced by additional diagnostics because the osseous status (X-ray/CT scan) mostly defines the treatment. But specific intraoperative diagnostics

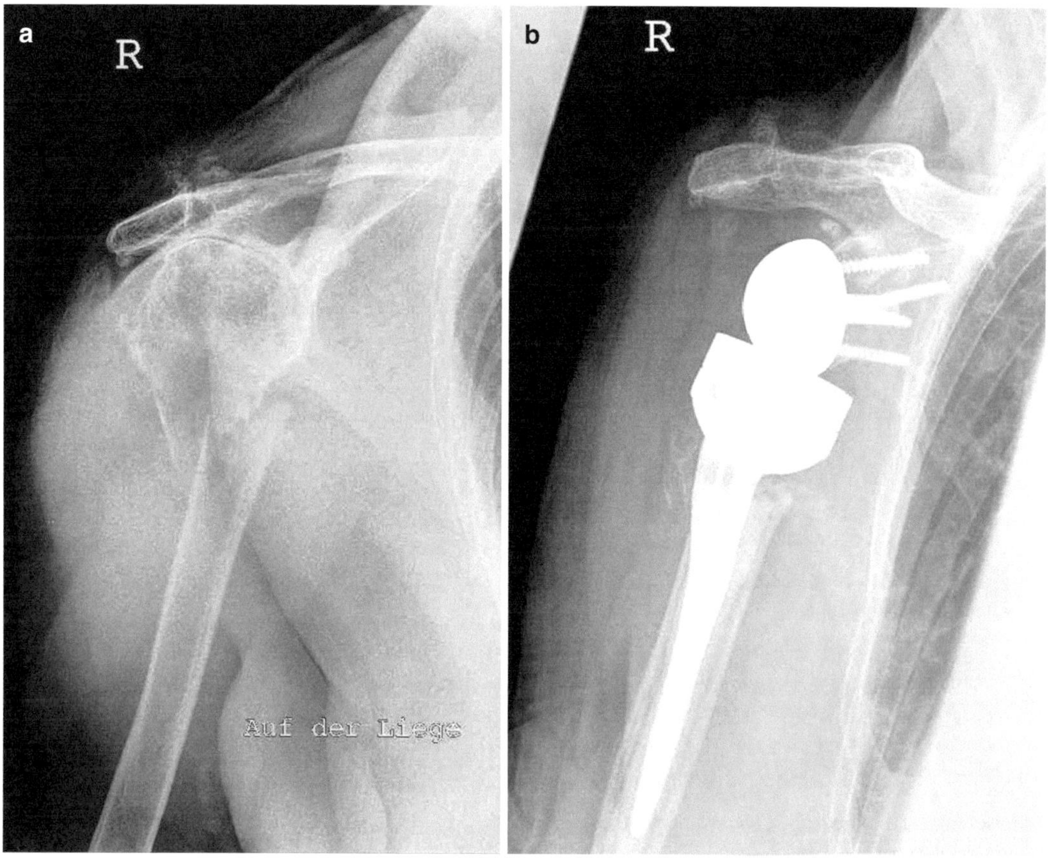

Fig. 11.6 Reverse Arthroplasty in a proximal humeral fracture (86 years, female) with a pre-existing rotator cuff arthropathy (Tornier, Aequalis reversed shoulder fracture stem with Bio RSA glenoid augmentation) (**a**) preoperative X-ray a.p. view (**b**) postoperative X-ray a.p. view (Courtesy of Dr. V. Braunstein, Munich)

(e.g. careful visualisation of parts of the RC) and technical decisions can be lead by detailed knowledge of the RC status. Current literature states the importance of the intact RC function for satisfying clinical results in all treatment modalities [1, 3, 21]. Wilmanns et al. evaluated 39 patients with proximal humeral fractures 6 months postoperatively clinically and with ultrasound. Patients with RCT showed a significantly inferior clinical outcome [3]. Bahrs et al. confirmed this conclusion in a larger series of 302 patients with a follow up of 53 months [1].

The most important information of additional preoperative imaging besides tear pattern and localization is the estimation of reparability of the tear. With both surgical approaches (osteosynthesis vs. anatomic shoulder arthroplasty) current case series show satisfying clinical outcome with additional rotator cuff reconstruction [4, 22]. But further studies of higher evidence levels are still missing.

In the case of prosthetic replacement the choice of implant defines the importance of rotator cuff integrity. While in anatomic shoulder replacement a dysfunction of the RC (tear, resorption of the tubercula) correlates with inferior clinical results [21] the shoulder function in reverse shoulder arthroplasty (RSA) is less dependant on RCT integrity. RSA gains growing interest in the treatment of the elderly patient with a complex fracture situation. Early clinical studies show satisfying postoperative results [5, 23]. In rotator cuff arthropathy an improved clinical outcome is found in patients with a remaining force couple, so that a stable refixation of the tubercula is strongly recommended. For the indication of RSA the sudden loss of function after 10–12 years postoperatively has to be considered especially in patients younger than 70 years [24] (Fig. 11.6).

Summary

Rotator cuff integrity is fundamental for a satisfying shoulder function after proximal humeral fractures. Patients' history, clinical examination and additional radiologic diagnostics (e.g. x-ray/CT) give information about the status of the RC and may influence the chosen treatment option. In all surgical techniques continuity of the RC (RSA – infraspinatus/teres minor/ subscapularis) should be one important goal of the treatment as clinical studies report herewith improved outcomes.

References

1. Bahrs C, Rolauffs B, Stuby F, Dietz K, Weise K, et al. Effect of proximal humeral fractures on the age-specific prevalence of rotator cuff tears. J Trauma. 2010;69:901–6.
2. Fjalestad T, Hole MO, Blucher J, Hovden IA, Stiris MG, et al. Rotator cuff tears in proximal humeral fractures: an MRI cohort study in 76 patients. Arch Orthop Trauma Surg. 2010;130:575–81.
3. Wilmanns C, Bonnaire F. Rotator cuff alterations resulting from humeral head fractures. Injury. 2002;33:781–9.
4. Fallatah S, Dervin GF, Brunet JA, Conway AF, Hrushowy H. Functional outcome after proximal humeral fractures treated with hemiarthroplasty. Can J Surg. 2008;51:361–5.
5. Tischer T, Rose T, Imhoff AB. The reverse shoulder prosthesis for primary and secondary treatment of proximal humeral fractures: a case report. Arch Orthop Trauma Surg. 2008;128:973–8.
6. Milgrom C, Schaffler M, Gilbert S, van Holsbeeck M. Rotator-cuff changes in asymptomatic adults. The effect of age, hand dominance and gender. J Bone Joint Surg Br. 1995;77:296–8.
7. Gallo RA, Sciulli R, Daffner RH, Altman DT, Altman GT. Defining the relationship between rotator cuff injury and proximal humerus fractures. Clin Orthop Relat Res. 2007;458:70–7.
8. Robinson CM, Page RS. Severely impacted valgus proximal humeral fractures. Results of operative treatment. J Bone Joint Surg Am. 2003;85-A: 1647–55.
9. Kim SH, Ha KI. Arthroscopic treatment of symptomatic shoulders with minimally displaced greater tuberosity fracture. Arthroscopy. 2000;16:695–700.
10. Schai PA, Hintermann B, Koris MJ. Preoperative arthroscopic assessment of fractures about the shoulder. Arthroscopy. 1999;15:827–35.
11. Melis B, Nemoz C, Walch G. Muscle fatty infiltration in rotator cuff tears: descriptive analysis of 1688 cases. Orthop Traumatol Surg Res. 2009;95:319–24.
12. Hamada K, Yamanaka K, Uchiyama Y, Mikasa T, Mikasa M. A radiographic classification of massive rotator cuff tear arthritis. Clin Orthop Relat Res. 2011;469:2452–60.
13. Shrader MW, Sanchez-Sotelo J, Sperling JW, Rowland CM, Cofield RH. Understanding proximal humerus fractures: image analysis, classification, and treatment. J Shoulder Elbow Surg. 2005;14:497–505.
14. Goutallier D, Postel JM, Bernageau J, Lavau L, Voisin MC. Fatty muscle degeneration in cuff ruptures. Pre- and postoperative evaluation by CT scan. Clin Orthop Relat Res. 1994:78–83.
15. Thomazeau H, Rolland Y, Lucas C, Duval JM, Langlais F. Atrophy of the supraspinatus belly. Assessment by MRI in 55 patients with rotator cuff pathology. Acta Orthop Scand. 1996;67:264–8.
16. Nanda R, Goodchild L, Gamble A, Campbell RS, Rangan A. Does the presence of a full-thickness rotator cuff tear influence outcome after proximal humeral fractures? J Trauma. 2007;62:1436–9.
17. Strobel K, Hodler J, Meyer DC, Pfirrmann CW, Pirkl C, et al. Fatty atrophy of supraspinatus and infraspinatus muscles: accuracy of US. Radiology. 2005;237:584–9.
18. Wall LB, Teefey SA, Middleton WD, Dahiya N, Steger-May K, et al. Diagnostic performance and reliability of ultrasonography for fatty degeneration of the rotator cuff muscles. J Bone Joint Surg Am. 2012;94:e83.
19. Gallo RA, Altman DT, Altman GT. Assessment of rotator cuff tendons after proximal humerus fractures: is preoperative imaging necessary? J Trauma. 2009;66:951–3.
20. Scheibel M. Humeral head fracture and cuff. Unfallchirurg. 2011;114:1075–8, 1081–2.
21. Young AA, Walch G, Pape G, Gohlke F, Favard L. Secondary rotator cuff dysfunction following total shoulder arthroplasty for primary glenohumeral osteoarthritis: results of a multicenter study with more than five years of follow-up. J Bone Joint Surg Am. 2012;94:685–93.
22. Aksu N, Aslan O, Kara AN, Isiklar ZU. Simultaneous repair of chronic full-thickness rotator cuff tears during fixation of proximal humerus fractures and clinical results. Acta Orthop Traumatol Turc. 2010;44:173–9.
23. Lenarz C, Shishani Y, McCrum C, Nowinski RJ, Edwards TB, et al. Is reverse shoulder arthroplasty appropriate for the treatment of fractures in the older patient? Early observations. Clin Orthop Relat Res. 2011;469:3324–31.
24. Favard L, Levigne C, Nerot C, Gerber C, De Wilde L, et al. Reverse prostheses in arthropathies with cuff tear: are survivorship and function maintained over time? Clin Orthop Relat Res. 2011;469:2469–75.

Osteoporosis and BMD of the Proximal Humerus

12

Ingo J. Banke

Introduction

The incidence of proximal humerus fractures rises rapidly with age. More than 70 % of fractures of the proximal humerus can be assigned to the age above 60 years showing the highest age-specific peak in 80–89 year old women [10]. Between the age of 30 and 60 years the distribution in men and women is equal. Afterwards the incidence for proximal humeral fractures in women compared to men increases by 4 times leading to an estimated overall male to female ratio of 3:7 [10]. This strong effect of advanced age and female sex underlines the significant association between proximal humerus fractures and osteoporosis. Due to this fracture and concomitant disability promoting effect osteoporosis has gained vast clinical and public health importance over the last decades [3]. Multicenter studies have demonstrated the major impact of osteoporotic proximal humeral fractures on reduction of subjective patient-perceived health and functional disability [1].

I.J. Banke
Clinic of Orthopedics and Sports Orthopedics, Klinikum rechts der Isar, Technical University of Munich, Munich, Germany
e-mail: ingo.banke@gmx.net

Bone Mineral Density and Osteoporosis

Bone mass decline with in consequence low bone mineral density (BMD) and neuromuscular function diminishment with increased risk to fall are the major predisposing factors for occurrence of proximal humerus fractures [2, 10]. In consequence after the menopause in women and, to a lesser extent, with advancing age in men low-energy traumas as a fall from standing height are sufficient as mechanism of injury for three-quarters of all proximal humerus fractures [3].

In the Western world osteoporosis, a chronic progressive disease with multifactorial etiology and silent course is the most common metabolic bone disease [3]. The main clinical manifestations are fragility fractures of the distal radius, proximal femur, thoracolumbar spine and proximal humerus. Significant increase of proximal humerus fracture incidence in osteoporotic bone has been shown in several studies [3, 10].

Osteoporosis and Proximal Humerus Fracture Surgery

Osteoporosis not only raises the frequency of proximal humerus fractures. A lower trabecular bone density also leads to a reduced biomechanical stability of the fractured bone [13] with in consequence a diminished mechanical stability of

P. Biberthaler et al. (eds.), *Fractures of the Proximal Humerus*, Strategies in Fracture Treatments,
DOI 10.1007/978-3-319-20300-3_12

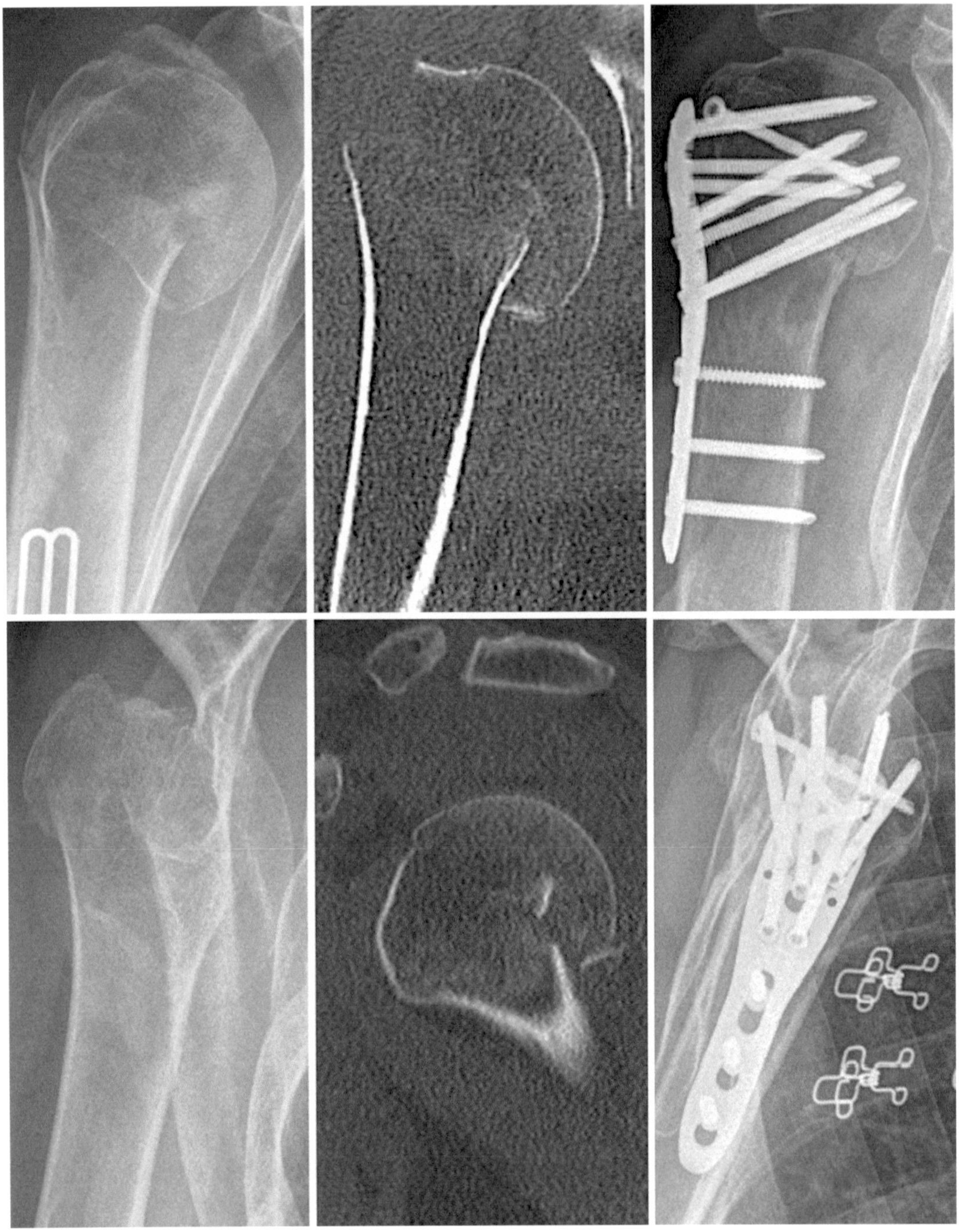

Fig. 12.1 Anatomic reduction of osteopenic dislocated Neer type 4 impacted varus fracture of the proximal humerus with precontoured low profile fixed-angle locking plate and rotator cuff suture fixation

internal (and external) fixation. Difficulty in surgical treatment and intra- as well as postoperative complications significantly increase [6]. In combination with local BMD additional risk factors as age, nonanatomic reduction and insufficient restoration of the medial cortical support further significantly rise the failure rate of internal fixation in unstable proximal humerus fractures [6].

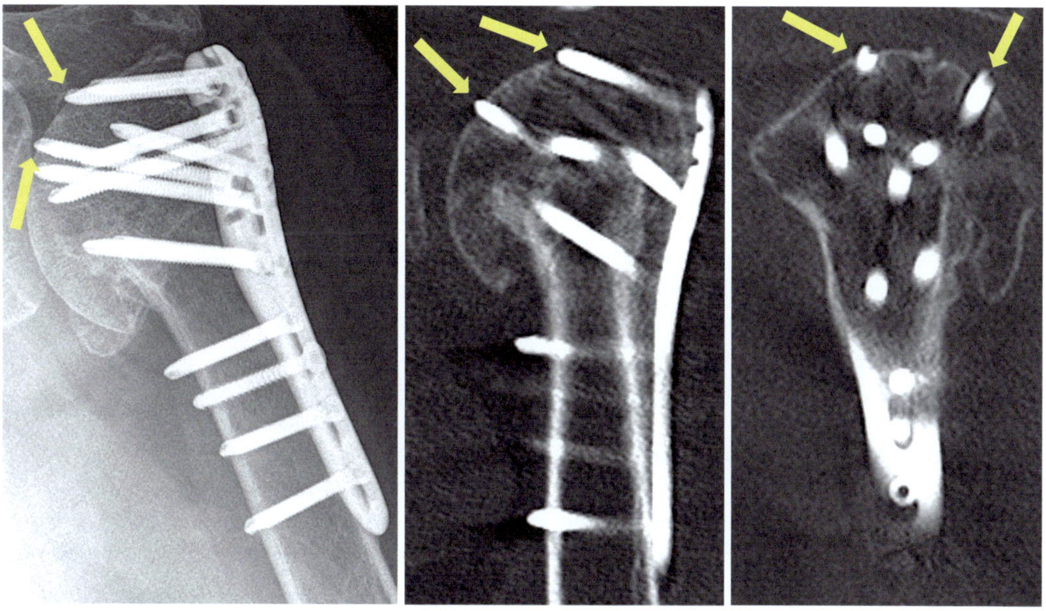

Fig. 12.2 Non-union with cranial screw cut out (indicated by *arrows*) of the osteopenic bone 9 months after anatomic proximal humerus fracture reduction

Various studies have shown that pullout strength of screws is highly dependent on BMD [12]. Conventional plate fixations with spherical head screws are highly sensible for low BMD due to predominantly axial pullout forces. In contrast internal fixators with fixed-angle or polyaxial locking screws interact with axial and bending loads (Fig. 12.1). This is advantageous particularly in low BMD due to the greater resistance against shear forces [12]. Screw positioning itself can influence the bone-to-implant biomechanical behavior as well, which is of special importance in low BMD [4].

Delayed healing, non-union or simply implant cut out of the osteopenic bone (Fig. 12.2) mostly result due to prevention of dynamic bone contact caused by too rigid implants [11]. The high initial stiffness of rather rigid implants such as intramedullary nails and conventional plates leads to an early loosening and failure of the implant-bone interface under biomechanical cyclic loading [8]. In contrast implants with low stiffness and flexible characteristics such as the newer precontoured locking plates with suture augmentation (Fig. 12.1) minimize the peak stresses at the bone-implant interface [9]. This rather dynamic fixation construct makes them favorable especially for osteoporotic bone fractures in the elderly population [8]. However despite the experimentally shown strong evidence of local osteoporosis on fracture fixation implant anchorage in clinical studies this impact could not be directly reproduced yet. Lack of missing complication definitions, correct osteoporosis assessment and unclear inclusion criteria are thought to be responsible for this. Prospective studies directly examining the correlation between local BMD and the fixation failure risk are needed [5].

In order to manage surgical difficulties and avoid intra- and postoperative complications associated with osteoporosis sufficient preoperative assessment of the local bone quality is of utmost importance. This facilitates decision-making in the surgical treatment of patients sustaining proximal humerus fractures leading to better results.

Diagnostical Workup

The cornerstones of the preoperative fragility fracture workup are strictly based on a clinical setting where the time-span between initial radiological diagnosis of a proximal humerus fracture and its surgical treatment should be kept as short as possible in terms of morbidity and outcome [10].

Trauma Mechanism

A history of low-energy trauma, especially in the elderly population is highly suspicious for an underlying osteoporotic fracture genesis.

Evaluation of Osteoporosis Risks

Beside age and gender, in the medical history individual risk factors as diseases or medications, alcohol usage or smoking contributing to a low BMD should be questioned. As osteoporosis itself has no symptoms, one should focus on consequences of osteoporosis like an increased risk of fragility fractures. The skeletal history should include fractures and their healing in the past. Also chronic pain may be attributed to chronic fragility fractures.

In the physical examination signs of fragility fractures like a vertebral collapse, possibly presenting with sudden back pain or radicular pain, hump or loss of height as well as deformities of the extremities or an impaired mobility could serve as a warning signal. As osteoporosis is a recognized complication in specific diseases and disorders also external signs of these co-morbidities such as malnutrition, endocrine disorders like Cushing's syndrome or hypogonadal states should be assessed.

Blood evaluation should be performed routinely for serum electrolytes, calcium, total protein, albumin, kidney and liver parameters and thyroid-stimulating hormone. For detection of potentially underlying causes of a low BMD in patients with a suspicious history it may be tailored enlarged with additional parameters such as phosphorus, magnesium, intact parathyroid hormone, 25-hydroxy vitamin D, serum testosterone and complete blood count. However in a clinical setting these additional parameters should not be routinely assessed.

Dual-energy X-ray absorptiometry (DXA) for quantitative assessment of BMD plays no role in a preoperative setting. Nevertheless DXA is considered the gold standard for osteoporosis diagnosis and should be employed postoperatively for further diagnosis and therapy.

Conventional Radiography

For preoperative assessment of osteoporotic changes in the proximal humerus plain radiography can be helpful. Prediction of local BMD via radiographs provides the most technically uncomplicated and cost-effective process for clinicians [10]. Thereby in anteroposterior radiographs the cortical thickness of the proximal humeral diaphysis may serve as a reliable predictor of local bone quality at the level of humeral head, surgical neck, greater and lesser tuberosity [14]. In general patients over 70 years show significantly lower cortical thickness and local BMD than those under 70 years [14]. However for decision making regarding operative and non-operative treatment (spiral) computed tomography imaging (CT) is more valuable [10].

Computed Tomography (CT)

Spiral CT is an established diagnostic tool for assessing local BMD in the spine. As CT scans display the preoperative imaging of choice in complex and/or low BMD proximal humeral fracture repairs they could be easily used at the same time for preoperative determination of local humeral BMD [10]. By calculating the average Hounsfield unit values in standardized regions of the proximal humerus and linear calibration equation to calculate from the obtained Hounsfield units to BMD, assessment of cancellous BMD of the proximal humerus is by principle possible with high intraobserver and interobserver reliability (intraclass correlation coefficient >0.9) [7]. In a clinical investigation with this method low local BMD has been shown to correlate with fracture fixation failure [6]. However it still remains to be determined whether CT based local BMD assessment can be easily reproduced and efficiently applied by clinicians in daily routine [10].

Preoperative Planning

When an underlying low BMD or osteoporosis in proximal humerus fracture is reasonably suspected or confirmed the thinking about correct treatment should deviate from standardized concepts. Especially in osteoporotic three- and four-part fractures of the proximal humerus treatment is difficult lacking a common consensus of the best technique leading to the best outcome in elderly patients. The preexisting reduced biological fracture healing potential (diminished periosteal blood supply, osteogenic activity and immune defense) should not be further harmed by the approach, surgical exposition, reduction technique or choice of implant. Secondly a more stable fixation is needed. (Low profile) locking plates with routinely performed suture fixation in the rotator cuff became more and more the treatment of choice even in cases with uncomplicated proximal humerus fracture (Fig. 12.3). However in osteoporosis minimally invasive reduction and implanting techniques should be favored. If percutaneous techniques with internal reduction are applied stability of fracture should not be neglected. Thirdly in the case of structural defects (biological) augmenting fixation may be indicated. Various tailored therapeutic augmentation concepts to fill the void in the humeral head are available from iliac crest bone graft, injectable resorbable calcium sulfate or phosphate and hydroxyapatite cement (Fig. 12.4), crushed cancellous allograft bone chips and intramedullary fibular grafts [10]. Finally in severely displaced three- and four-part fractures or even comminuted fractures with high risk of humeral head necrosis due to an underlying low BMD and other comorbidities primary arthroplasty should be considered as well. If preoperative planning already involves organization of postoperative treatment range-of-motion exercises producing a bending stress and avoiding axial stress should be favored early after operation [4].

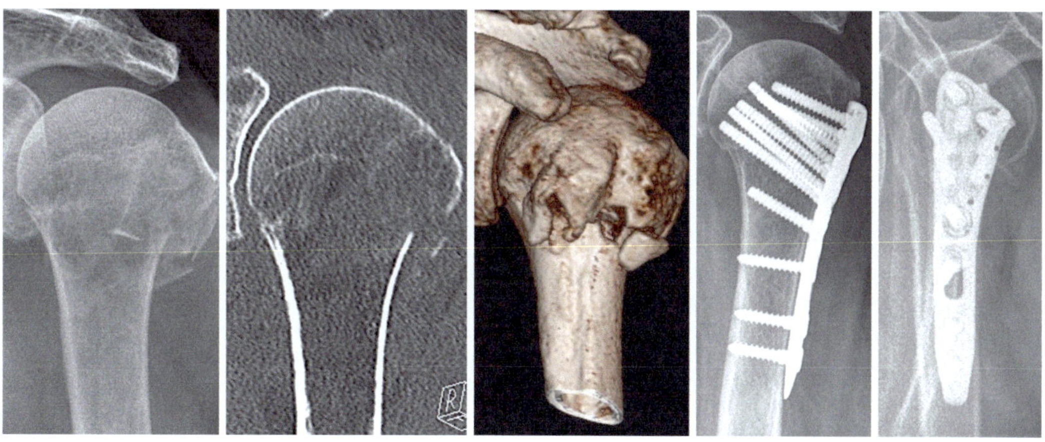

Fig. 12.3 Anatomic reduction of osteopenic uncomplicated impacted valgus fracture of the proximal humerus with precontoured low profile polyaxial locking plate and rotator cuff suture fixation

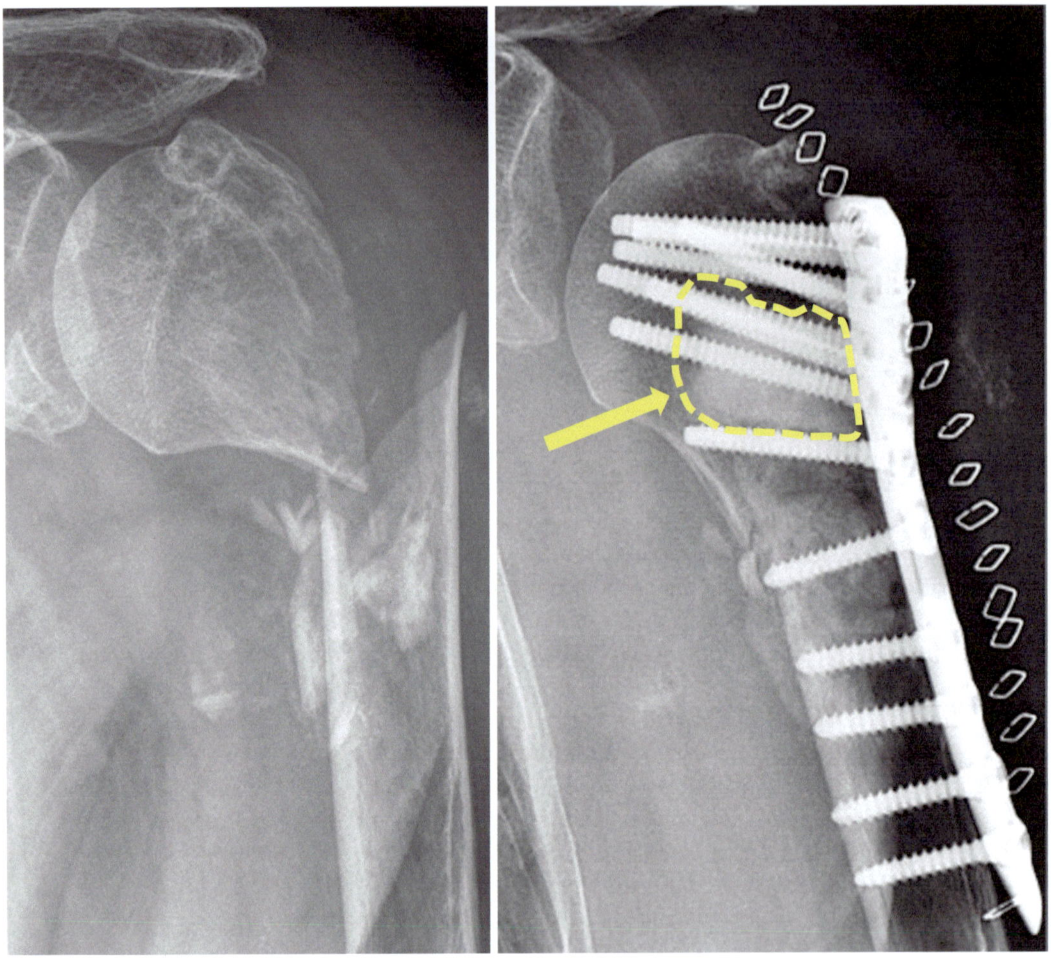

Fig. 12.4 Augmentation of highly osteoporotic humeral head void (for better visualization highlighted by *arrows* and *broken line*) with injectable resorbable calcium sulfate and hydroxyapatite bioceramic augmentation in anatomic proximal humerus fracture reduction

Summary

The osteoporotic proximal humeral fracture is challenging and the risk of insufficient fixation with in consequence poor outcome evident. Fragility fracture workup with local BMD assessment is of utmost importance for the choice of the best patient tailored fracture management. Preoperative determination of local BMD may be helpful especially regarding the need of additional (biological) augmentation. However if successful surgical fixation of the osteoporotic proximal humerus fracture is highly questioned or even not possible due to lacking anatomic reduction without medial cortical support repair primary arthroplasty should be chosen.

References

1. Calvo E, Morcillo D, Foruria AM, et al. Nondisplaced proximal humeral fractures: high incidence among outpatient-treated osteoporotic fractures and severe impact on upper extremity. J Shoulder Elbow Surg. 2011;20(5):795–801.
2. Court-Brown CM, Caesar B. Epidemiology of adult fractures: a review. Injury. 2006;37:691–7.
3. Cummings SR, Melton LJ. Epidemiology and outcomes of osteoporotic fractures. Lancet. 2002; 359(9319):1761–7.

4. Fankhauser F, Schippinger G, Weber K, et al. Cadaveric-biomechanical evaluation of bone-implant construct of proximal humerus fractures (Neer type 3). J Trauma. 2003;55:345–9.
5. Goldhahn J, Suhm N, Goldhahn S, et al. Influence of osteoporosis on fracture fixation – a systematic literature review. Osteoporos Int. 2008;19(6):761–72.
6. Krappinger D, Bizzotto N, Riedmann S, et al. Predicting failure after surgical fixation of proximal humerus fractures. Injury. 2011;42(11):1283–8.
7. Krappinger D, Roth T, Gschwentner M, et al. Preoperative assessment of the cancellous bone mineral density of the proximal humerus using CT data. Skeletal Radiol. 2012;41:299–304.
8. Lill H, Hepp P, Korner J, et al. Proximal humeral fractures: how stiff should an implant be? A comparative mechanical study with new implants in human specimens. Arch Orthop Trauma Surg. 2003;123(2–3): 74–81.
9. Namdari S, Lipman AJ, Ricchetti ET, et al. Fixation strategies to prevent screw cut-out and malreduction in proximal humeral fracture fixation. Clin Orthop Surg. 2012;4:321–4.
10. Namdari S, Voleti PB, Mehta S. Evaluation of the osteoporotic proximal humeral fracture and strategies for structural augmentation during surgical treatment. J Shoulder Elbow Surg. 2012;21(12):1787–95.
11. Sadowski C, Riand N, Stern R, et al. Fixation of fractures of the proximal humerus with the PlantTan Humerus Fixator Plate: early experience with a new implant. J Shoulder Elbow Surg. 2003; 12(2):148–51.
12. Seebeck J, Goldhahn J, Stadele H, et al. Effect of cortical thickness and cancellous bone density on the holding strength of internal fixator screws. J Orthop Res. 2004;22:1237–42.
13. Silva MJ. Biomechanics of osteoporotic fractures. Injury. 2007;38 Suppl 3:S69–76.
14. Tingart MJ, Apreleva M, von Stechow D. The cortical thickness of the proximal humeral diaphysis predicts bone mineral density of the proximal humerus. J Bone Joint Surg Br. 2003;85(4):611–7.

Surgical Decision Making 13

Gunther H. Sandmann

Non-operative Treatment

The fracture of the proximal humerus accounts for 5 % of all fractures and the typical trauma mechanism in young patients is high energy trauma often associated with neurovascular affection. In the elderly with osteoporotic alterations of the proximal humerus the main trauma mechanism is a fall from standing height in terms of a low energy trauma [1].

The decision for operative or conservative treatment depends on several factors including the biological age of the patient, concomitant diseases and the associated potential risks of anaesthesia, the patient´s compliance and the existing bone stock. In addition, the type of fracture is an important factor in the decision making regarding conservative versus surgical therapy. In general, all minimally displaced fractures with a fragment dislocation <5 mm, a deviation of the axis <20° and a displacement of the tubercula <2 mm are suitable for conservative treatment. It has to be pointed out that a short immobilization period for 1 week is often necessary, but physical therapy should be started as soon as the pain level allows it.

In this context Koval et al. [2] could show that the beginning of physical therapy within 14 days after the incident leads to improved results. In addition, a dynamic evaluation of the fracture under fluoroscopic guidance is recommended to be able to distinguish relatively stable impacted fractures from unstable fracture types.

In our University setting the shoulder is immobilized in a sling for 1 week along with physical therapy of elbow and wrist. Consecutively depending on the pain, back an forth swinging of the arm is allowed. Finally passive and active-assisted mobilization of the arm up to 90° abduction and flexion is performed for the first 6 weeks after trauma unless exercises with free range of motion can be performed. In their series of 125 valgus-impacted fractures treated conservatively Court-Brown et al. [3] showed that 80 % of the elderly patients had good to excellent results though residual deficits in strength and range of motion were noticed. Therefore in case of an active, high demanding patient at an age >60 years suffering from only slightly displaced fractures we would tend to recommend surgical intervention to avoid an immobilization period as described for the conservative treatment regime above and a potentially faster recovery.

G.H. Sandmann
Department of Traumatology,
Technical University of Munich,
Munich, Germany
e-mail: drsandmann@icloud.com

P. Biberthaler et al. (eds.), *Fractures of the Proximal Humerus*, Strategies in Fracture Treatments,
DOI 10.1007/978-3-319-20300-3_13

Operative Treatment

Surgical intervention in proximal humerus fractures is recommended for all types of displaced fractures as long as operative treatment is possible. Concerning the tubercula a displacement greater than 2 mm is inacceptable as secondary impingement might arise. According to Neer [4] those fractures running through the surgical neck along with an ad latus dislocation of 10 mm and a retroversion up to 45° would be suitable for conservative treatment. However, our own algorithm for treating proximal humerus fractures only accepts a maximal displacement of 5 mm ad latus and a retroversion of the humeral head of 20°. Further absolute indications for operative treatment comprise fractures with multiple metaphyseal fragments, fractures running through the anatomical neck, head-split fractures and fractures with concomitant dislocation of the shoulder or affection of vessels/nerves.

For the operative intervention there are various different treatment options available reaching from reconstructive procedures like implanting minimal invasive K-wires [5, 6], locking plates [7–9], or proximal humerus nails [10, 11] to performing arthroplasty either in terms of implanting an anatomic [12, 13] or reverse prosthesis [14–16]. Thus the surgeon needs to carefully evaluate the patient's fracture data to be able to find the best treatment option in terms of operative treatment for the individual patient.

In this context it should be mentioned that the percutaneous treatment of fractures using K-wires for fracture reduction is soft tissue sparing, but the reduction of the fracture might be difficult and the fixation of the fracture by K-wires is often not stable enough for early mobilization, so that we do not recommend this technique.

In our setting locking plates are used on a routine basis to treat humeral head fractures [17, 18]. As standard approach a modified deltoideopectoral approach is recommended, using the anatomic interval between the Deltoid and the Pectoralis major muscle. Therefore this approach is soft- tissue sparing and does neither endanger the axillary nerve nor the deltoid function. However, nowadays still several publications exist, which could not find an affection of the deltoid muscle in the treatment of humeral head fractures using the delta split approach [19]. The fracture is reduced and the plate itself might be used as a tool for the reduction of the displaced head. Cortical screws are used to fix the plate on the shaft and then in a next step the displaced humeral head is reduced against the plate. It is appropriate and in most of the cases important to use additional cerclages to fix the tubercula against the plate. The position of the plate and the length of the screws need to be checked on x-ray to avoid a secondary impingement or an affection of the glenoid.

In contrast, implanting a proximal humerus nail via a delta split approach the rotator cuff needs to be incised along the fibers. This implant can be useful in the treatment of fractures with metaphyseal fragments. Nevertheless, the removal of proximal humeral nails might be sometimes difficult and concomitant injuries of the rotator cuff are described. Still, the results of humeral head fractures treated with plates or with nails are similar and so the use of the implant depends on the surgeons' preferences and skills.

Over the past decade there have been controversies about the need of surgical treatment of 3- and 4-part humeral head fractures and a renaissance of conservative treatment can be noticed. This is mainly based on studies by Olerud et al. [20] showing no advantages of the surgical compared to non-operative treatment of humeral head fractures. Nevertheless, this work offers some limitations since the used implants do not seem to be appropriate for the treatment of complex humeral head fractures. Still, up to date there is no sufficient data indicating that operative treatment-independently from the chosen implant-might lead to an improved outcome compared to non-operative treatment [21]. So future research and prospective-randomized trials are necessary to find the best possible treatment option for humeral head fractures.

Timing of Treatment

In general fractures of the proximal humerus do not present or do not require an emergency operation and thus can be planned in most of the cases for the next days. Those fractures with reconstructive potential have a higher priority compared to displaced fractures – e.g. head split fractures – in which only the implantation of a prosthesis remains.

Still, there are cases, where urgent operative treatment is necessary including the rare open fractures of the proximal humerus, dislocated fractures where a closed reduction is not possible [22] and fractures with concomitant nerve [23] or vessel [24] affections. Especially in dislocated fractures with displaced fragments in the axillary groove and pressure by the fragments on the axillary nerve or the plexus an urgent open reduction is necessary. These cases should be referred – if possible – to a trauma center as the reconstruction of the proximal humerus might fail and the implantation of a prosthesis becomes necessary over the course of the treatment.

References

1. Krappinger D, Roth T, Gschwentner M, et al. Preoperative assessment of the cancellous bone mineral density of the proximal humerus using CT data. Skeletal Radiol. 2012;41(3):299–304.
2. Koval KJ, Gallagher MA, Marsicano JG, Cuomo F, McShinawy A, Zuckerman JD. Functional outcome after minimally displaced fractures of the proximal part of the humerus. J Bone Joint Surg Am. 1997;79(2):203–7.
3. Court-Brown CM, Cattermole H, McQueen MM. Impacted valgus fractures (B1.1) of the proximal humerus. The results of non-operative treatment. J Bone Joint Surg Br. 2002;84(4):504–8.
4. Neer 2nd CS. Displaced proximal humeral fractures. II. Treatment of three-part and four-part displacement. J Bone Joint Surg Am. 1970;52(6):1090–103.
5. Bogner R, Hubner C, Matis N, Auffarth A, Lederer S, Resch H. Minimally-invasive treatment of three- and four-part fractures of the proximal humerus in elderly patients. J Bone Joint Surg Br. 2008;90(12):1602–7.
6. Bahrs C, Badke A, Rolauffs B, et al. Long-term results after non-plate head-preserving fixation of proximal humeral fractures. Int Orthop. 2010;34(6):883–9.
7. Roderer G, Erhardt J, Graf M, Kinzl L, Gebhard F. Clinical results for minimally invasive locked plating of proximal humerus fractures. J Orthop Trauma. 2010;24(7):400–6.
8. Sudkamp N, Bayer J, Hepp P, et al. Open reduction and internal fixation of proximal humeral fractures with use of the locking proximal humerus plate. Results of a prospective, multicenter, observational study. J Bone Joint Surg Am. 2009;91(6):1320–8.
9. Hirschmann MT, Fallegger B, Amsler F, Regazzoni P, Gross T. Clinical longer-term results after internal fixation of proximal humerus fractures with a locking compression plate (PHILOS). J Orthop Trauma. 2011;25(5):286–93.
10. Mittlmeier TW, Stedtfeld HW, Ewert A, Beck M, Frosch B, Gradl G. Stabilization of proximal humeral fractures with an angular and sliding stable antegrade locking nail (Targon PH). J Bone Joint Surg Am. 2003;85-A Suppl 4:136–46.
11. Gradl G, Dietze A, Kaab M, Hopfenmuller W, Mittlmeier T. Is locking nailing of humeral head fractures superior to locking plate fixation? Clin Orthop Relat Res. 2009;467(11):2986–93.
12. Fialka C, Stampfl P, Arbes S, Reuter P, Oberleitner G, Vecsei V. Primary hemiarthroplasty in four-part fractures of the proximal humerus: randomized trial of two different implant systems. J Shoulder Elbow Surg. 2008;17(2):210–5.
13. Cadet ER, Ahmad CS. Hemiarthroplasty for three- and four-part proximal humerus fractures. J Am Acad Orthop Surg. 2012;20(1):17–27.
14. Valenti P, Katz D, Kilinc A, Elkholti K, Gasiunas V. Mid-term outcome of reverse shoulder prostheses in complex proximal humeral fractures. Acta Orthop Belg. 2012;78(4):442–9.
15. Garrigues GE, Johnston PS, Pepe MD, Tucker BS, Ramsey ML, Austin LS. Hemiarthroplasty versus reverse total shoulder arthroplasty for acute proximal humerus fractures in elderly patients. Orthopedics. 2012;35(5):e703–8.
16. Rasmussen JV, Jakobsen J, Brorson S, Olsen BS. The Danish Shoulder Arthroplasty Registry: clinical outcome and short-term survival of 2,137 primary shoulder replacements. Acta Orthop. 2012;83(2):171–3.
17. Kettler M, Biberthaler P, Braunstein V, Zeiler C, Kroetz M, Mutschler W. Treatment of proximal humeral fractures with the PHILOS angular stable plate. Presentation of 225 cases of dislocated fractures. Unfallchirurg. 2006;109(12):1032–40.
18. Tepass A, Blumenstock G, Weise K, Rolauffs B, Bahrs C. Current strategies for the treatment of proximal humeral fractures: an analysis of a survey carried out at 348 hospitals in Germany, Austria, and Switzerland. J Shoulder Elbow Surg. 2013;22(1):e8–14.

19. Martetschlager F, Siebenlist S, Weier M, et al. Plating of proximal humeral fractures. Orthopedics. 2012; 35(11):e1606–12.
20. Olerud P, Ahrengart L, Ponzer S, Saving J, Tidermark J. Internal fixation versus nonoperative treatment of displaced 3-part proximal humeral fractures in elderly patients: a randomized controlled trial. J Shoulder Elbow Surg. 2011;20(5):747–55.
21. Handoll HH, Ollivere BJ, Rollins KE. Interventions for treating proximal humeral fractures in adults. Cochrane Database Syst Rev. 2012;(12): CD000434.
22. Simpson NS, Schwappach JR, Toby EB. Fracture-dislocation of the humerus with intrathoracic displacement of the humeral head. A case report. J Bone Joint Surg Am. 1998;80(6):889–91.
23. Bono CM, Grossman MG, Hochwald N, Tornetta P 3rd. Radial and axillary nerves. Anatomic considerations for humeral fixation. Clin Orthop Relat Res. 2000;4(373):259–64.
24. Gorthi V, Moon YL, Jo SH, Sohn HM, Ha SH. Life-threatening posterior circumflex humeral artery injury secondary to fracture-dislocation of the proximal humerus. Orthopedics. 2010;33(3):200–2.

Part IV

Conservative Treatment

14 Non-operative Management of Proximal Humerus Fractures

Ashesh Kumar and James P. Waddell

Introduction

The management of proximal humeral fractures has been discussed in surgical textbooks for greater than 3000 years. Detailed descriptions of reduction and splinting are found in surgical texts from both Ancient Egypt and Greece [1]. Today, proximal humeral fractures account for up to 5 % of all fractures treated [2]. Between 50 and 80 % of these can be treated non-operatively and are non-displaced or minimally displaced 2-part fractures [3–8]. Three- and four-part fractures represent 15 % of all proximal humeral fractures. Seventy percent of three- and four-part fractures are seen in patients over 60 years old and 50 % of such fractures are seen in those over 70 years old [2]. The elderly are more susceptible to this type of fracture due to co-morbid conditions that predispose these patients to low energy falls. Such co-morbid conditions include poor vision, balance problems, loss of protective reflexes, and polypharmacy. Furthermore, poor bone quality in the elderly population accounts for a greater severity of injury with more complex fracture patterns in spite of little mechanical insult. With a growing elderly population, the rate of proximal humeral fractures has increased by an average of 13 % per year between 1970 and 2002 [2, 9–12]. The number of these fractures in the elderly population is expected to triple by 2030 [6].

Treating orthopaedic surgeons seldom need be reminded of the tremendous effect of these fractures on patients. Many patients are left with the inability to care for themselves at the most fundamental level. Dressing, bathing, toileting, feeding, and even the ability to leave the house may all be affected. Previously independent patients can become quite dependent and the period of dependence may last for several months. Indeed, approximately 6 months to 1 year is needed for good or very good recovery, with better results being obtained from the recovery of non-displaced versus displaced fractures [3, 5, 13–19].

It is imperative that treating orthopaedic surgeons have a thorough understanding of this common problem. However, there is a great deal of variability and heterogeneity among studies and treatment algorithms that investigate proximal humeral fractures. Differences in treatment manifest at all levels of the therapeutic chain. The relative influence and consideration of patient-related factors such as age, functional demand, and co-morbid conditions varies amongst surgeons in treating proximal humerus fractures. Similarly, there is considerable variance in standard imaging for diagnosis, splinting options for initial immobilization, and rehabilitation protocols between surgeons, institutions, and regions [20–22]. Finally, there is controversy regarding surgical versus conservative

A. Kumar, MD, MSc, FRCSC (✉)
J.P. Waddell, MD, FRCSC
Division of Orthopaedics,
St. Michael's Hospital, Toronto, ON, Canada
e-mail: dr.ashesh.kumar@gmail.com;
WADDELLJ@smh.ca

P. Biberthaler et al. (eds.), *Fractures of the Proximal Humerus*, Strategies in Fracture Treatments,
DOI 10.1007/978-3-319-20300-3_14

management of three- and four- part proximal humerus fractures [23]. Consequently, there is a need for a clear evidence-based consensus on how to manage these challenging and complex fractures. A thorough understanding of the natural history of conservative treatment is especially important to establish a baseline for which to compare the usefulness of emerging operative technologies.

Diagnosis

Our treatment algorithm starts with good quality radiographs. See Fig. 14.1. We use a trauma series which includes a true anteroposterior (AP) and a scapular Y views perpendicular and parallel to the plane of the scapula respectively. An axillary lateral view is also taken to asses the reduction of the humeral head within the glenoid. If radiographs are insufficient to understand the fracture morphology and identify all the components of the fracture then a CT scan is indicated. A CT scan can further aid in the diagnosis by giving information regarding fracture morphology, bone stock of the humeral head and tuberosities, degree of comminution, size of the fragments amenable to fixation, and the length of the posteromedial metaphyseal extension.

Proper imaging allows the determination of both fracture displacement and angulation. Both are helpful in deciding if non-operative treatment is appropriate. Neer has previously described acceptable displacement to be 1 cm and acceptable angulation of 45° [24]. Clinical and/or fluoroscopic image intensification can be used to determine the stability of the head and shaft. If the head and shaft move as a single unit then the fracture is deemed impacted and thus stable. If there is significant motion between the head and shaft then the fracture is deemed unstable.

Stable fractures respond well to short term immobilization to allow time for swelling and pain to resolve. While unstable fractures are often treated operatively the decision to operate must take into account other patient factors. Displaced fractures in patients in whom surgery may not be warranted include: elderly; low demand; uncooperative due to mental illness or substance abuse; significant co-morbid conditions; and those patients with active infections elsewhere. This group of patients with unstable fractures can be still be treated non-operatively. However, they often require a prolonged period of immobilization ranging from 2 to 4 weeks.

Initial Immobilization

The goal of initial immobilization is to provide mechanical support. Supporting the fracture acutely prevents fracture displacement and promotes fracture consolidation while pain and swelling resolve. Short term immobilization can take on a variety of forms. Splinting options include but are not limited to the broad arm sling, collar and cuff, sling and swath, shoulder immobilizer, Gilchrist bandage, and the shoulder abduction cushion. There is limited evidence for the superiority of one type of immobilization device over another. In 1993 Rommens et al. compared the Desault bandage against the Gilchrist bandage in 28 patients with a proximal humerus fracture. There was no effect on fracture healing or functional outcome. However, the Gilchrist-bandage appeared to cause less pain and skin irritation. In our opinion, there is not enough evidence to advocate for one sling over another as long as the goal of providing mechanical support is adhered to. Our preferred splinting methods include a simple collar and cuff or a Velpeau sling both of which are shown in Fig. 14.2.

Rehabilitation

Recommendations for the adequate time required for the initial period of immobilization varies from a few days to more than 3 weeks. Recommendations prior to the 90s were based on clinical experience and uncontrolled case studies [16, 18, 25–29]. Controlled clinical trials that examine when to begin mobilization of the injured arm started to appear in the 1990s and continue to be a topic of current interest.

The principal goal of rehabilitation is to restore functional range of motion to levels that

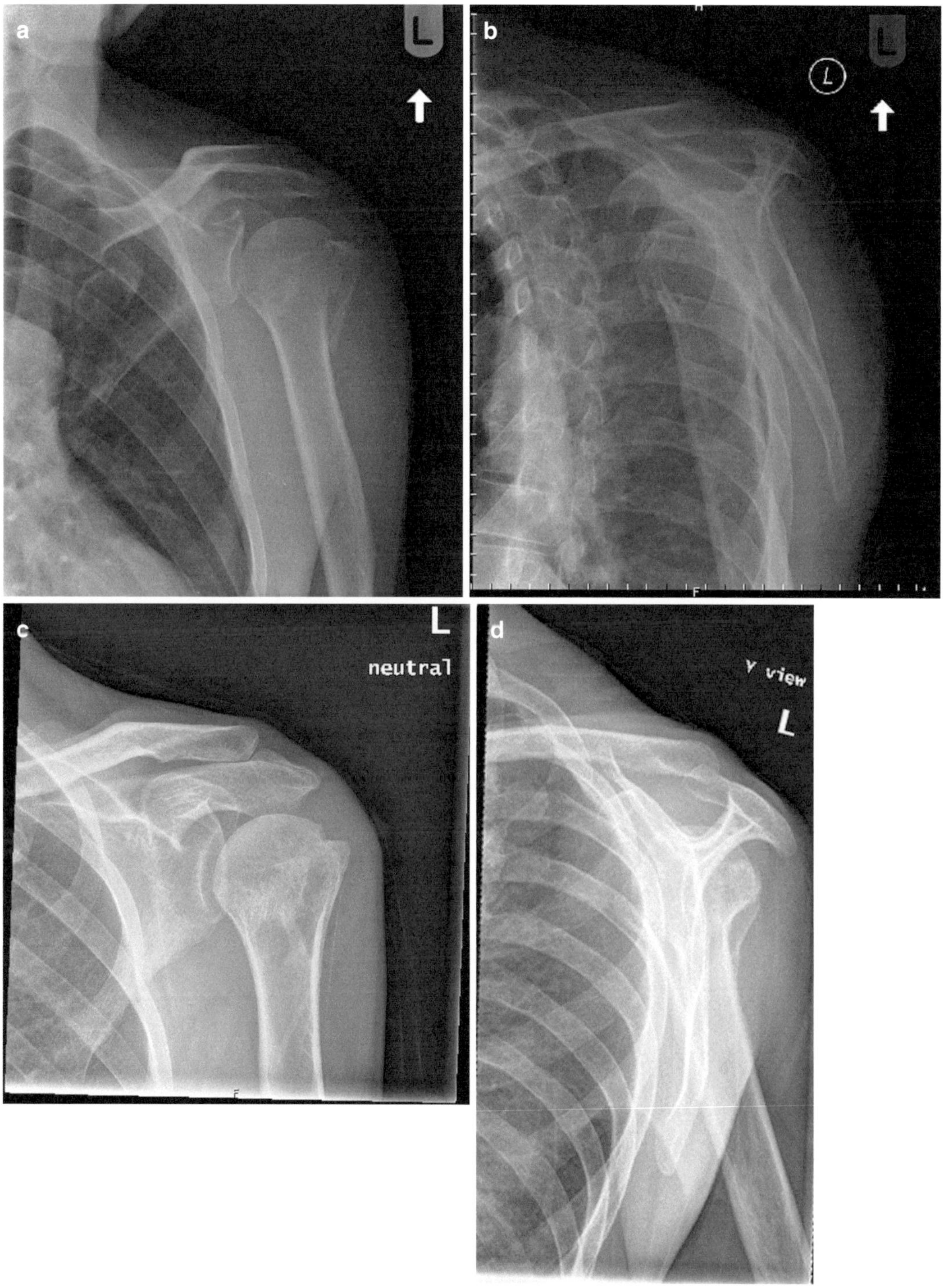

Fig. 14.1 Radiographs of a 3-part proximal humerus fracture. (**a**, **b**) AP, and scapular Y views on presentation to the emergency room. (**c**, **d**) AP and scapular Y views of healed 3-part proximal humerus fracture after non-operative management

closely approximate a patient's pre-injury status. However, rehabilitation regimens vary a great deal between surgeons, institutions, regions, and patient's personal resources. The recommended duration of immobilization, timing of first physiotherapy session, intensity and frequency of sessions, and setting for therapy be it home or hospital/private centre all play into this variability [30]. Furthermore, the experience level of the therapist and accessory modalities of treatment offered by therapists create further heterogeneity.

It is generally accepted that prolonged immobilization is complicated by shoulder stiffness and thus patients tend to have poorer outcomes. At our institution we emphasize self-performed early movement exercises after a short course of immobilization to ameliorate loss of function as shown

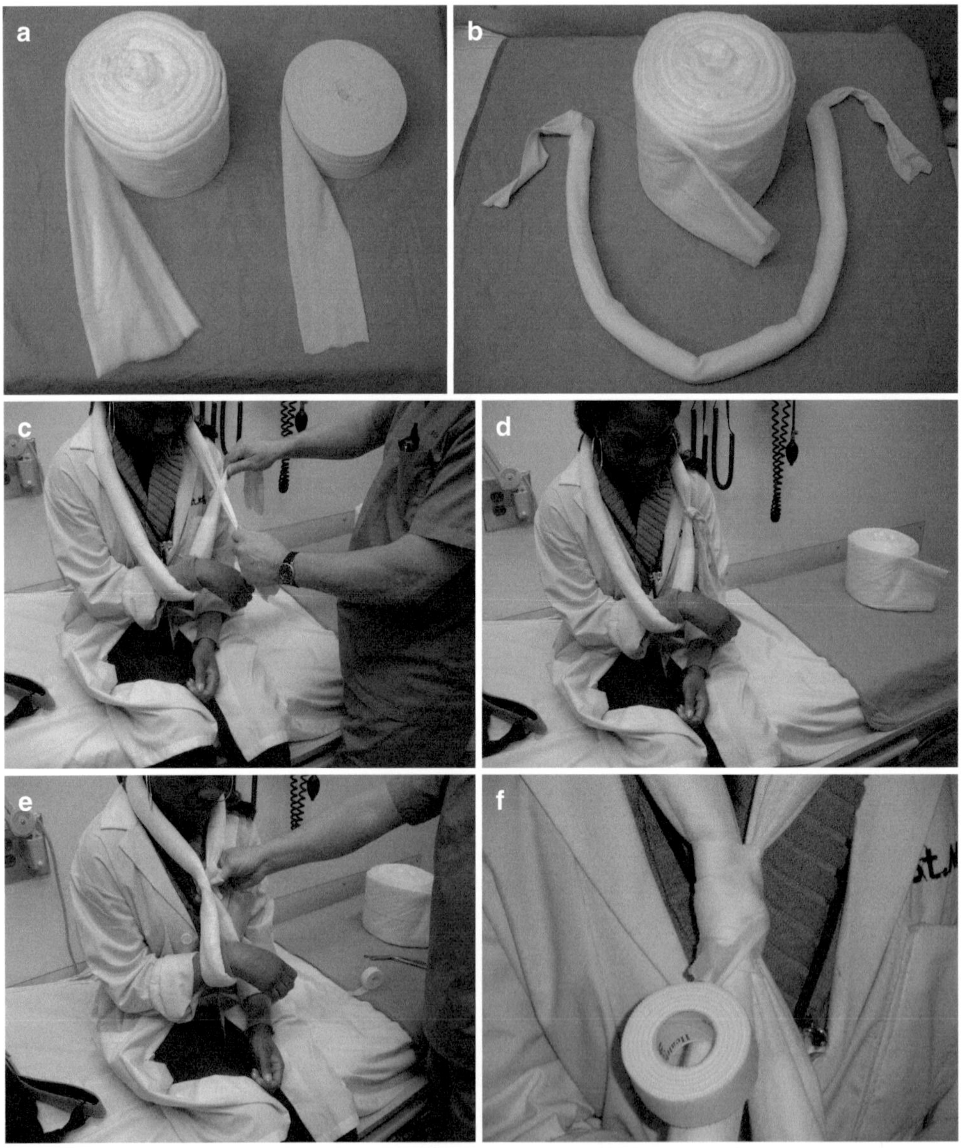

Fig. 14.2 Splint application. (**a**) Materials required are an 8″ ABD roll pictured on the left and a 3″ stockinette pictured right. (**b**) A length of ABD is cut and used to pad a cut length of stockinette. (**c**, **d**) The padded stockinette is used to support the wrist of the injured extremity, wrapped around the neck, and then tied off in a simple double knot as shown. (**e**, **f**) The knotted side and unknotted side are pinched together to form a cuff and tape is applied to secure it. (**g**) Completed collar-and-cuff style splint. (**h**) Velpeau sling pictured from the front and (**i**) back

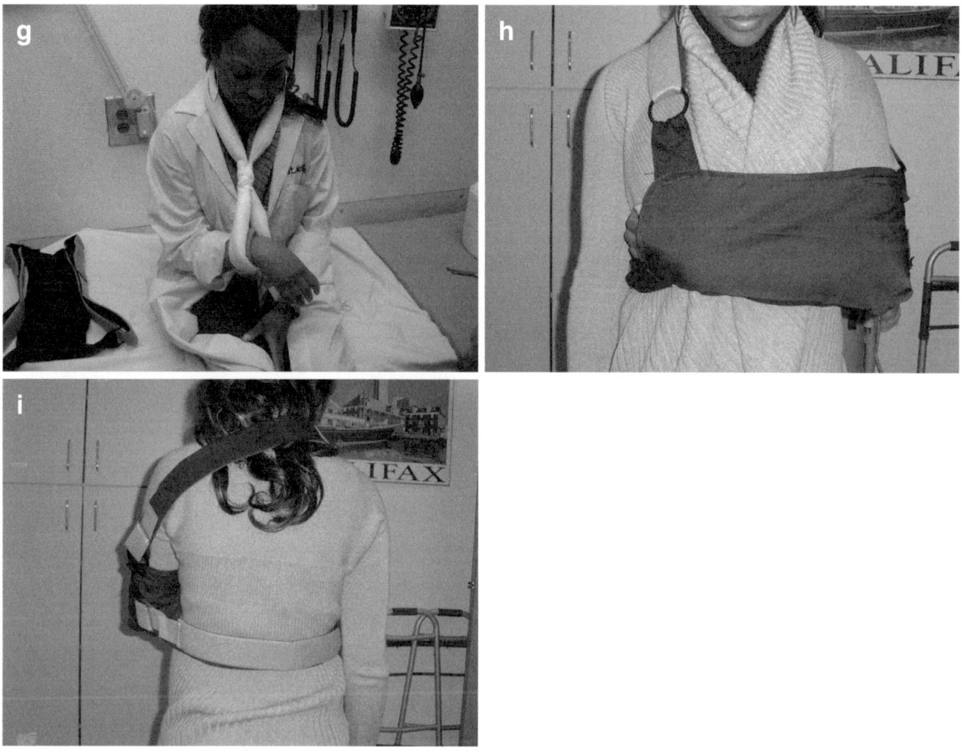

Fig. 14.2 (continued)

in Fig. 14.3. Rehabilitation generally follows two stages. Passive/assisted range of motion exercises followed by progressive resistance exercises.

Brostrom is credited as being the first to hypothesize that immediate mobilization following proximal humeral fracture would lead to faster recovery of functional mobility [18]. His brief report of 97 proximal humeral fractures found good or excellent results in 59 fractures treated with immediate passive mobilization on the fourth day following injury and active range of motion initiated 9–11 days following injury. Brostrom graded range of motion on a 100 point scale with good outcomes having a score of 75 or greater.

More recent studies have supported Brostrom's historical findings [13, 31]. Hodgson performed a prospective randomized controlled trial examining 86 minimally displaced two-part proximal humeral fractures comparing two rehabilitation regimens. Immediate physiotherapy within 1 week of injury was undertaken in one group and compared to a conventional 3 week period of immobilization in the other group. This study found better shoulder function in the group of patients mobilized immediately at the 8 and 16 week follow-up visits as measured by the Constant score. However, a statistical difference between the groups disappeared by 52 weeks. Importantly, patients mobilized immediately also reported less pain over the course of their treatment.

Hodgson's results were supported by an earlier study performed by Kristiansen in 1989 [14]. This study was a prospective randomized controlled trial which randomly allocated 85 patients with proximal humeral fractures to start mobilization exercises at 1 week or 3 weeks. Using a modified Neer's score [24, 32], they found that patients mobilized early had statistically significant better scores of overall shoulder function largely as a result of a reduction in their sensation of pain over the first 3 months. The effect disappeared at 6 months and both groups continued with similar outcomes over follow-ups for the 2 year duration of the study.

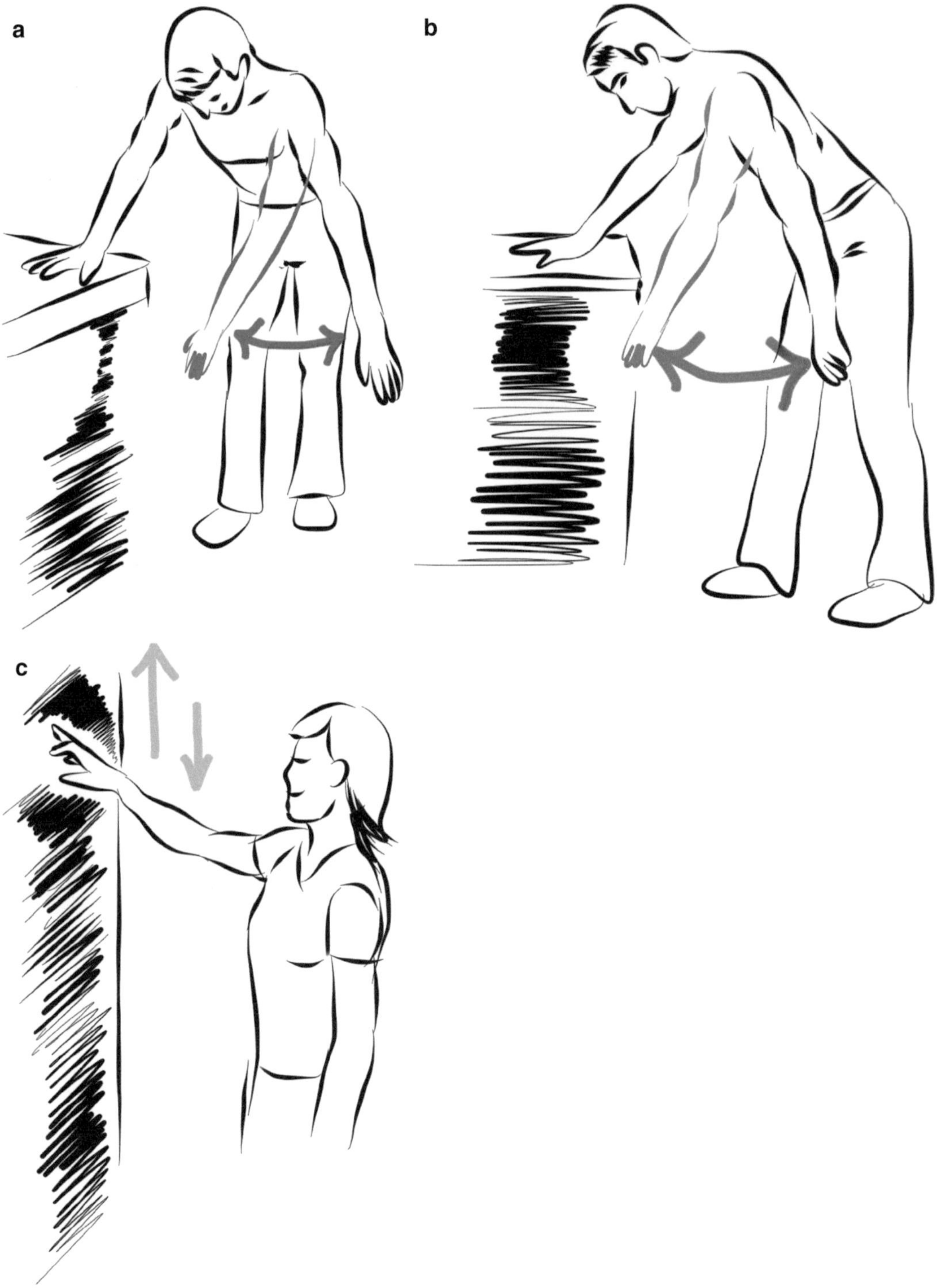

Fig. 14.3 Examples of selected self-rehabilitation exercises. (**a**, **b**) Pendulum swings. (**c**) Patient 'walks' fingers up wall as high as possible to increase shoulder flexion range of motion

Most recently, Lefevre-Colau performed a single institution RCT in 2007 [15]. In this trial, 74 patients with impacted proximal humeral fractures were randomized to either early mobilization regimens, beginning within 72 h of injury, or conventional mobilization regimens which immobilized fractures for 3 weeks. The primary outcome measure recorded was the patient's Constant score at 3 months. Secondary outcomes measured were: reduction in pain intensity; differences in active and passive range of motion as compared to the un-injured shoulder. Their results echo previous studies in that patients in the early mobilization group had significantly better Constant scores, reduction in pain intensity, and superior mobilization early during the course of treatment . However, statistical significance between the two groups was not seen after the 6 months.

Of great interest, the authors also pooled their data with other studies including those previously described above to examine the safety of early mobilization. Both fracture non-union and fracture displacement were considered. Studies that evaluated a conventional regimen of 3 weeks of fracture immobilization reported 4 patients out of a total of 373 with either a non-union or fracture displacement requiring surgical intervention [5, 7, 15, 29]. Studies that evaluated early mobilization within 1 week of injury failed to find a single case of non-union or fracture displacement out of a total of 165 patients [13, 15, 31]. The authors conclude these proportions are not statistically different when assessed with the Fisher exact test ($P=0.32$).

Overall, it appears that early mobilization reduces the subjective experience of pain early in the course of treatment. However, the outcomes between early and late mobilizers seem to equalize after a period of 6 months to a year. This data might suggest that longer periods of immobilization for more complicated fractures may not worsen the final outcome and thus may be an appropriate treatment option for those patients who are not suitable surgical candidates due to medical co-morbid conditions.

However, currently there is insufficient evidence to definitively state when to begin rehabilitation. In a Cochrane database systematic review, Handoll and Olliviere explain the difficulties and dangers of trying to establish a general consensus for treatment with small, single institution trials [33]. Furthermore, trial heterogeneity prohibits the pooling of results in a meaningful manner. The need for large-scale and high-quality clinical trials with robust methodology is apparent.

Non-operative Treatment Outcomes

There has been recent interest in identifying those subgroups of proximal humeral fractures that can be successfully managed non-operatively. It is generally agreed that non-displaced and minimally displaced two-part fractures do well with conservative treatment [5, 7, 19, 34, 35] (Also 2,3,4 of Zyto paper). However, management of displaced three- and four-part fractures remains controversial and is an area of current scientific debate [17, 28, 36]. With the growing prevalence of operative care for three- and four part fractures, there is a need for an understanding of the natural history of these fractures when treated non-operatively.

Valgus impacted fractures account for the most common type of proximal humerus fracture presenting to orthopaedic surgeons [37]. The identifying deformity of these fractures is the impaction of the humeral head on the proximal region of the metaphysis [38]. Often studies group together valgus three-part fractures with conventional Neer three-part fractures [5, 24, 39, 40]. The neglected distinction is that Neer's three-part fractures are displaced and include rotation of the humeral head as part of the pathoanatomy [41].

Court-Brown et al. studied the outcomes of non-operative management of different variants of B1.1 valgus impacted fractures of the proximal humerus [5]. Hundred and twenty-five consecutive valgus impacted fractures were analyzed over the course of a year. Most of these were in elderly patients. They found 80 % had a good to excellent result according to Neer's outcome criteria. The same study compared valgus impacted three-part fractures to the conventional Neer three-part fracture with rotation of the humeral head. Their findings suggest a better prognosis at 1 year for the valgus impacted group based on the mean Neer and Constant scores.

A systematic review of the literature was conducted in 2009 to consolidate the outcomes and summarize the complication rates of non-operative management of proximal humeral fractures [42]. Data was captured pertaining to fracture pattern, radiographic healing, clinical outcomes, and treatment complications. Predictably, one- and two-part fractures responded well to non-operative treatment with the best prognosis. The radiographic union rate was 100 % and patients achieved an average functional flexion range of motion of 151°.

With respect to three- and four-part fractures, it is important to first understand that the prevalence of operative care is growing. Patient demand is partly responsible for driving this trend. There are increasing numbers of more mobile elderly patients with greater demands of better functional outcome [43]. Advances in operative care are also driving this trend. The advent of fixed-angle plate fixation promised surgeons greater control over comminuted osteoporotic fractures. Consequently, there has been a renewed interest in the surgical management of patients with low-quality bone stock [44–46]. Prosthetic replacement is also being performed with greater interest in the light of addressing concerns regarding avascular necrosis, poor bone healing, and limited range of motion that is often thought to accompany conservative treatment [47].

Iyengar's systematic review also investigated three- and four-part fractures and found these demonstrated a 98 % rate of radiographic union but were also associated with a complication rate of 48 % [42]. Complications reported were: varus malunion (23 %, 15 cases); and avascular necrosis (14 %, 9 cases). The authors caution that conservative treatment carries a significant complication rate but also warn that the current literature is unclear as to whether or not operative treatment produces better outcomes or diminishes the aforementioned complication rate in these patients. Furthermore, operative treatment carries it's own inherent set of risks and complications [47–49]. Overall, the results support a high rate of healing and satisfactory outcomes with non-operative management of three- and four-part proximal humeral fractures.

Conclusion

Well designed prospective studies are clearly needed to assess the treatment effect, complications, outcomes, and cost effectiveness of operative management compared to non-operative management for displaced proximal humeral fractures. Future prospective studies should ideally include complete demographic information, long-term follow up, a validated shoulder outcome measurement tool, compiled range of motion data, and a thorough summary of complications [42]. Currently there are three such trials with published protocols [50–52]. Such studies will be the next step in guiding effective treatment for this challenging group of fractures.

References

1. Brorson S. Management of fractures of the humerus in ancient Egypt, Greece, and Rome: an historical review. Clin Orthop Relat Res. 2008;467(7):1907–14.
2. Horak JJ, Nilsson BEB. Epidemiology of fracture of the upper end of the humerus. Clin Orthop Relat Res. 1975;112:250–3.
3. Rasmussen S, Hvass I, Dalsgaard J, Christensen BS, Holstad E. Displaced proximal humeral fractures: results of conservative treatment. Injury. 1992;23(1):41–3.
4. Palvanen M, Kannus P, Niemi S, Parkkari J. Update in the epidemiology of proximal humeral fractures. Clin Orthop Relat Res. 2006;442:87–92.
5. Court-Brown CM, Cattermole H, McQueen MM. Impacted valgus fractures (B1.1) of the proximal humerus. The results of non-operative treatment. J Bone Joint Surg Br. 2002;84(4):504–8.
6. Court-Brown CM, Garg A, McQueen MM. The epidemiology of proximal humeral fractures. Acta Orthop Scand. 2001;72(4):365–71.
7. Court-Brown CMC, McQueen MMM. The impacted varus (A2.2) proximal humeral fracture: prediction of

outcome and results of nonoperative treatment in 99 patients. Acta Orthop Scand. 2004;75(6):736–40.
8. Fjalestad T, Strømsøe K, Blücher J, Tennøe B. Fractures in the proximal humerus: functional outcome and evaluation of 70 patients treated in hospital. Arch Orthop Trauma Surg. 2005;125(5):310–6.
9. Lauritzen JBJ, Schwarz PP, Lund BB, McNair PP, Transbøl II. Changing incidence and residual lifetime risk of common osteoporosis-related fractures. Osteoporos Int. 1993;3(3):127–32.
10. Bengnér UU, Johnell OO, Redlund-Johnell II. Changes in the incidence of fracture of the upper end of the humerus during a 30-year period. A study of 2125 fractures. Clin Orthop Relat Res. 1988;(231): 179–82.
11. Kristiansen BB, Christensen SWS. Proximal humeral fractures. Late results in relation to classification and treatment. Acta Orthop Scand. 1987;58(2):124–7.
12. Kannus P, Palvanen M, Niemi S, Parkkari J, Järvinen M, Vuori I. Increasing number and incidence of osteoporotic fractures of the proximal humerus in elderly people. BMJ. 1996;313(7064):1051–2.
13. Hodgson SA, Mawson SJ, Stanley D. Rehabilitation after two-part fractures of the neck of the humerus. J Bone Joint Surg. 2003;85(3):419–22.
14. Kristiansen B, Angermann P, Larsen TK. Functional results following fractures of the proximal humerus. A controlled clinical study comparing two periods of immobilization. Arch Orthop Trauma Surg. 1989;108(6):339–41.
15. Lefevre-Colau MM, Babinet A, Fayad F, Fermanian J, Anract P, Roren A, et al. Immediate mobilization compared with conventional immobilization for the impacted nonoperatively treated proximal humeral fracture. A randomized controlled trial. J Bone Joint Surg. 2007;89(12):2582–90.
16. Clifford PC. Fractures of the neck of the humerus: a review of the late results. Injury. 1980;12(2):91–5.
17. Zyto K, Ahrengart L, Sperber A, Törnkvist H. Treatment of displaced proximal humeral fractures in elderly patients. J Bone Joint Surg Br. 1997;79(3): 412–7.
18. Brostrom F. Early mobilization of fractures of the upper end of the humerus. Arch Surg Am Med Assoc. 1943;46(5):614.
19. Koval KJ, Gallagher MA, Marsicano JG, Cuomo F, McShinawy A, Zuckerman JD. Functional outcome after minimally displaced fractures of the proximal part of the humerus. J Bone Joint Surg Am. 1997;79(2):203–7.
20. Poeze M, Lenssen AF, Van Empel JM, Verbruggen JP. Conservative management of proximal humeral fractures: can poor functional outcome be related to standard transscapular radiographic evaluation? J Shoulder Elbow Surg. 2010;19(2):273–81.
21. Guy P, Slobogean GP, McCormack RG. Treatment preferences for displaced three- and four-part proximal humerus fractures. J Orthop Trauma. 2010;24(4): 250–4.
22. Bell JE, Leung BC, Spratt KF, Koval KJ, Weinstein JD, Goodman DC, et al. Trends and variation in incidence, surgical treatment, and repeat surgery of proximal humeral fractures in the elderly. J Bone Joint Surg. 2011;93(2):121–31.
23. Resch H. Proximal humeral fractures: current controversies. J Shoulder Elbow Surg. 2011;20(5):827–32.
24. Neer CS. Displaced proximal humeral fractures. I. Classification and evaluation. J Bone Joint Surg Am. 1970;52(6):1077–89.
25. Heppenstall RB. Fractures of the proximal humerus. Orthop Clin North Am. 1975;6(2):467–75.
26. Kessel L, Bayley I. Clinical disorders of the shoulder. Edinburgh/New York: Churchill Livingston; 1986.
27. Post M. Fractures of the upper humerus. Orthop Clin North Am. 1980;11(2):239–52.
28. Mills HJH, Horne GG. Fractures of the proximal humerus in adults. J Trauma. 1985;25(8):801–5.
29. Young TB, Wallace WA. Conservative treatment of fractures and fracture-dislocations of the upper end of the humerus. J Bone Joint Surg Br. 1985;67(3): 373–7.
30. Hodgson S. Proximal humerus fracture rehabilitation. Clin Orthop Relat Res. 2006;442:131–8.
31. Correard RP, Balatre J, Calcat P. Results in fractures of the surgical neck of the humerus treated by immediate mobilization. A series of 54 cases in patients over 50. Ann Chir. 1969;23(25):1323–6.
32. Neer CS. Displaced proximal humeral fractures. II. Treatment of three-part and four-part displacement. J Bone Joint Surg Am. 1970;52(6):1090–103.
33. Handoll HH, Ollivere BJ. Interventions for treating proximal humeral fractures in adults. Cochrane Database Syst Rev. 2010;(12):CD000434.
34. Tejwani NC, Liporace F, Walsh M, France MA, Zuckerman JD, Egol KA. Functional outcome following one-part proximal humeral fractures: a prospective study. J Shoulder Elbow Surg. 2008;17(2):216–9.
35. Hanson B, Neidenbach P, de Boer P, Stengel D. Functional outcomes after nonoperative management of fractures of the proximal humerus. J Shoulder Elbow Surg. 2009;18(4):612–21.
36. Cofield RHR. Comminuted fractures of the proximal humerus. Clin Orthop Relat Res. 1988;(230):49–57.
37. Resch H, Beck E, Bayley I. Reconstruction of the valgus-impacted humeral head fracture. J Shoulder Elbow Surg. 1995;4(2):73–80.
38. Brooks CH, Revell WJ, Heatley FW. Vascularity of the humeral head after proximal humeral fractures. An anatomical cadaver study. J Bone Joint Surg Br. 1993;75(1):132–6.
39. Boileau P, Walch G. The three-dimensional geometry of the proximal humerus. Implications for surgical technique and prosthetic design. J Bone Joint Surg Br. 1997;79(5):857–65.
40. Iannotti JP, Gabriel JP, Schneck SL, Evans BG, Misra S. The normal glenohumeral relationships. An anatomical study of one hundred and forty shoulders. J Bone Joint Surg Am. 1992;74(4):491–500.

41. Robinson CM, Page RS. Severely impacted valgus proximal humeral fractures. J Bone Joint Surg Am. 2004;86-A(Suppl 1 (Pt 2)):143–55.
42. Iyengar JJ, Devcic Z, Sproul RC, Feeley BT. Nonoperative treatment of proximal humerus fractures: a systematic review. J Orthop Trauma. 2011; 25(10):612–7.
43. Manton KG, Gu X, Lamb VL. Change in chronic disability from 1982 to 2004/2005 as measured by long-term changes in function and health in the U.S. elderly population. Proc Natl Acad Sci U S A. 2006;103(48): 18374–9.
44. Drosdowech DSD, Faber KJK, Athwal GSG. Open reduction and internal fixation of proximal humerus fractures. Orthop Clin North Am. 2008;39(4): 429–39, vi.
45. Anglen JJ, Kyle RFR, Marsh JLJ, Virkus WWW, Watters WCW, Keith MWM, et al. Locking plates for extremity fractures. J Am Acad Orthop Surg. 2009; 17(7):465–72.
46. Ricchetti ET, DeMola PM, Roman D, Abboud JA. The use of precontoured humeral locking plates in the management of displaced proximal humerus fracture. J Am Acad Orthop Surg. 2009;17(9):582–90.
47. Kontakis GG, Koutras CC, Tosounidis TT, Giannoudis PP. Early management of proximal humeral fractures with hemiarthroplasty: a systematic review. J Bone Joint Surg Br. 2008;90(11):1407–13.
48. Sudkamp N, Bayer J, Hepp P, Voigt C, Oestern H, Kaab M, et al. Open reduction and internal fixation of proximal humeral fractures with use of the locking proximal humerus plate. Results of a prospective, multicenter, observational study. J Bone Joint Surg Am. 2009;91(6):1320–8.
49. Thanasas C, Kontakis G, Angoules A, Limb D, Giannoudis P. Treatment of proximal humerus fractures with locking plates: a systematic review. J Shoulder Elbow Surg. 2009;18(6):837–44.
50. Handoll H, Brealey S, Rangan A, Torgerson D, Dennis L, Armstrong A, et al. Protocol for the ProFHER (PROximal Fracture of the Humerus: Evaluation by Randomisation) trial: a pragmatic multi-centre randomised controlled trial of surgical versus non-surgical treatment for proximal fracture of the humerus in adults. BMC Musculoskelet Disord. 2009;10:140.
51. Brorson SS, Olsen BSB, Frich LHL, Jensen SLS, Johannsen HVH, Sørensen AKA, et al. Effect of osteosynthesis, primary hemiarthroplasty, and non-surgical management for displaced four-part fractures of the proximal humerus in elderly: a multi-centre, randomised clinical trial. Trials. 2009; 10:51.
52. Den Hartog D, Van Lieshout EMM, Tuinebreijer WE, Polinder S, Van Beeck EF, Breederveld RS, et al. Primary hemiarthroplasty versus conservative treatment for comminuted fractures of the proximal humerus in the elderly (ProCon): a multicenter randomized controlled trial. BMC Musculoskelet Disord. 2010;11:97.

Part V

Surgical Management

15 Intraoperative Considerations

Sebastian Siebenlist

Pre-operative Assessment

Severity as well as morphology of proximal humeral fractures, concomitant injuries and patient's general conditions (age, quality of bone and soft tissues, level of activity) have to be considered for both, the surgical approach and the technical procedure.

Whereas non-dislocated or slightly dislocated two or three part fractures may be addressed through a percutaneous or minimal-invasive approach depending on the surgeon's preference, four part fractures or dislocated fractures should be managed using the delto-pectoral approach. Especially for complex fracture types, the availability of fracture arthroplasty (anatomic or reversed proximal humeral replacement) has to be checked to extend surgical procedure if necessary. As well, the operating team, the time of operation (particularly in case of patients with multiple injuries), and the surgeon's experience have to be taken into account before surgery. Based on patient's constitution, accompanying fractures of the shoulder girdle (glenoid or clavicle) should be surgically managed in the same operative procedure.

S. Siebenlist, MD
Department of Trauma Surgery, Klinikum rechts der Isar, Technical University Munich, Munich, Germany
e-mail: sebastian.siebenlist@gmx.de

Patient Positioning

Patient positioning is of great importance to ensure optimal surgical exposure. Therefore, this procedure should be performed by the surgeon himself.

For proximal humeral fractures, the patient is placed on a standard operating table in the so-called "beach-chair position". A supine position is chosen ensuring that buttocks and great trochanter are positioned at the main break of the operating table. Then the patient is slid laterally to the edge of the table on the operative side and the back of the table is elevated between 30° and 45° depending on the surgeon's preference (Fig. 15.1). A wedge-pad underneath the thighs should be used to facilitate the sitting position to avoid slouching during the operative procedure with the patient's feet slightly lowered. The knees have to be placed using pillows and/or padding to avoid peroneal nerve pressure injuries. Patient's chest and legs have to be secured using padded straps. For positioning of the patient's head care must be taken as well, thus fixing it in a neutral position in both, the coronal and the sagittal plane, to avoid lateral flexion or hyperextension of the neck that may cause airway obstruction, cerebral vascular insults, stretching of the cervical roots or brachial plexus traction [8, 13, 20, 21]. An elastofoam is used to gently secure the head in this neutral position. Commercially available head positioners can also be used.

P. Biberthaler et al. (eds.), *Fractures of the Proximal Humerus*, Strategies in Fracture Treatments,
DOI 10.1007/978-3-319-20300-3_15

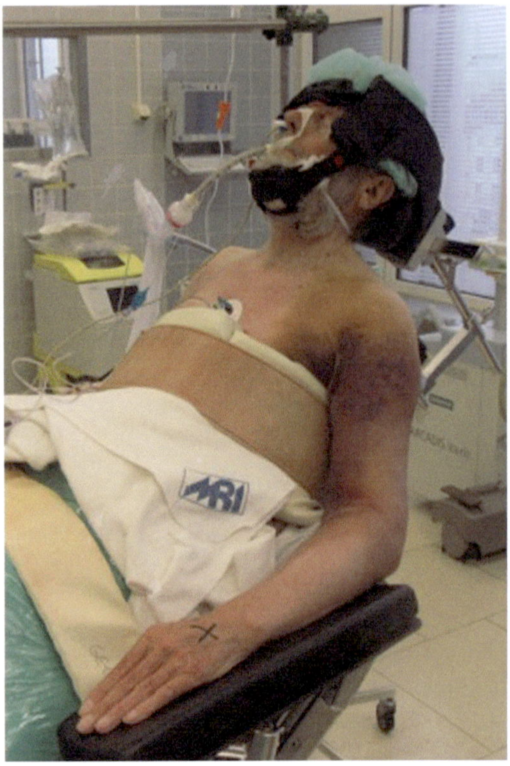

Fig. 15.1 The patient is positioned on a standard operating table in the 45° beach-chair position. A simple arm support is used to keep the arm in neutral position of forearm rotation

To simplify an appropriate intraoperative fluoroscopy, the patient needs to be positioned in a sufficiently lateral position on the operating table and the arm needs to be dropped freely downwards aside of the table. The entire shoulder, including the scapula, should be in a sufficiently lateral position on the operating table to allow for a complete extension of the humerus and external rotation of the arm up to 90°. The operating table may be turned into the room to facilitate the access to the anterior, lateral, and posterior aspects of the shoulder.

As standard, a simple arm support is used to keep the arm (90° flexion elbow joint) in a neutral position regarding forearm rotation during the surgical approach (Fig. 15.1). In this position the arm can be moved in any direction by the surgeon. However, the arm has to be secured by the assistant surgeon during surgery. Alternatively, a commercially available positioner system for arm support can be used to relieve the operating team and to allow the assistant to fully concentrate on the procedure. Therefore, the patient's arm is secured at a padded arm rest using sterile straps. Before surgery, it has to be made sure that the assist system allows for the patient's arm being accurately positioned and exactly fixed where it is needed (Fig. 15.2).

Moreover, the surgeon should evaluate the range of motion of the shoulder including internal and external rotation under general anesthesia. The hand and the forearm should be wrapped in a sterile stockinette. To warrant the sterile field the axilla should be separated by self-adhesive surgical drapes. After covering, the image intensifier fluoroscopy (C-arm) is placed for intraoperative radiographs in a.p and axial direction (Fig. 15.2).

During patient's positioning care has to be taken to prevent excessive traction. In terms of neurologic complications, the brachial plexus and the axillary nerve are mostly affected [19, 22, 31, 33]. Thus, positions of extreme extension and abduction should be avoided to not stretch the nerval structures. Moreover, cerebral ischemia and vasovagal episodes are reported related to beach chair positioning [14, 32].

Surgical Approach

Functional outcome after surgical treatment of proximal humeral fractures was evaluated in many studies over the last decade [2, 5, 16, 17, 27, 29]. Nevertheless, the discussion about the surgical approach with special respect to the delto-pectoral and deltoid-splitting approach is still controversial.

Hepp et al. [11] were the only ones who reported on approach-related results following proximal humeral plating. In 39 patients with an anterolateral deltoid-splitting approach, the authors observed less pain and higher activity levels of daily living scores the early follow-up. On the other hand, the 44 patients treated by a deltopectoral approach obtained higher Constant scores after 12 months of follow-up. Based on their findings, Hepp and colleagues [11] concluded that the choice of surgical approach may influence the functional shoulder outcome.

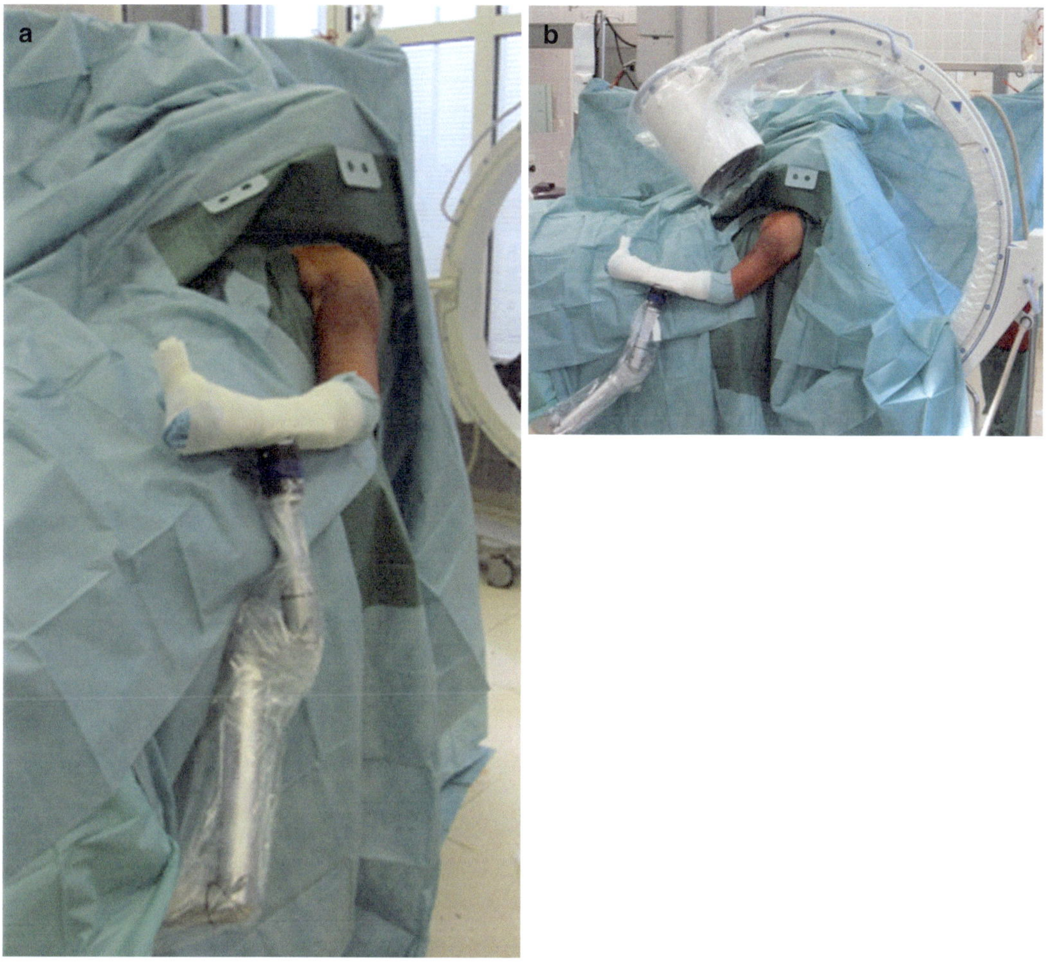

Fig. 15.2 The patient is placed in the beach-chair position and the arm is fixed using an assist system (TRIMANO 3D support arm, MAQUET GmbH & Co. KG, Rastatt, Germany) (**a**). This sterile-covered arm support system can be connected to every operating table and allows to move and securely fix the arm at any position during operation. After covering, the image amplifier (sterile-covered C-arm) is integrated in the operating set-up for intraoperative fluoroscopy (**b**)

Deltopectoral Approach

For proximal humeral fractures, most upper extremity surgeons recommend the delto-pectoral approach, especially in cases of comminuted or dislocated fracture types.

A 10–12 cm skin incision is made starting from the coracoid process to the distal insertion of the deltoid muscle (Fig. 15.3). The deltopectoral interval is blunt dissected from medially to the cephalic vein, followed by a blunt dissection of the subdeltoid and subpectoral spaces. Superiorly, the incision reaches the clavicle and a Hohmann-retractor can be placed above the acromiohumeral ligament for a wider exposition, if necessary. The deltopectoral groove is opened distally until the insertion of the pectoralis muscle. The clavipectoral fascia is split vertically just lateral to the conjoined tendons and up to the coracoacromial ligament to expose the fracture by internal and external rotation. One must consider that the coracoacromial ligament remains intact to avoid cranial glenohumeral instability. The upper insertion of the pectoralis major muscle can be cut for about 1–2 cm to allow better exposure of the metaphyseal region of the humerus or the inferior aspect of the glenohumeral joint. While putting the arm in abduction

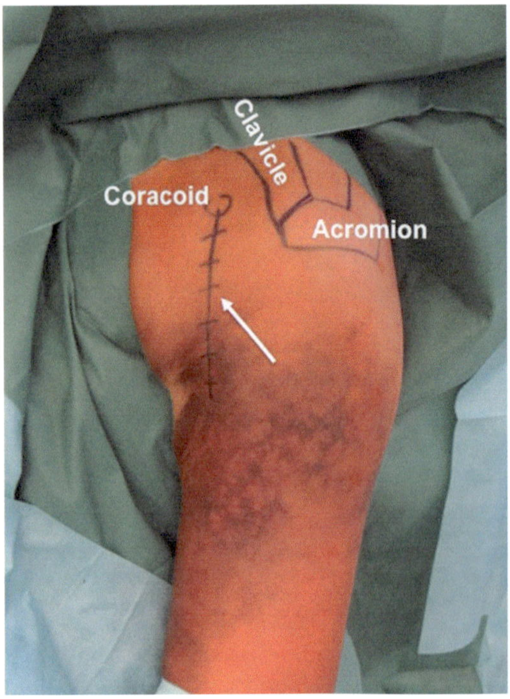

Fig. 15.3 Deltopectoral approach (*arrow*)

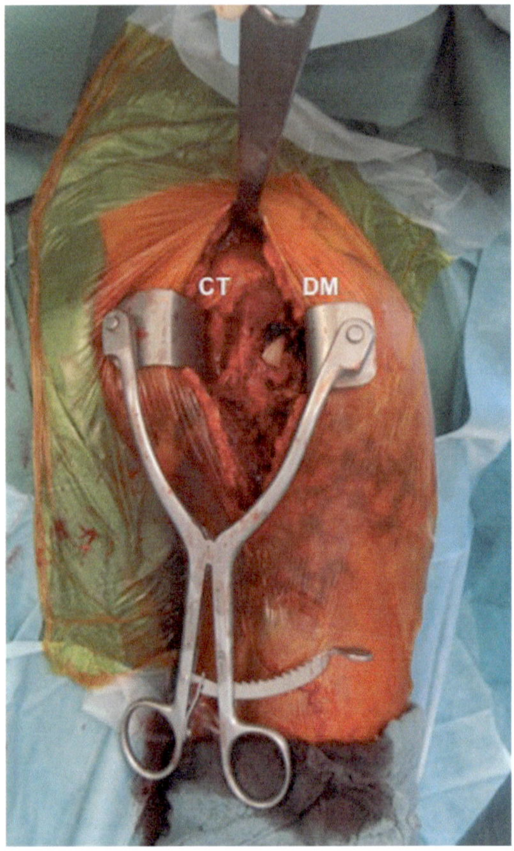

Fig. 15.4 View to the deltopectoral interval. The conjoint tendons (*CT*) and the deltoid muscle (*DM*) is retracted by a self-retaining, symmetric retractor

and internal rotation, a partial release of the deep surface of the deltoid can be performed to facilitate drilling and plate positioning [10]. Medially, the conjoint tendon is freed and retracted using a self-retaining, symmetric retractor that simultaneously retracts the deltoid muscle at the lateral side (Fig. 15.4). If the arm is anteverted with the elbow flexed during this procedure the conjoint tendon is relaxed, and thereby, the placement of the retractor is facilitated. Alternatively, a Hohmann-retractor can be placed around the humeral shaft to retract the deltoid muscle. After resection of the subdeltoid bursa, the subscapularis muscle is exposed, and following the anterior humeral circumflex vessels (at the inferior border of the subscapularis muscle) as well as the axillary nerve, both should be palpated in an effort to prevent iatrogenic injury during further preparation.

Several surgeons, however, note that this approach may not be the appropriate method for angular stable plate fixaton of proximal humeral fractures [4, 6, 28]. They note that it is difficult to gain the correct drill angle, possibly leading to slight anterior plate placement, and subsequently criticize the substantial soft tissue dissection, the retraction of the deltoid muscle as well as the humeral manipulation to access the lateral aspect of the humerus. To obtain the correct drill angle using a standard deltopectoral appraoch, the partial release of the humeral insertion of the deltoid muscle is described [10]. Certainly, this procedure has to be carefully considered because a release of more than one fifth of the deltoid insertion is reported to probably deteriorate anterior deltoid function [3, 15]. Furthermore, this approach may negatively influence postoperative outcomes due to devascularization of fracture fragments during dissection and plating or disruption of the critical blood supply to the humeral head [5, 7, 18]. According to Hertel et al. [12], the most relevant predictors of humeral head ischemia are the length of the dorsomedial metaphyseal extension, the integrity of the medial hinge, and the basic fracture type itself. Therefore, care must be taken with the deltopectorial approach to not deteriorate the initial situation of blood supply preventing an avascular necrosis of the humeral head.

Deltoid-Splitting Approach

In recent years the originally developed for rotator cuff surgery and intramedullary nailing of humeral shaft fractures deltoid-splitting (antero-lateral) approach has become more and more popular for plate osteosynthesis of the proximal humerus [5, 9, 24, 25, 29].

The first skin incision of this less-invasive approach starts from the antero-lateral tip of the acromion extending 5 cm distally in line with the arm. For superficial dissection, the deltoid muscle is split in line with its fibers (in the avascular raphe between the anterior and middle head) no more than 5 cm distal to the acromion to protect the axillary nerve. The subacromial bursa should be resected to reveal the underlying rotator cuff and the proximal humerus. Then, the axillary nerve is identified by palpation and consequently protected during the further procedure. After fracture reduction, the plating implant is inserted along the humeral shaft and positioned at the upper end of the greater tuberosity and approximately 2 mm posterior to the bicipital groove. Using the antero-lateral approach the lateral plating zone can be directly accessed with minimized muscle retraction. Then, the second skin incision is performed over the distal 3 holes of the plate following fluoroscopic control. After blunt dissection, the distal ending of the plate is displayed for fixation to the humeral shaft.

The risk of iatrogenic axillary nerve injury is often reported as disadvantage of the deltoid-splitting approach. The anatomic course of the axillary nerve, however, is reliably predictable as proven in various anatomical studies [1, 26, 30]. Moreover, diverse clinical outcome studies verified no lesions to the axillary nerve using the antero-lateral approach for plate fixation of proximal humeral fractures [4, 5, 11, 16, 23]. These authors agree that the deltoid-splitting approach may be a safe alternative when correctly implemented with palpating or visualizing the axillary nerve before plate insertion. Additionally, they suggest the use of a longer plate (min. 5 holes) to insert the screws at a certain distance above and below the lateral branch of the axillary nerve. Moreover, proponents of the deltoid-splitting approach argue with potential benefits for fracture healing due to a lower rate of avascular necrosis of the humeral head [4, 11, 28]. In addition, Gardner et al. [6] reported that a minimal-invasive, anterolateral approach allows for direct access to the appropriate plating zone, a bare spot between the humeral head-penetrating vessels from the anterior and posterior circumflex system. Furthermore, they summarized that this approach avoids exposure of the humeral head blood supply, precludes deltoid release, and may minimize further vascular compromise of fracture fragments during reduction and fixation.

Surgical Equipment/Fixation Devices

In the following, the surgical instruments and special devices (Fig. 15.5) required for operative management of proximal humeral fractures are listed in alphabetical order:

- Backhaus clamps
- Bankart clamps
- Browne-type Deltoid Retractor (radiolucent carbon fiber)
- Curettes
- Evans Reverse Hohmann Retractor
- Hohmann retractors
- Kocher clamps
- Kölbel self-retaining deltopectoral retractor with various pairs of snap-in, freely pivoting blades blades
- K-wires
- Luer
- Needle holders
- Raspatorium
- Surgical retractor (Weitlaner)
- Verbrügge clamps
- Scalpel
- Surgical scissors

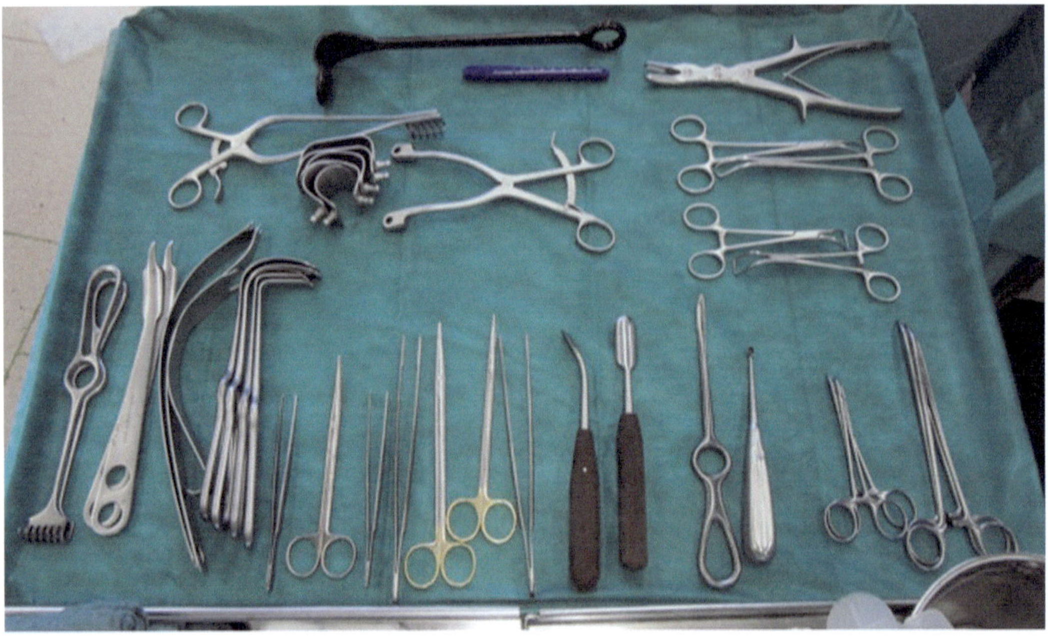

Fig. 15.5 Surgical equipment for proximal humeral fracture management

References

1. Apaydin N, Tubbs RS, Loukas M, Duparc F. Review of the surgical anatomy of the axillary nerve and the anatomic basis of its iatrogenic and traumatic injury. Surg Radiol Anat. 2010;32:193–201.
2. Fankhauser F, Boldin C, Schippinger G, et al. A new locking plate for unstable fractures of the proximal humerus. Clin Orthop Relat Res. 2005;430:176–81.
3. Gagey O, Hue E. Mechanics of the deltoid muscle. A new approach. Clin Orthop. 2000;375:250–7.
4. Gardner MJ, Boraiah S, Helfet DL, et al. The anterolateral acromial approach for fractures of the proximal humerus. J Orthop Trauma. 2008;22:132–7.
5. Gardner MJ, Griffith MH, Dines JS, et al. The extended anterolateral acromial approach allows minimally invasive access to the proximal humerus. Clin Orthop Relat Res. 2005;434:123–9.
6. Gardner MJ, Voos JE, Wanich T, et al. Vascular implications of minimally invasive plating of proximal humerus fractures. J Orthop Trauma. 2006;20:602–7.
7. Gerber C, Schneeberger AG, Vinh TS. The arterial vascularization of the humeral head. An anatomical study. J Bone Joint Surg Am. 1990;10:1486–94.
8. Habe K, Kawasaki T, Horishita T, et al. Airway problem during the operation with beach-chair position: a case of arytenoid dislocation and the relationship between intra-cuff pressure of endotrachial tube and the neck position. Masui. 2011;60:682–5.
9. Habermeyer P, Lehmann L. Rotatorenmanschette, Rotatorenintervall und lange Bizepssehne. In: Habermeyer P, editor. Schulterchirurgie. Munich: Urban & Fischer; 2002. p. 333–74.
10. Hawkins RJ, Kiefer GN. Internal fixation techniques for proximal humeral fractures. Clin Orthop Relat Res. 1987;223:77–85.
11. Hepp P, Theopold J, Voigt C, et al. The surgical approach for locking plate osteosynthesis of displaced proximal humeral fractures influences the functional outcome. J Shoulder Elbow Surg. 2008;17(1):21–8.
12. Hertel R, Hempfing A, Stiehler M, Leunig M. Predictors of humeral head ischemia after intracapsular fracture of the proximal humerus. J Shoulder Elbow Surg. 2004;13(4):427–33.
13. Hynson JM, Tung A, Guevara JE, et al. Complete airway obstruction during arthroscopic shoulder surgery. Anesth Analg. 1993;76:875–8.
14. Kahn RL, Hargett MJ. Beta-adrenergic blockers and vasovagal episodes during shoulder surgery in the sitting position under interscalene block. Anesth Analg. 1999;88(2):378–81.
15. Klepps S, Auerbach J, Calhon O, et al. A cadaveric study on the anatomy of the deltoid insertion and its relationship to the deltopectoral approach to the proximal humerus. J Shoulder Elbow Surg. 2004;13(3):322–7.
16. Laflamme GY, Rouleau DM, Berry GK, et al. Percutaneous humeral plating of fractures of the proximal humerus: results of a prospective multicenter clinical trial. J Orthop Trauma. 2008;22(3):153–8.
17. Martetschläger F, Siebenlist S, Weier M, et al. Plating of proximal humeral fractures. Orthopedics. 2012;35(11):e1606–12.

18. Meyer C, Alt V, Hassanin H, et al. The arteries of the humeral head and their relevance in fracture treatment. Surg Radiol Anat. 2005;27(3):232–7.
19. Mullins RC, Drez Jr D, Cooper J. Hypoglossal nerve palsy after arthroscopy of the shoulder and open operation with the patient In the beach-chair position. A case report. J Bone Joint Surg Am. 1992;74(1):137–9.
20. Pohl A, Cullen OJ. Cerebral Ischemia during shoulder surgery in the upright position: a case series. J Clin Anesth. 2005;17:463–9.
21. Rhee YG, Cho NS. Isolated unilateral hypoglossal nerve palsy after shoulder surgery in beach-chair position. J Shoulder Elbow Surg. 2008;17:e28–30.
22. Rodeo SA, Forster RA, Weiland AJ. Neurological complications due to arthroscopy. J Bone Joint Surg Am. 1993;75:917–26.
23. Röderer G, Abouelsoud M, Gebhard F, et al. Minimally invasive application of the non-contact-bridging (NCB) plate to the proximal humerus: an anatomical study. J Orthop Trauma. 2007;21:621–7.
24. Rommens PM, Blum J, Runkel M. Retrograde nailing of humeral shaft fractures. Clin Orthop Relat Res. 1998;350:26–39.
25. Rouleau DM, Laflamme GY, Berry GK, et al. Proximal humerus fractures treated by percutaneous locking plate internal fixation. Orthop Traumatol Surg Res. 2009;95:56–62.
26. Smith J, Berry G, Laflamme Y, et al. Percutaneous insertion of a proximal humeral locking plate: an anatomic study. Injury. 2007;38(2):206–11.
27. Solberg BD, Moon CN, Franco DP, Paiement GD. Surgical treatment of three and four-part proximal humeral fractures. J Bone Joint Surg Am. 2009;91(7):1689–97.
28. Sturzenegger M, Fornaro E, Jakob RP. Results of surgical treatment of multifragmented fractures of the humeral head. Arch Orthop Trauma Surg. 1982;100(4):249–59.
29. Suedkamp N, Bayer J, Hepp P, et al. Open reduction and internal fixation of proximal humeral fractures with use of the locking proximal humerus plate. Results of a prospective, multicenter, observational study. J Bone Joint Surg Am. 2009;91(6):1320–8.
30. Traxler H, Surd R, Laminger KA, et al. The treatment of subcapital humerus fracture with dynamic helix wire and the risk of concommitant lesion of the axillary nerve. Clin Anat. 2001;14(6):418–23.
31. Uno A, Baln GI, Mehta JA. Arthroscopic relationship of the axillary nerve to the shoulder joint capsule: an anatomic study. J Shoulder Elbow Surg. 1999;8(3):226–30.
32. Villevieille T, Delaunay L, Gentili M, Benhamou D. Arthroscopic shoulder surgery and ischemic cerebral complications. Ann Fr Anesth Reanim. 2012;31(11):914–8.
33. Weber SC, Abrams JS, Nottage WM. Complications associated with arthroscopic shoulder surgery. Arthroscopy. 2002;18(2 Suppl 1):88–95.

Two and Three Part Fractures

16

Volker Braunstein

Introduction

According to Codman's observation from 1934 [1] fractures of the proximal humerus produce a combination of 4 segments including greater tuberosity, lesser tuberosity, articular surface and the humeral shaft. Considering this observation all potential two-part and three part fractures can be identified. Numerous classifications base upon Codman's conclusion result in heterogeneous recommendations regarding conservative and operative treatment. Beside fracture morphology the evaluation of factors like bone quality, blood supply of the humeral head and fracture fragments, lesions of the rotator cuff and patient demands are essential for adequate treatment [2]. The incidence of displaced proximal humeral fractures, particularly two-part and three-part patterns, requiring surgical intervention is relatively low [3].

In case of two-part surgical neck fractures impaction or dislocation of the metaphyseal zone and the degree of displacement an angulation are essential to find the adequate treatment option. Patient's functional outcomes following non-operative management of two-part surgical neck fractures are generally good [4].

V. Braunstein
OrthoPlus Muenchen / Munich, Lenbachplatz 2a, 80333, Muenchen / Munich, Germany
e-mail: vbraunstein@mac.com

Isolated fractures of the greater tuberosity account for approximately 20 % of all proximal humeral fractures. They are often associated with anterior glenohumeral dislocation or can result a shear injury against the lower surface of the acromion or superior glenoid [5].

Operative treatment of greater tuberosity fracture is recommended by most authors in case of a dislocation of more than 5 mm, due to the risk of impingement and malunion resulting in impairment of glenohumeral joint motion [6].

Isolated lesser tuberosity fractures are exceedingly rare. They only account for approximately 2 % of all proximal humeral fractures [7]. The majority of authors recommend operative treatment in case of more than 5 mm displacement or 45° of angulation, mechanical block to internal rotation, continued pain, and weakness of terminal internal rotation [7]. However, due to the risk of late displacement and possible involvement of the bicipital groove Ogawa et al. [8] prefer to fix even minimally displaced lesser tuberosity fractures.

Three part fractures usually include a surgical neck and greater tuberosity fracture. The combination of surgical neck and lesser tuberosity fracture is uncommon. Operative treatment is required in case of tuberosity dislocation of more than 5 mm and in cases without metaphyseal impaction.

P. Biberthaler et al. (eds.), *Fractures of the Proximal Humerus*, Strategies in Fracture Treatments,
DOI 10.1007/978-3-319-20300-3_16

Open Management of Two Part and Three Part Fractures

Open management of two part and three part fractures will allow good exposure for reduction and fixation. However, soft tissue damage could influence the blood supply of the fractured bone fragments resulting in an impairment of bone healing.

The deltopectoral approach is the working horse for open fracture management of humeral head fractures. Respecting the integrity of the deltoid muscle is the major advantage of this approach. However, some authors are impaired by the potential small exposure, especially in case of superior and posterior dislocation of the grater tuberosity.

Therefore some authors prefer to split the deltoid muscle (e.g. using the Mackenzie or the transdeltoid lateral approach). The advantage of this kind of approach is the good exposure and visualization of displaced bone fragments. Though, beside the potential damage of the deltoid muscle the course of the axillary nerve must be kept in mind.

In case of isolated greater tuberosity fractures a large variation of approaches and fixation techniques are described in literature. Open management could be necessary in case of small fragments, comminution, and distinct dislocation [7]. Biomechanical studies proved superior primary mechanical stability for tension banding using heavy non-absorbable sutures and for two cancellous screws when compared to transosseous sutures [9].

The subscapularis tendon and the bone fragment unit will need to be mobilized and fibrous tissue removed frequently in case of isolated lesser tuberosity fractures. Therefore, open fractures management will be necessary in almost all cases. As the approach should consider the involvement of the medial wall of the intertubercular groove and the integrity of the tendon of the long head of the biceps the choice is limited to deltopectoral approaches for most cases. Cannulated screws with or without washers [10], heavy suture, and cerclage wire [11] are used for the fixation of the lesser tuberosity.

Open management of three part fractures is recommended whenever satisfactory reduction or fixation is not achieved by closed or limited open approaches. Locking plates and locking nails are mainly used for fixation. For both implants comparable short and long term results are found in literature [12]. Although no benefit could be found for interfragmentary motion in biomechanical studies [13], additional cerclages wires will be at least a intraoperative helpful tool for mobilization and reduction.

Percutaneous Management of Two and Three Part Fractures

Beside cosmetic aspects the crucial advantage of percutaneous management of two and three part fractures are minimal soft-tissue damages resulting in less scar tissue while fracture healing [14]. However, there is no exposure for reduction of fracture fragments. Therefore, reduction can only be achieved by closed reduction maneuvers and the surgeon needs to be skilled at these techniques. Furthermore, an exact analysis of the fracture is necessary to understand which reduction maneuvers will be efficient for a sufficient reduction. Hirzinger et al. established a classification to analyze specific fracture patterns [15] including varus and valgus, impacted and distracted fractures. The resulting differentiation of these specific fractures types is a helpful an efficient tool to get an idea which reduction technique could be efficient for the particular dislocated fracture.

The axillary nerve, which lies approximately 6 cm below the lateral edge of the acromion, could be at risk while using percutaneous osteosynthesis techniques. Hence, k-wires should not be inserted in this region.

K-wires or threaded pins could be inserted in fracture fragments to use them in joystick techniques for fracture reduction. Especially in osteoporotic bone this technique could be unsatisfactory.

K-wires or threated pins will be helpful for temporary fixation. Definitive osteosynthesis could be performed using also K-wires or threated pins which can be additionally blocked at the humeral shaft (Humerusblock respectively Resch-Block) [16], cannulated screws or a combination of both.

Literature

1. Codman EA, Akerson IB. The pathology associated with rupture of the supraspinatus tendon. Ann Surg. 1931;93(1):348–59.
2. Murray IR, Amin AK, White TO, Robinson CM. Proximal humeral fractures: current concepts in classification, treatment and outcomes. J Bone Joint Surg Br. 2011;93(1):1–11.
3. Park MC, Murthi AM, Roth NS, Blaine TA, Levine WN, Bigliani LU. Two-part and three-part fractures of the proximal humerus treated with suture fixation. J Orthop Trauma. 2003;17(5):319–25.
4. Court-Brown CM, Garg A, McQueen MM. The epidemiology of proximal humeral fractures. Acta Orthop Scand. 2001;72(4):365–71.
5. Mattyasovszky SG, Burkhart KJ, Ahlers C, Proschek D, Dietz S-O, Becker I, et al. Isolated fractures of the greater tuberosity of the proximal humerus: a long-term retrospective study of 30 patients. Acta Orthop. 2011;82(6):714–20.
6. Bono CM, Renard R, Levine RG, Levy AS. Effect of displacement of fractures of the greater tuberosity on the mechanics of the shoulder. J Bone Joint Surg Br. 2001;83(7):1056–62.
7. Gruson KI, Ruchelsman DE, Tejwani NC. Isolated tuberosity fractures of the proximal humerus: current concepts. Injury. 2008;39(3):284–98.
8. Ogawa K, Takahashi M. Long-term outcome of isolated lesser tuberosity fractures of the humerus. J Trauma. 1997;42(5):955–9.
9. Braunstein V, Wiedemann E, Plitz W, Muensterer OJ, Mutschler W, Hinterwimmer S. Operative treatment of greater tuberosity fractures of the humerus – a biomechanical analysis. Clin Biomech. 2007;22(6):652–7.
10. van Laarhoven HA, te Slaa RL, van Laarhoven EW. Isolated avulsion fracture of the lesser tuberosity of the humerus. J Trauma. 1995;39(5):997–9.
11. Hayes PRL, Klepps S, Bishop J, Cleeman E, Flatow EL. Posterior shoulder dislocation with lesser tuberosity and scapular spine fractures. J Shoulder Elbow Surg. 2003;12(5):524–7.
12. Handoll HHG, Ollivere BJ, Rollins KE. Interventions for treating proximal humeral fractures in adults (Review). Cochrane Database Syst Rev. 2012;12:CD000434.
13. Voigt C, Hurschler C, Rechi L, Vosshenrich R, Lill H. Additive fiber-cerclages in proximal humeral fractures stabilized by locking plates: no effect on fracture stabilization and rotator cuff function in human shoulder specimens. Acta Orthop. 2009;80(4):465–71.
14. Bogner R, Hübner C, Matis N, Auffarth A, Lederer S, Resch H. Minimally-invasive treatment of three- and four-part fractures of the proximal humerus in elderly patients. J Bone Joint Surg Br. 2008;90(12):1602–7.
15. Hirzinger C, Tauber M, Resch H. Proximal humerus fracture: new aspects in epidemiology, fracture morphology, and diagnostics. Unfallchirurg. 2011;114(12):1051–8.
16. Resch H, Povacz P, Fröhlich R, Wambacher M. Percutaneous fixation of three- and four-part fractures of the proximal humerus. J Bone Joint Surg Br. 1997;79(2):295–300.

3- and 4-Part Fractures

17

Chlodwig Kirchhoff and Peter Biberthaler

Introduction

A dynamic variation of the incidence of proximal humerus fractures has been described by several authors between 1965 and 1989 with rates between 56 and 69/100,000 [1]. However, current epidemiologic studies refute an further increase, presenting an incidence rate of 63/100,000 in 2006 [2] and 61/100,000 in 2008 [3]. In this context in the literature an incidence rate of 21 % of 3- and 4 part fractures of the proximal humerus are reported [2]. Regarding age about 70 % occur in patients >60 years of age. Also an increase of fracture complexity along with the patients' age was noticed.

In this context the quality of bone is of great importance regarding the resulting type of fracture. Conceiving the same trauma mechanism younger patients <40 years of age suffer from a shoulder dislocation since their bone quality is superior to capsule-ligamentous stability whereas patients >65 years of age experience a proximal humeral fracture and in patients with an age between 40 and 65 years of age trauma results in a combination of injuries in terms of dislocation and fracture [2]. However, the most problematic fracture type is without doubt the fracture of the proximal humerus in patients >65 years. Therefore regarding the choice of the adequate treatment special consideration need to be paid to several criteria such as age, comorbidities, operability, previous osteoporotic fractures compliance and requirements of the patient. A careful indication has to be made whether there is an adequate chance of surgical restoration of the natural joint using ORIF or the need for implantation of a primary arthroplasty. However, in the elderly patient primary reversed arthroplasty seems to present an adequate alternative [4, 5].

Three Part Fractures

Basically these fractures are compression fracture types since the joint supporting humeral head fragment is pressed into the metaphyseal area [2]. In line with this fracture type both tuberosities might fracture as well but not necessarily displace. Consecutively three fracture line develop, one in the surgical and one in the anatomical humeral head respectively and the third in between both tuberosities. Regarding the extent of fragment dislocation but also regarding prognostic criteria for humeral head perfusion

C. Kirchhoff (✉)
Klinikum rechts der Isar, Technical University Munich, Munich, Germany
e-mail: dr.kirchhoff@mac.com

P. Biberthaler
Department for Trauma Surgery, Klinikum rechts der Isar, Technical University Munich, Munich, Germany
e-mail: Peter.Biberthaler@mri.tum.de

P. Biberthaler et al. (eds.), *Fractures of the Proximal Humerus*, Strategies in Fracture Treatments,
DOI 10.1007/978-3-319-20300-3_17

the periosteal conjunction plays an important role so that in case of a 3-part fracture along with fracture of the greater tuberosity due to the strong traction of the subscapularis muscle and complete periosteal decoupling an additional rotational defective position occurs.

Four Part Fractures

Regarding prognosis of four part fractures a distinct differentiation between impacted fractures with valgus malpositioning with and without horizontal shift. In case of a four part fracture a dislocation of the calotte is displaced >6 mm the treating surgeon can assume that the humeral head fragment does not hold any soft tissue conjunction so that not only perfusion is compromised but also the reduction of the uncoupled calotte fragment remains difficult up to impossible [2]. If the initial radiograph does not provide sufficient information on the extent of the fracture the performance of CT including 3D reformats is obligatory for fracture understanding and treatment planning. CT allows for the exact identification of each fragment and the corresponding interfragmentary capsule- and periosteal conjunctions being essential for the evaluation of the humeral head perfusion. So in general the humeral head perfusion depends extremely on the position of the calotte fragment to the stem fragment, of the greater tuberosity to the stem fragment, as well as of the minor tuberosity to the head fragment whereas not only the distance but also the direction of dislocation is of importance. Regarding impacted four part fractures in valgus malposition the medial as well as the lateral periosteum might be damaged whereas the lateral periosteum is usually only torn longitudinally with a persisting conjunction between greater tuberosity and stem.

Prognostic criteria for three and four-part fractures are the length of the postero-medial calotte fragment, tilting of the calotte and its horizontal displacement respectively, dislocation of the tuberosities and the presence f fracture dislocation and/or head split fracture.

Indications for Surgery and Surgical Treatment

Intentions to treat of performing surgery are an anatomic reduction and stable retention. An anatomic reduction is in any case desirable since in case of secondary humeral head necrosis correctly healed tuberosities provide good original conditions for two-stage humeral head prosthesis considered as precondition for comparable results to primary fracture endoprosthesis. Stable retention until fracture healing is done presents another basis for good results.

However, even very experienced shoulder surgeons are afflicted with a rather high rate of humeral head necrosis of 1/3 when it comes to complex humeral head fractures [2]. In this context the authors Hente et al. [2] report on rather low rates of humeral head necrosis using locking plates for treating multi fragment fractures. The authors state as reason the surgery technique preserving the perfusion anatomy along with high primary stability allowing for a revascularization of the humeral head.

In any case the interpretation of humeral head necrosis is in this context critically to be discussed.

Basically the spectrum of implants comprises bone sutures/cerclages, locking k-wires, screw fixation and locking plates as well as nailing. However, in performing osteosynthesis of complex humeral head fractures an additional tension band wiring is recommended entailing a certain antagonism of the rotator cuff for postoperative functional treatment.

In general the indication for osteosynthetic versus endoprosthetic treatment depends on fracture morphology, patient's age, extent of osteoporosis, general status, compliance and demands of the patient as well as experience of treating surgeon.

In contrast more or less absolute indications for performing humeral head endoprosthesis are non-reconstructable fractures in old patients, head split fracture, fracture dislocation of old patients and dorsally hocked dislocation fracture with a destruction of >50 % of the bearing area.

Three part fractures along with fracture of the greater tuberosity are most favorable treated by anatomic reduction of the stem to the humeral head, derotation and valgization of the humeral head.

Preoperative Evaluation

- It is crucial to document the preoperative integrity to the axillary nerve
- Plain radiographs in 1st true anteroposterior (AP) view and 2nd lateral view are basically required (see Fig. 17.1). We recommend in any kind of complex fracture pattern (2-part, metaphyseal comminution; 3-part and 4-part) a CT-scan of the affected shoulder (see Fig. 17.2).

Positioning

- We recommend placing the patient in Beach chair position
- Essential is an unobstructed intraoperative C-arm view of the proximal humerus
- We use a TRIMANO armholder (Arthrex, Naples) in a standardized fashion, allowing for excellent intraoperative manipulation and stabilization of the arm (see Fig. 17.3).

Anatomy and Exposure

- We strongly recommend a deltopectoral approach, starting between the coracoid and the AC-Joint extending to the lateral axillary line (see Fig. 17.4). The deltopectoral interval has to be thoroughly identified, usually landmarked by the cephalic vein. The cephalic vein can be either lateralized or medialized.

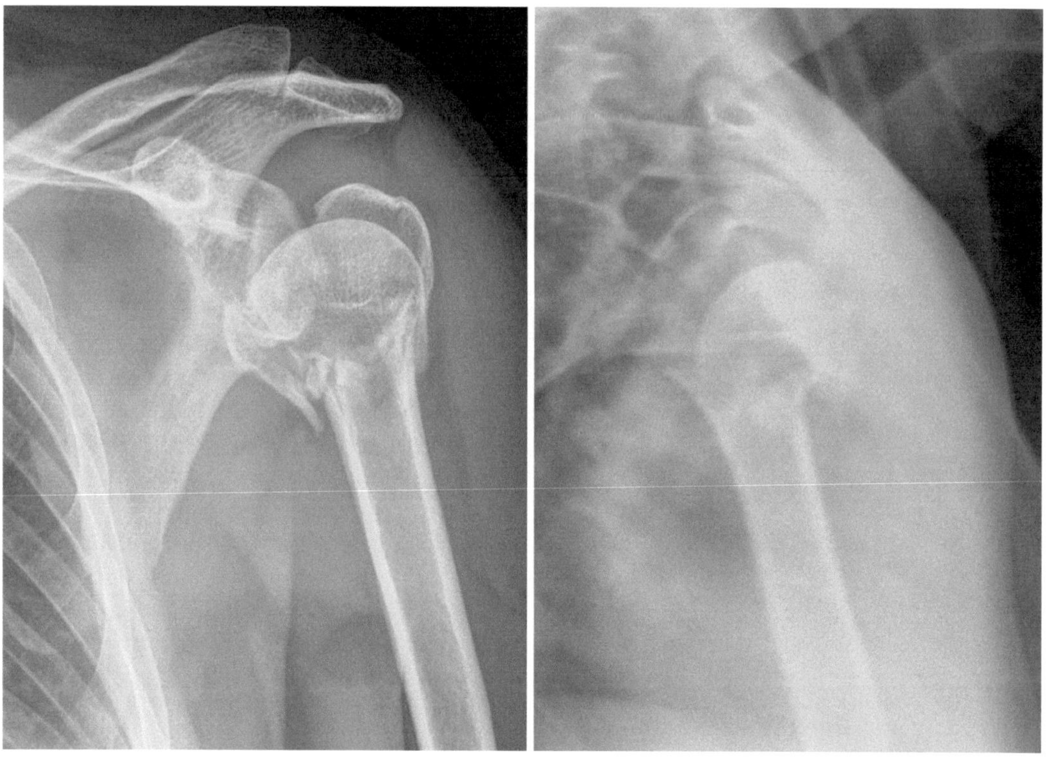

Fig. 17.1 The figure demonstrates X-rays in ap and axial view of a left shoulder. Depicted is a Neer IV.4 fracture

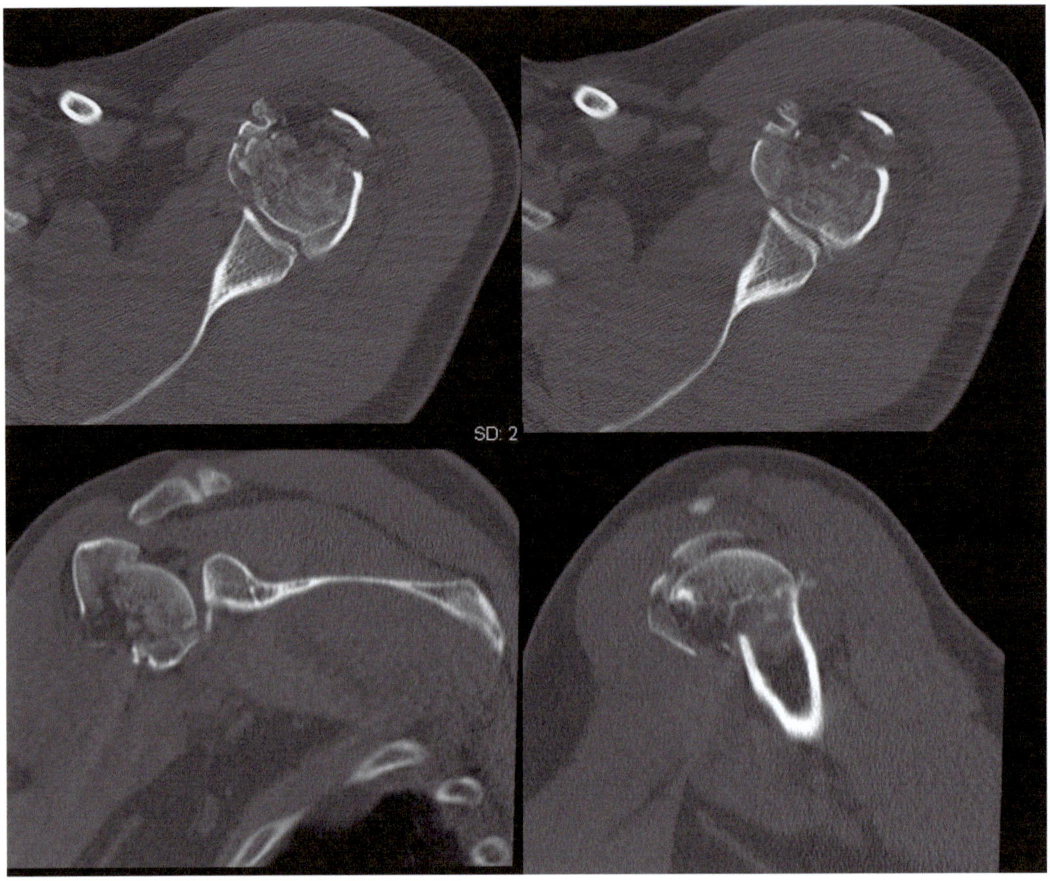

Fig. 17.2 The figure depicts axial as well as multiplanar reconstructions of the left shoulder from Fig. 17.1. CT reveals additional information regarding the extent of the fracture and the integrity of the joint surface

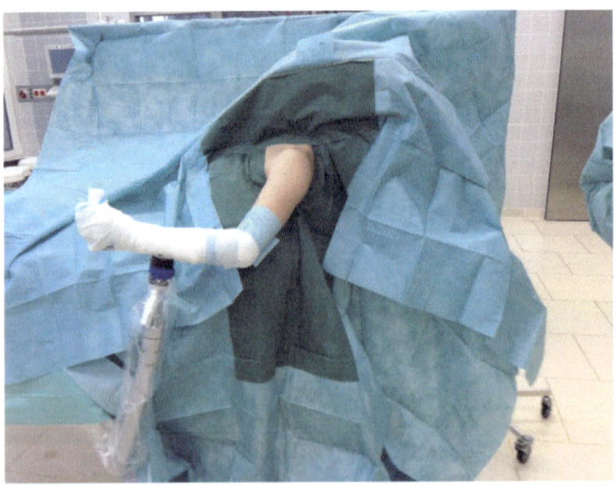

Fig. 17.3 The figure depicts the situs after disinfection and draping. The arm is hold on a Trimano armholder

- The deltoid muscle is retracted either a self spanning shoulder retractor or a Brown retractor. We use a carbon Brown retractor (Innomed, Switzerland), allowing for intraoperative C-arm control without the need for instrument removal.
- The medial border of the dissection is marked by the conjoined tendons
- For identification of the lesser tuberosity the long head of the biceps has to be found medial to the pectoralis major insertion. In about 80 % of head fractures a signification injury of the LHB can be found, requiring tenotomy throughout the rotator interval and subpectoral tenodesis of the LHB.

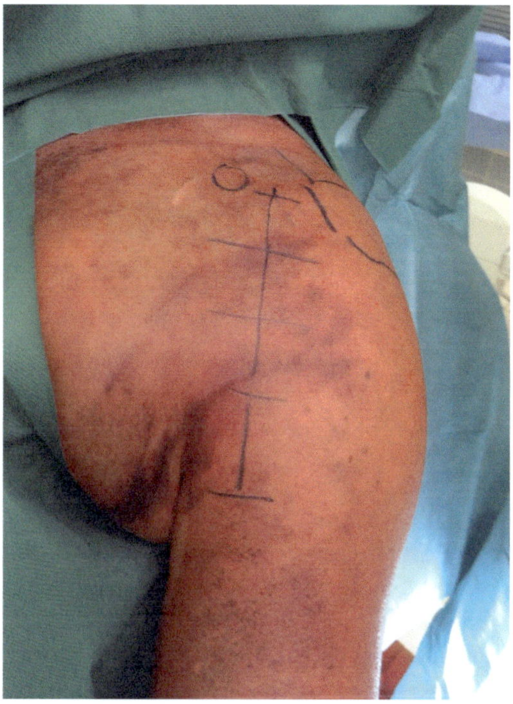

Fig. 17.4 A view onto the shoulder. The surgical landmarks regarding coracoid, acromion as well as the deltopectoral approach are drawed in

- Fracture hematoma is removed by irrigation, followed by blunt adhesiolysis in the subacromial (SA) space after identification of the coracoacromial (CA) ligament. Sometimes a Fukuda retractor within the SA space is useful.
- The GT fragment and the facets of the supraspinatus, infraspinatus, and teres minor and the corresponding rotator cuff attachments must be identified.
- In a first step we recommend applying a heavy traction sutures (Nr. 5 FiberWire, Arthrex, Naples) to the lesser tuberosity in a modified Mason Allen stitch.
- In a second step one or two traction sutures are placed within the greater tuberosity. Usually the arm therefor has to be internally rotated to at least 30° and abducted to 45°.
- In case of posterior damage to the greater tuberosity with affection of the infraspinatus insertion a fourth traction suture has to be placed at the posterior aspect of the greater tuberosity.
- In case of significant affection of the joint line an opening of the rotator interval can be necessary. In case of fracture of the lesser tuberosity the joint can even be visualized by reflection of the lesser tuberosity.
- In a next step the fracture has to be reduced by 1st pulling on the traction sutures.
- Most 3- and 4-part fracture tends to a valgus impaction. Therefore an elevator can be used to lever the head component into varus throughout the fracture line within the greater tuberosity.
- After adjusting the head to an anatomic position, the result should be temporary stabilized using 2.0 K-wires. Subsequently a verification using fluoroscopy has to be done.
- Some patients with highly osteoporotic bone and an epiphyseal void require either bone grafting or augmentation.
- In a next step an adequate locking plate is selected. Within the shaft a minimum of three bicortical screws is required.
- The plate can be provisionally fixed using K-Wires. The proximal ap-positioning has to be carefully adjusted to the fracture lines of the greater tuberosity. A to high or to proximal positioning of the plate has to be avoided as otherwise hardware related subacromial impingement my result.
- After fluoroscopic verification of proper placement the plate is fixed by a first bicortical, non-locking screw within the long hole.
- After an anew check of plate positioning subsequential drilling and screwing of the head component follow.
- We recommend a careful and slow drilling, as perforation of the head has to be carefully avoided.
- In osteoporotic bone usually the depth gauge can be positioned directly to the subchondral bone.

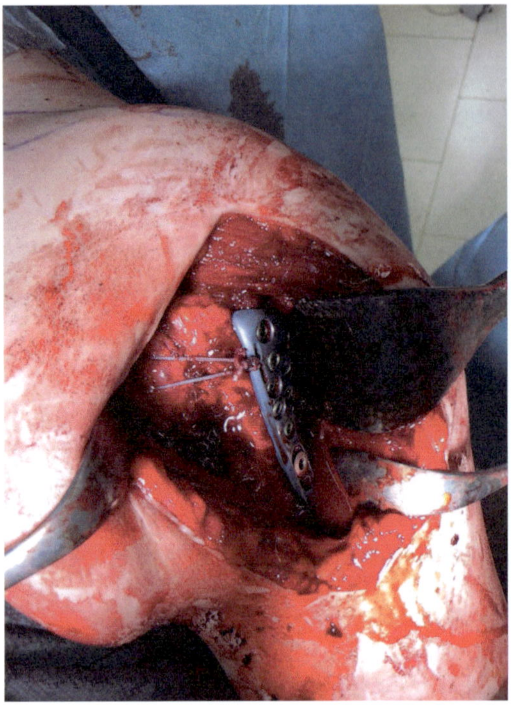

Fig. 17.5 A view from ap onto the situs after reconstruction of the humeral head using a locking plate. Clearly visible is the traction suture within the lesser tuberosity, being sutured to the plate

- After completion of the head osteosynthesis the construct is completed by two bicortical locking screws within the shaft.
- Finally the traction sutures are threaded through the dedicated holes within the plate and interlaced using eight half stitches (see Fig. 17.5).
- At the end of the procedure a careful C-arm control in different angles is mandatory for excluding screw perforation.
- Finally we recommend placement of a suction drain, closure of the deltopectoral interval and placement of the arm in a sling.

Postoperative Care and Rehabilitation Protocol

- The patient is seen at 6 weeks, 12 weeks, 6 months and 12 months postoperatively.
- Radiographs in true anteroposterior (AP) view, 2nd lateral view and 3rd axillary view are taken at each visit (see Fig. 17.6).
- The exact rehabilitation protocol is based on the intraoperative findings regarding bone

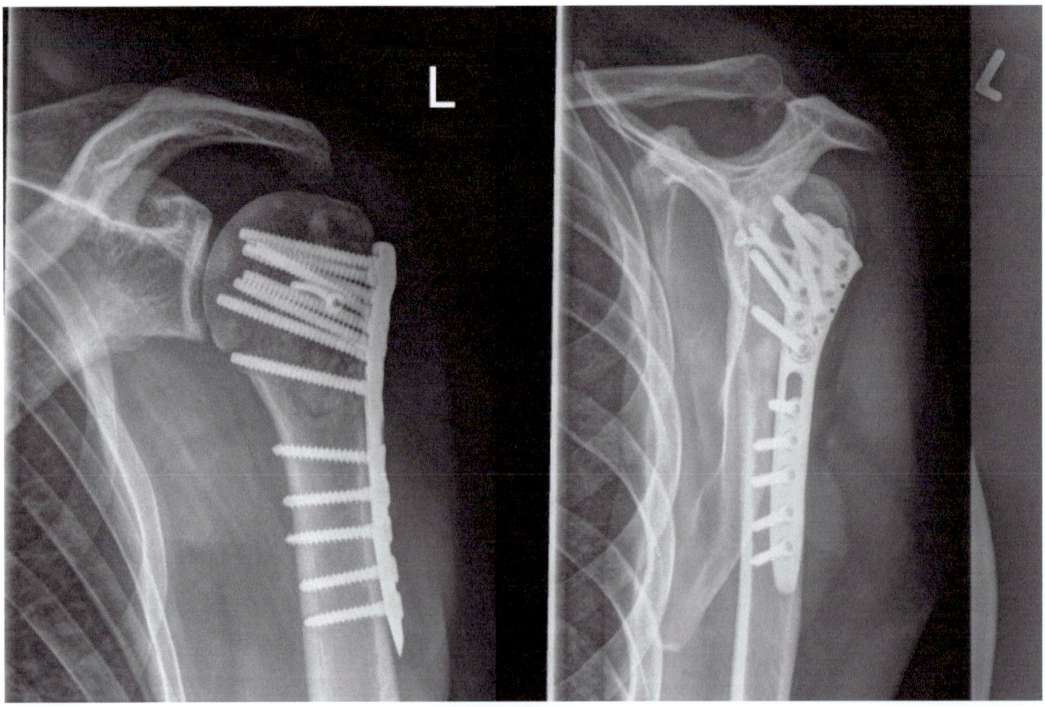

Fig. 17.6 X-rays in ap and sagittal orientation of the shoulder 6 weeks after surgery

quality and affection of the rotator cuff insertion. Usually we allow only passive motion until 90° of flexion and extension and 30° of external/internal rotation. In case of tenodesis of the LHB active elbow motion against resistance is not allowed for the first 6 weeks.

- Active-assisted motion starts after 6 weeks.

References

1. Lind T, Kroner K, Jensen J. The epidemiology of fractures of the proximal humerus. Arch Orthop Trauma Surg. 1989;108(5):285–7.
2. Court-Brown CM, Caesar B. Epidemiology of adult fractures: a review. Injury. 2006;37(8):691–7.
3. Kim SH, Szabo RM, Marder RA. Epidemiology of humerus fractures in the United States: nationwide emergency department sample, 2008. Arthritis Care Res (Hoboken). 2012;64(3):407–14.
4. Young SW, Segal BS, Turner PC, Poon PC. Comparison of functional outcomes of reverse shoulder arthroplasty versus hemiarthroplasty in the primary treatment of acute proximal humerus fracture. ANZ J Surg. 2010;80(11):789–93.
5. Krappinger D, Bizzotto N, Riedmann S, Kammerlander C, Hengg C, Kralinger FS. Predicting failure after surgical fixation of proximal humerus fractures. Injury. 2011;42(11):1283–8.

Part VI

Current Standards and Future Trends in Arthroscopy

Arthroscopic Options for Treatment of Proximal Humeral Fractures

18

Helen Vester, Andreas Lenich, and Andreas B. Imhoff

All-Arthroscopic Management of Tuberosity Fractures

Introduction

Traditionally, fractures of the proximal humerus are treated with open reduction and internal fixation. Generally, surgery is undertaken through a standard deltopectoral approach or through a deltoid-splitting approach to obtain anatomical reduction and to secure internal fixation. This method shows satisfying results as reported by several authors [16, 26, 29]. Park et al. reported excellent results in 80–90 % of the cases in a series of proximal humeral fractures including 13 greater tuberosity fractures treated with open reduction and internal fixation. Flatow et al. evaluated a series of 12 isolated greater tuberosity fractures treated with open reduction and internal fixation: they demonstrated six excellent and six good results at a 5-year follow-up. However, extensive dissection of the deltoid muscle for visualization of the fracture fragments may contribute to the morbidity of the deltoid muscle, to create a risk of injury to the axillary nerve or shoulder stiffness [21, 24, 25].

Open reduction and the cannulated screw or plate fixation technique have been commonly used to treat displaced greater tuberosity fractures. Although being a well-established method, it can lead to associated morbidities such as further migration of the fracture fragment as well as poor fixation. Moreover in patients with severe osteoporosis or poor bone quality in general, anchoring may pose a severe problem [11]. Fortunately, minimally invasive techniques for reduction and fixation of greater tuberosity fractures may solve these problems.

Thus, arthroscopic methods for reduction and fixation of greater tuberosity fractures are recommended to avoid extensive dissection and associated morbidity resulting from the surgical procedure [16, 26]. The arthroscopic approach bears several advantages such as less injury to the surrounding soft tissue including muscles and faster regeneration. Moreover, no implant removal is necessary. Apart from that, the arthroscopic approach offers a refixation of the rotator cuff, which allows for an early mobilization and physiotherapy. Open reduction and refixation of the bone needs more time for bone healing.

Nevertheless, the indications for an arthroscopic approach are rare. The following chapter gives an overview of possible indications for arthroscopic treatment and technical details.

H. Vester
Department of Trauma Surgery, Klinikum rechts der Isar, Technical University of Munich, Munich, Germany
e-mail: Vester@uchir.me.tum.de

A. Lenich • A.B. Imhoff (✉)
Department of Sports Orthopaedics, Klinikum rechts der Isar, Technical University of Munich, Munich, Germany
e-mail: a.imhoff@lrz.tum.de, imhoff@tum.de

P. Biberthaler et al. (eds.), *Fractures of the Proximal Humerus*, Strategies in Fracture Treatments,
DOI 10.1007/978-3-319-20300-3_18

Greater Tuberosity Fractures

Greater tuberosity fractures may occur as components of proximal humeral fractures or as own entity. The prevalence of isolated greater tuberosity fractures has been estimated to be 20 % of all proximal humeral fractures [9].

Isolated greater tuberosity fractures result from direct impact or indirectly by avulsion and shearing. This fracture can be described as an avulsion fracture of the rotator cuff. Usually, the fracture line is transverse or longitudinal with or without displacement. As a result of the pull of the supraspinatus muscle, the fractured greater tuberosity can be displaced in a superior or posterior direction, and usually the displacement is >10 mm (sometimes even up to the subacromial space). Greater tuberosity fractures healing in an anatomical position will not affect shoulder function. However, without appropriate management, displaced fractures can lead to malunion, pain, and loss of function. Thus, conservative treatment is not recommended for displaced fractures with the risk of malunion, pain and secondary arthritis.

Open reduction and internal fixation is recommended for greater tuberosity fractures, if fragments are displaced >10 mm. If greater tuberosity fragments are displaced ≥2 mm they should be anatomically reduced and only minimally displaced fractures (<2 mm) should be treated nonsurgically [18]. Healing of greater tuberosity fractures with even a small amount of superior displacement (>2 mm) could result in subacromial impingement and shoulder dysfunction; in particular with limited abduction and external rotation [18].

Different Methods Used for Arthroscopic Refixation of Greater Tuberosity Fractures

Suture-Bridge Technique

For this technique, two single loaded medial-row suture anchors (e.g. Bio-Corkscrews 5.5 Arthrex, Naples FL) are placed on the articular margin of the humeral head in 45° orientation. The second medial anchor is inserted 1.5 cm posterior to the first one. Then the non-absorbable sutures (e.g. Fiberwire,

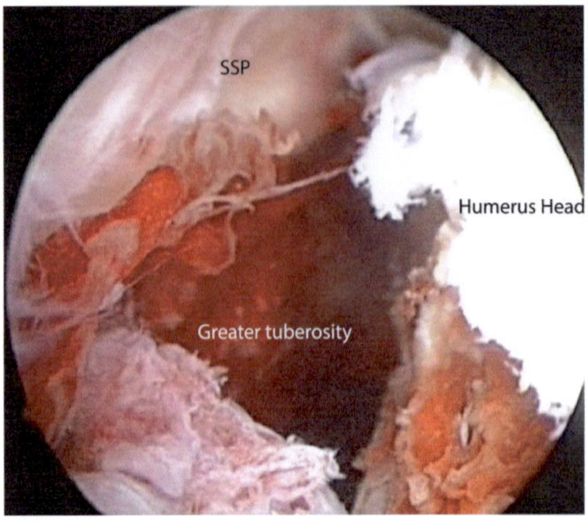

Fig. 18.1 Here the fracture area is depicted (Reprinted with permission from Lorenz and Lenich [18])

Arthrex) are passed through the intact rotator cuff attached to the greater tuberosity fragment.

The medial mattress sutures are tied. The pilot holes for a knotless suture anchor are prepared directly in line with the medial anchors and approximately 5 mm distal to the lateral edge of the greater tuberosity fragment. A suture limb from each medial suture anchor is then threaded through the PushLock (Arthrex) eyelet on the distal end of the driver. With constant tension applied, two PushLock anchors are inserted into the pilot hole using the suture-bridge technique (Fig. 18.1).

Speedbridge Technique

The speedbridge-technique is a totally knotless transosseous fixation of greater tuberosity fractures by laminar fixation of the rotator cuff. It is performed with a Swivel Lock anchor (Arthrex) with a Screw (Bio-Corkscrew, Arthrex) and a non-absorbable suture (Fiber Chain, Arthrex). There are various configuration possibilities for this technique, such as single row, double row, the V- or W- (so called Cassiopeia) configuration. Depending on the type of fracture and/or the bone quality a stronger fixation may be needed.

For the origin speedbridge technique, two Swivel Lock anchors are placed at the medial part of the rotator cuff footprint with a distance of 1.5–3 cm depending on the fracture and corresponding rotator cuff rupture. Then the non-absorbable sutures (Fiber Tapes, Arthrex) are passed through the intact cuff attached to the greater tuberosity fragment. Fiber Tapes are crossed (Fig. 18.2) and intraosseous fixation with Bio Swivel lock anchors is performed at the lateral edge of the greater tuberosity fragment.

The bone quality of the medial part of the humeral head is often poor, complicating the screw fixation. Therefore, a V-shaped or even a Cassiopeia configuration of the speedbridge technique may be indicated. The V shape technique is an alternative for the original single row technique. In contrast to the original single row speedbridge technique all four Fiber Tapes of the medial anchors are fixed with a single Bio Swivel Lock anchor at the lateral edge of the greater tuberosity fragment (Fig. 18.3). This is of advantage in case of poor bone quality at the medial part of the humeral head.

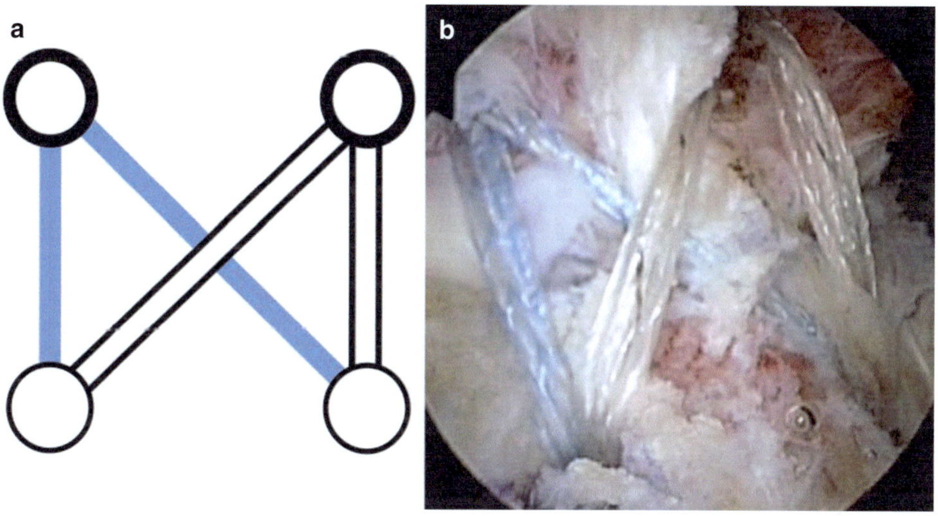

Fig. 18.2 (**a**) Configuration of the original speedbridge technique. (**b**) Intraoperative view of the double row speedbridge technique fixed with four bio anchors (Bio Cork Screws, Arthrex, Naples) and Fiber Tapes [3, 4] (Reprinted with permission from Banke et al. [4])

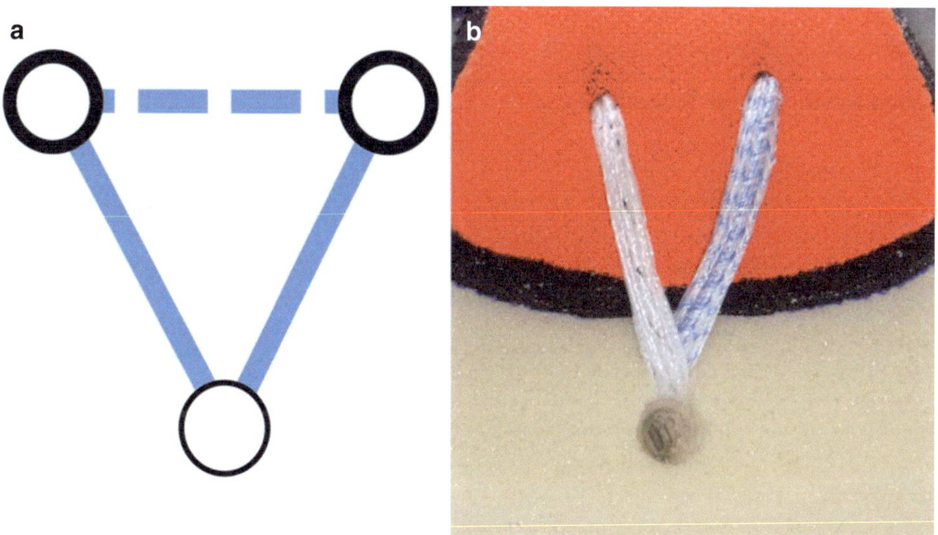

Fig. 18.3 (**a**, **b**) V-configuration of the speedbridge technique with Fiber Tape and bioresorbable anchors [3, 4] (Reprinted with permission from Banke et al. [4])

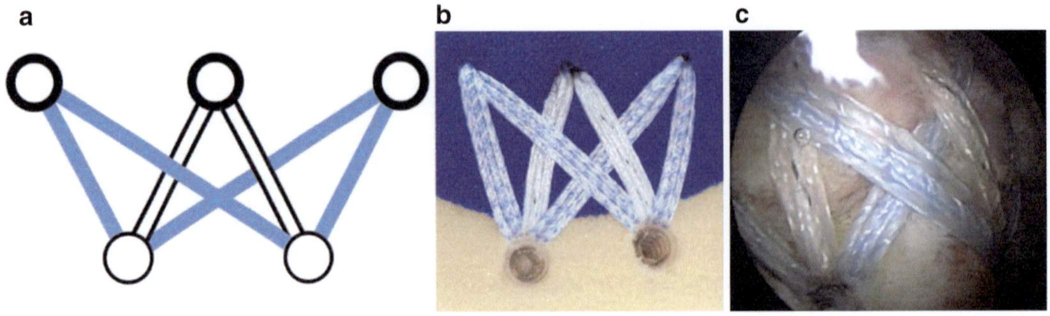

Fig. 18.4 (**a**, **b**) W- Cassiopeia-Configuration of the speedbridge technique (*bold circles* mark the medial edge, *light circles* mark the lateral edges). (**c**) Intraoperative refixation in crossed double row technique with three Fiber Tapes (2× *blue*, 1× *white*) and 5 bio resorbable anchors [3, 4] (Reprinted with permission from Banke et al. [4])

Moreover, in case of greater tuberosity fractures with a large fragment or corresponding extensive damage or rupture of the rotator cuff, the Cassiopeia technique can be used. In contrast to the original speedbridge technique three Swivel Lock anchors are used and fixed with the rotator cuff at the medial edge of the fragment. The Fiber Tapes are crossed and fixed with two Bio Swivel Lock anchors at the lateral edge in a W-configuration ("Cassiopeia", Fig. 18.4).

Biomechanical studies and case reports could detect a minimal advantage of the double-row suture anchor fixation and suture-bridge technique compared to the two-screw fixation technique regarding loading force of 3 and 5 mm displacement as well as maximum failure load [15, 17].

Fractures of the Lesser Tuberosity

Among proximal humeral fractures, isolated fractures of the greater tuberosity are rare and fractures of the lesser tuberosity are exceedingly rare. Isolated avulsion fractures of the lesser tuberosity represent an extremely rare injury that occurs mainly in younger patients [27].

Due to the functional environment including the coracoid process and acromial edge, only marginal dislocations of fractured tuberosities should be tolerated. Due to the insertion of the rotator cuff, displacement of either tuberosity leads to biomechanical changes in the inserting tendons and consecutive degenerative changes in the corresponding muscles. Operative fixation is widely recommended in cases of 5 mm dislocation or even with 3 mm dislocation of the greater tuberosity in overhead workers and athletes. In fractures of the lesser tuberosity, operative treatment is recommended for even minor displacement [2, 26]. In general, operative therapy of the lesser tuberosity must be considered beneficial in comparison with conservative approaches [22].

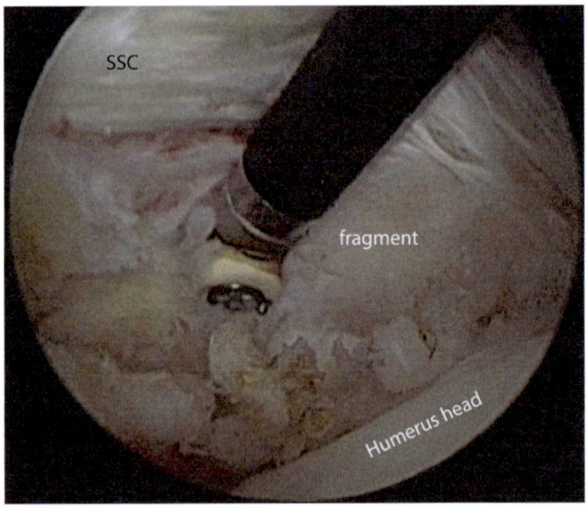

Fig. 18.5 Intraoperative view of a lesser tuberosity fracture (Reprinted with permission from Lorenz and Lenich [18])

Arthroscopic fracture fixation consists of diagnostic arthroscopy for detection of other pathologies (Figure 18.5). A typical intraarticular pathology is for example a lesion of the biceps pulley system. After debridement of the fracture one or two suture anchors are placed at the medial rim of the fracture. The subscapularis tendon is fixed with strong sutures (e.g. Fiber Tape,

Arthrex) lateral of the fracture creating a constant surface pressure of the fragment [18].

Problems Occurring During Arthroscopy

At present, certain difficulties are associated with arthroscopic methods for reduction and fixation of greater tuberosity fractures. Results from case studies and case reports suggest that arthroscopic methods for reduction and fixation of this type of fracture are associated with the same difficulties as arthroscopic repair of rotator cuff tears. First, there are many muscles around the shoulder joint. Hence, the distance from the skin to the joint cavity is relatively long and makes arthroscopic procedures more difficult. Second, a tourniquet cannot be used in this type of surgery, so bleeding affects visualization and increases the difficulty of the procedure. This bleeding can be reduced by regulation of the blood pressure. Third, a lateral position and traction of the shoulder can increase the joint space, resulting in difficulties in identifying the anatomical position of the shoulder. Finally, arthroscopic treatment of greater or lesser tuberosity fractures requires a long learning curve. Therefore, this method should be reserved for surgeons experienced and routinized with shoulder arthroscopy and rotator cuff repair.

Arthroscopically Assisted Management of Humeral Head Fractures

Generally, humeral head fractures are managed by open reduction (with a deltopectoral approach for example) and internal fixation, e.g. with a plate. With an arthroscopic approach normally, the fracture cannot be properly reduced and fixed as the operation situs is too confusing. Nevertheless, apart from the above mentioned fracture of the greater or lesser tuberosity, arthroscopy can be performed first to identify possible accompanying intra- articular pathologies. Nevertheless, there are few reports about arthroscopical management of humeral head fractures. Dawson et al. for example [7] reported about a 4-part fracture-dislocation treated by arthroscopically assisted reduction of the humeral head and percutaneous pinning. This technique avoids the need for a deltopectoral approach, preserving soft tissue coverage of the humeral head fragment. Fracture was treated by arthroscopic assisted percutaneus pinning. The authors report that the visualization obtained was sufficient to perform the entire procedure without significant fluid extravasation into the soft tissue.

A posterior and lateral arthroscopic portal was used and the glenoid served as sufficient anatomic reference to perform the procedure. Intra-articular evaluation of the joint showed the biceps tendon and the cancellous bone of the dislocated humeral head, anterior to the glenoid. Only the anterior and inferior parts of the head fragment remained with soft tissue coverage. No soft tissue was seen in the posterior portion of the head fragment. Using a lateral arthroscopic portal, a 7-mm cannulated screw was introduced being used as "joystick" to obtain reduction of the humeral head under arthroscopic assistance. Once the reduction was obtained, the screw was withdrawn Three K-wires were percutaneously inserted from the diaphysis to the proximal humeral head, using a motor drill.

Through a small lateral approach, the greater tuberosity was reduced and fixed on the humeral head by means of a 4.0-mm cancellous screw. In this case, no signs of avascular necrosis of the head were noted at 7 months of follow-up evaluation. The arthroscopic findings of only anterior and inferior soft tissue attached to the humeral head fragment are relevant, because any attempt to reduce the humeral head using a deltopectoral approach could have damaged the limited irrigitation of it. Hepp et al. compared functional outcome and humeral head necrosis after open reduction and internal fixation by a deltopectoral (DP) or deltoid-splitting [6] approach in 83 patients. They observed one case of avascular necrosis in group DS and three in group DP [10]. Stable osteosynthesis is important, but the outcome of operatively treated proximal humeral fractures is dependent on soft tissue management as well.

Nevertheless, humeral head fractures are generally treated by open reduction and internal fixation. Arthroscopy can be beneficial regarding better intra-articular evaluation, improved soft-tissue management and detection of potential accompanying pathologies.

Arthroscopic Management of Proximal Humerus Malunion

Malunion of the proximal humeral fracture is an often debilitating and painful injury, which is a challenge of treatment.

These deformities need to be distinguished regarding their basic pathology. One classification can be found in the current literature. Beredjiklian et al. named three subtypes which are malposition of the tuberosities (type 1), articular surface incongruity (type 2) and articular fragment malposition (type 3) [5]. Moreover, soft tissue pathologic changes play a major role in the limited movement seen in proximal humeral malunion cases. Generally, malunion of proximal humeral fractures are treated by osteotomy and open reduction through an anteriosuperior approach using screws, sutures or suture anchors. Nevertheless, many components of the pathology complex, like soft tissue changes, injuries of the rotator cuff, intraarticular changes, etc. can be better addressed arthroscopically. Arthroscopy is used as an evaluation tool to assess the soft tissue contractures and intra-articular bony abnormalities. Malposition of the tuberosities is a deformity that can and should be addressed arthroscopically as well for displacements <10 mm.

Malunion of the greater tuberosity is usually located posterosuperior. This displacement is due to the deforming forces of the inserting rotator cuff. Displacement of the greater tuberosity of more than 2 mm may lead to subacromial impingement and limitation of abduction and external rotation.

Then the patients present with typical subacromial impingement signs, pain and limitated motion. During arthroscopy a debridement of the subacromial bursa and synovia and arthroplasty can be performed. The rotator cuff is detached from its insertion at the greater tuberosity. The greater tuberosity is then reshaped creating a smooth surface without any prominent and impinging bone. Afterwards the rotator cuff is repaired using the suture-bridge or double row anchor fixation technique (see chapter before) [19].

Only few reports on arthroscopic treatment of the lesser tuberosity fracture malunion exist in the current literature. While the pathology after dislocation and malunion of the greater tuberosity fracture often consists of subacromial impingement and malfunction of the rotator cuff, a displacement of lesser tuberosity fracture leads to an impingement of the glenoid rim or loss of function of the subscapularis muscle. The arthroscopic treatment includes search for soft tissue pathologies, reshaping of the lesser tuberosity and refixation or debridement. Possible problems caused by the glenoid labrum can be detected. Moreover, the biceps tendon can be examined [12].

Arthroscopic treatment of proximal humeral fracture malunion is described even for treatment of a three-part fracture. After failure of the conservative treatment of a three-part fracture of the proximal humerus, the patient suffered 3 years later from limited internal rotation limiting his work and lifestyle. The reason for the limited internal rotation was a significant step in the articular humeral surface. This could be smoothed and reduced during arthroscopy [1].

Although arthroplasty is common for treatment of proximal humeral fracture malunion there are some indications, which are suitable for arthroscopic treatment. During arthroscopy concomitant pathologies, such as soft tissue changes or bony bumps invisible by plain x-rays can be examined and treated. Major dislocations or malunions still have to be treated by open reduction and fixation. Nevertheless, arthroscopic treatment gets more important and is a good alternative if the basic pathology includes soft tissue changes, intraarticular pathologies or minor dislocation.

Arthroscopic Implant Removal

The proximal humeral fracture is a typical fracture of the elderly patient. Open reduction and internal fixation is usually recommended and presents a commonly performed procedure. Locking plate fixation is a well-established surgical option with good results [14, 20, 23, 28]. Nevertheless, implant removal is often necessary due to pain, restricted range of motion or implant impingement. So far, open implant removal is the standard procedure. However, open removal with subacromial and subdeltoideal arthrolysis is an extensive surgery for the patient, the motor branch of the axillary nerve is at risk and infection risk is also increased. Therefore, arthroscopic implant removal seems to be a promising approach. However, up to now, only few case reports exist [8, 13, 30].

Surgical Technique

The arthroscopic procedure is performed under general anaesthesia with the patient in a beach chair position. Generally, the posterior, anteroinferior, anterolateral standard portals are used. Apart from that, three more portals at the lateral humerus proximal in the lane of the plate for screw removal are needed. Surgery starts with a standard diagnostic arthroscopy to detect potential intraarticular concomitant pathologies, like partial lesions of the rotator cuff or the long biceps tendon or even chondral lesions. In case of a limited range of motion due to arthrofibrosis, a subacromial and periglenoidal artholysis can be performed. The anterolateral portal is created directly inferior to the lateral margin of the acromion 1 cm posterior of the anterior acromial edge. Subacromial bursectomy is performed until the superior margin of the plate can be defined. The plate is debrided with a shaver or a small rasparatorium. It is imperative to remove all soft tissue from screw head cones to reassure a good grip of the screwdriver, preventing a deformation of the cones.

Then, under abduction and rotation of the arm, the proximal head screws, except the calcar screws, have to be positioned directly below the anterolateral portal, so that they can be taken out with a small-fragment-screwdriver through this portal. Losening of the screws in the soft tissue should be avoided. Three more skin excisions have to be performed on the lateral proximal humerus for removal of the calcar and shaft screw. A needle can localize the optimal height. Scar tissue and adhesions around the plate or even ossifications can be eliminated by a small chisel over the anterolateral portal. In the same fashion, the plate can be loosened and lifted. Afterwards, the anterolateral portal hast to be enlarged to approximately 2 cm. During the whole procedure, extraordinary care has to be taken for the axillary nerve. Depending on the initial approach, be it a deltopectoral or extended anterolateral approach, the nerve is closer to the scar and has to be exposed during arthroscopy. Finally the plate is extracted through this portal by a hook. The skin incisions are closed and a sterile bandage is applied. A post surgery x-ray is recommended for documentation of complete metal removement.

Arthroscopic implant removal provides the same benefits as open removal of hardware with a potential decrease in the associated risks. Additionally, it allows for routine evaluation and treatment of the glenohumeral joint pathologies. Advantages are a minimal soft tissue trauma, a minimal blood loss, a reduced risk of postoperative infections or adhesions, a complete glenohumeral inspection and treatment of concomitant intraarticular injuries.

The limits of this technique are seen in patients with adipositas per magna, locking plates being implanted several years ago and covered by massive ossifications, or some fused locking screws, which cannot be grasped by a left-hand thread. Nevertheless, arthroscopic plate removal is a valuable new opportunity for implant removal with all the advantages of minimally invasive surgery. Thus it is recommended for all surgeons being familiar with arthroscopic surgery.

Summary

All-Arthroscopic Management of Tuberosity Fractures

All-arthroscopic management of tuberosity fractures might be superior to the open approach as intraarticular pathologies can be detected and treated and also soft tissue can be treated with care. Most important is at least, that the arthroscopic approach represents a possibility for refixation of the rotator cuff respecting the functional role of the tuberosities allowing for an earlier physiotherapy treatment. The open or percutaneous fixation, in contrast, addresses solely the bone healing.

Arthroscopically-Assisted Management of Head Fractures

Humeral head fractures are generally treated by open reduction and internal fixation. So far, only few cases of arthroscopic treatment are published. The complication of humeral head necrosis or axillary nerve damage could be avoided by arthroscopical treatment.

Arthroscopic Management of Proximal Humerus Malunion

Proximal humerus fracture malunions are commonly treated by arthroplasty. Major dislocations or malunions still have to be treated with open reduction and fixation. Nevertheless, there are some indications, which are suitable for arthroscopic treatment. During arthroscopy concomitant pathologies, such as soft tissue changes or bony bumps invisible by plain x-rays can be examined and treated. Nevertheless, arthroscopic treatment gets more important and is a good alternative if the basic pathology includes soft tissue changes, intraarticular pathologies or minor dislocation.

Arthroscopic Implant Removal

Arthroscopic implant removal provides the same benefits as open removal of hardware with a potential decrease in the associated risks. Additionally, it allows for routine evaluation and treatment of intraarticular pathologies. Several advantages, such as less peri- and postoperative morbidity, minimal soft tissue trauma, minimal blood loss, reduced risk of postoperative infections or adhesions, etc. are limited in patients with adipositas per magna, locking plates, which are implanted several years ago and covered from massive ossifications, etc. Nevertheless, arthroscopic plate removal is a valuable new opportunity for implant removal with all the advantages of minimally invasive surgical procedure.

Acknowledgements Figures were kindly provided by Dr. Ingo Banke and PD Dr. Stephan Lorenz, Dpt. of sports orthopaedics, Munich.

References

1. As'ad M, Thet MM, Chambler AF. Arthroscopic treatment for malunion of a head-splitting proximal humeral fracture: the need for adequate initial radiologic investigation. J Shoulder Elbow Surg. 2007;16:e1–2.
2. Bahrs C, Lingenfelter E, Fischer F, et al. Mechanism of injury and morphology of the greater tuberosity fracture. J Shoulder Elbow Surg. 2006;15:140–7.
3. Banke JJ. Knotless and laminar repair of rotator cuff lesions with the tailored Speedbridge-Technique. OUP. 2012;1:244–8.
4. Banke JJ, Pedersen S, Braun S, Imhoff A. Potential of the Speedbridge technique. Arthroskopie. 2012; 25(2):99–102.
5. Beredjiklian PK, Iannotti JP, Norris TR, et al. Operative treatment of malunion of a fracture of the proximal aspect of the humerus. J Bone Joint Surg Am. 1998;80:1484–97.
6. Birkedal-Hansen H, Moore WG, Bodden MK, et al. Matrix metalloproteinases: a review. Crit Rev Oral Biol Med. 1993;4:197–250.
7. Dawson FA. Four-part fracture dislocation of the proximal humerus: an arthroscopic approach. Arthroscopy. 2003;19:662–6.
8. Dines JS, Hettrich CM, Kelly BT, et al. Arthroscopic removal of proximal humerus locking plates. Knee Surg Sports Traumatol Arthrosc. 2010;18:409–11.
9. Gruson KI, Ruchelsman DE, Tejwani NC. Isolated tuberosity fractures of the proximal humeral: current concepts. Injury. 2008;39:284–98.
10. Hepp P, Theopold J, Voigt C, et al. The surgical approach for locking plate osteosynthesis of displaced proximal humeral fractures influences the functional outcome. J Shoulder Elbow Surg. 2008;17:21–8.
11. Herscovici Jr D, Saunders DT, Johnson MP, et al. Percutaneous fixation of proximal humeral fractures. Clin Orthop Relat Res. 2000;375:97–104.
12. Hinov V, Wilson F, Adams G. Arthroscopically treated proximal humeral fracture malunion. Arthroscopy. 2002;18:1020–3.

13. Katthagen JC, Jensen G, Hennecke D, et al. Arthroscopic implant removal after fixed-angle plate osteosynthesis of the proximal humerus. Technique and initial results in comparison to open implant removal. Unfallchirurg. 2012;115:47–54.
14. Kumar C, Gupta AK, Nath R, et al. Open reduction and locking plate fixation of displaced proximal humerus fractures. Indian J Orthop. 2013;47:156–60.
15. Lee SU, Jeong C, Park IJ. Arthroscopic fixation of displaced greater tuberosity fracture of the proximal humerus. Knee Surg Sports Traumatol Arthrosc. 2012;20:378–80.
16. Lill H, Katthagen C, Jensen G, et al. Arthroscopic fracture management in proximal humeral fractures. Unfallchirurg. 2013;116:296–304.
17. Lin CL, Hong CK, Jou IM, et al. Suture anchor versus screw fixation for greater tuberosity fractures of the humerus--a biomechanical study. J Orthop Res. 2012;30:423–8.
18. Lorenz S, Lenich A. Fractures of the greater and lesser tuberosity of the humerus. Suture anchor fixation. Arthroskopie. 2012;25:134–8.
19. Martinez AA, Calvo A, Domingo J, et al. Arthroscopic treatment for malunions of the proximal humeral greater tuberosity. Int Orthop. 2010;34:1207–11.
20. Matejcic A, Vidovic D, Ivica M, et al. Internal fixation with locking plate of 3- and 4-part proximal humeral fractures in elderly patients: complications and functional outcome. Acta Clin Croat. 2013;52:17–22.
21. Neer 2nd CS. Displaced proximal humeral fractures: part I. Classification and evaluation. 1970. Clin Orthop Relat Res. 2006;442:77–82.
22. Ogawa K, Takahashi M. Long-term outcome of isolated lesser tuberosity fractures of the humerus. J Trauma. 1997;42:955–9.
23. Ong CC, Kwon YW, Walsh M, et al. Outcomes of open reduction and internal fixation of proximal humerus fractures managed with locking plates. Am J Orthop (Belle Mead NJ). 2012;41:407–12.
24. Park MC, Murthi AM, Roth NS, et al. Two-part and three-part fractures of the proximal humerus treated with suture fixation. J Orthop Trauma. 2003;17:319–25.
25. Park TS, Choi IY, Kim YH, et al. A new suggestion for the treatment of minimally displaced fractures of the greater tuberosity of the proximal humerus. Bull Hosp Jt Dis. 1997;56:171–6.
26. Pauly S, Herrmann S, Perka C, et al. Arthroscopic refixation of a combined fracture of the greater and lesser tuberosity of the proximal humerus. Knee Surg Sports Traumatol Arthrosc. 2012.
27. Scheibel M, Martinek V, Imhoff AB. Arthroscopic reconstruction of an isolated avulsion fracture of the lesser tuberosity. Arthroscopy. 2005;21:487–94.
28. Sudkamp N, Bayer J, Hepp P, et al. Open reduction and internal fixation of proximal humeral fractures with use of the locking proximal humerus plate. Results of a prospective, multicenter, observational study. J Bone Joint Surg Am. 2009;91:1320–8.
29. Taverna E, Sansone V, Battistella F. Arthroscopic treatment for greater tuberosity fractures: rationale and surgical technique. Arthroscopy. 2004;20:e53–7.
30. Voigt C, Geisler A, Lill H. Arthroscopic locking plate removal after proximal humeral fractures. Arch Orthop Trauma Surg. 2010;130:391–5.

Pathological Fracture of the Humerus

19

Andreas Toepfer, Ulrich Lenze, Florian Pohlig, and Rüdiger von Eisenhart-Rothe

Introduction

In general usually pathological fractures are caused by an inadequate trauma to the bone, which is impaired by the underlying disease. Pathologic fractures can be caused by a variety of local and systemic disorders. Aggressive neoplastic or pseudo tumor-like bone lesions present the second most common reason for pathologic fractures following osteoporosis. In this context the bony lesions can be divided into benign, primary malignant and secondary malignant tumorous lesions such as sarcoma and bone metastases respectively. Referring to the location of these bony lesions the humerus is considered as one of the most common localization of benign bone tumors as well as of sarcomas (osteosarcoma, chondrosarcoma, Ewing's sarcoma). Several primary tumors metastasize primarily in the liver and lungs but also very often in the skeletal system. The most frequently affected locations are the spine and pelvis followed by proximal parts of humerus and femur. Concludingly, besides the spine and the femur the humerus is one of the most common localizations of pathologic tumor associated fractures [1]. The proximal humerus is particularly prone to pathologic fractures because of its long arm of lever, high rotational forces of the surrounding muscles and the mostly spongiform metaphyseal bone [2]. A profound knowledge on the different causes of pathologic fractures, on diagnostics and therapeutical options is necessary for a successful treatment of this heterogenic disorder. This book predominately deals with pathologic fractures of neoplastic genesis because of the high incidence of tumor associated pathologic fractures.

Definition and Classification

Often the term "pathologic fracture" is solely used for tumor-associated fracture. But there are numerous reasons, which can be responsible for pathologic fractures beside bone tumors. Basically all fractures are considered as pathological fractures if they occur in systemically or locally damaged, thus less resistant to load bones, without adequate trauma. In contrast fractures occuring without any external trauma are called spontaneous fractures [4]. Nevertheless, adequate trauma possibly causing fractures does not necessarily exclude the diagnosis of a pathologic fracture. Therefore multiple parameters are relevant to diagnose a pathologic fracture e.g. injury type, underlying malignant disease, appearance on imaging [4]. Pathological transformations leading or predisposing to a pathologic fracture are caused be intrinsic

A. Toepfer (✉) • U. Lenze • F. Pohlig
R. von Eisenhart-Rothe
Klinik für Orthopädie und Sportorthopädie, Klinikum rechts der Isar Technische Universität München, Ismaningerstr. 22, Munich 81675, Germany
e-mail: andreastoepfer@t-online.de; uli_lenze@web.de; florian_pohlig@t-online.de; r_veisenhart@yahoo.de

P. Biberthaler et al. (eds.), *Fractures of the Proximal Humerus*, Strategies in Fracture Treatments,
DOI 10.1007/978-3-319-20300-3_19

and extrinsic factors and processes [5, 6]. Intrinsic reasons for example might be tumorous or inflammatory genesis as well as congenital or acquired bone metabolism disorders (e.g. Osteoporosis). Extrinsic processes, which could affect the bone quality negatively, can be medical radiotherapy (Fig. 19.1) and medications among others. Surgical interventions on bones, considerably increasing the risk of fractures are in a broader sense associated with the group of extrinsic processes. Therefore typical examples are biopsies and all types of continuity preserving partial bone resections such as excision biopsies, intralesional and marginal tumor resections as well as en-bloc resection (Fig. 19.2). Osteosynthetical procedures and drilling to the bone might also facilitate the occurrence of a fracture.

The so-called insufficiency fracture is a subtype of the pathologic fracture and is characterized by a break of the diseased bone under physiological loading.

In general this term is exclusively used for osteoporotic fractures [7]. Accordingly insufficiency fractures are most often found at load bearing parts of the skeleton, particularly the pelvis and sacrum, the proximal femur and also the thoraco-lumbar transition of the spine. In contrast the so-called stress fracture is defined as a break of

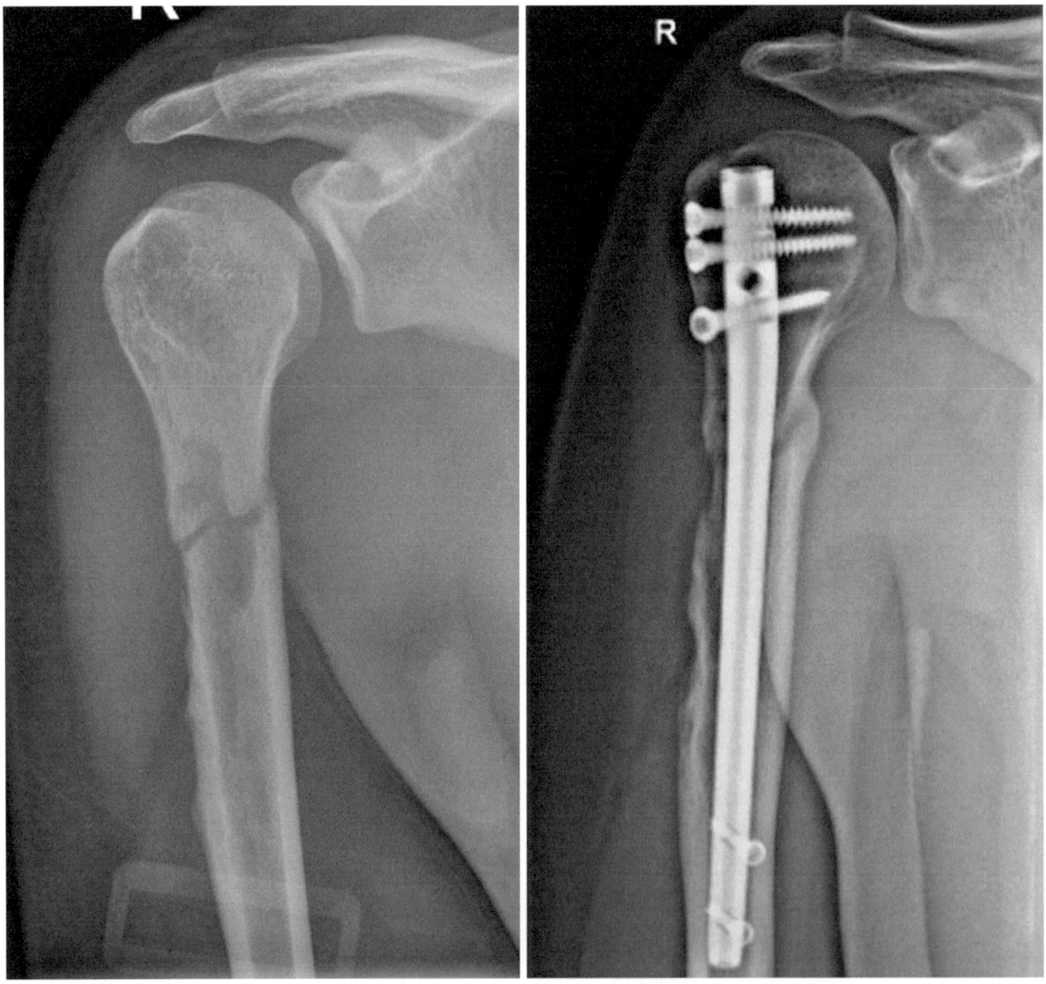

Fig. 19.1 Radiogenic fracture of the proximal humerus of a 11-year old male patient. After complete surgical removal (R0) of a recurrent Desmoid-type fibromatosis local radiotherapy with 60 Gy was administered after repeated recurrence. Six month after completion of radiotherapy, pathologic fracture of the proxial humerus occured while swimming (*left picture*). Bony consolidation is noticed 5 month after intramedullary nailig (*right picture*)

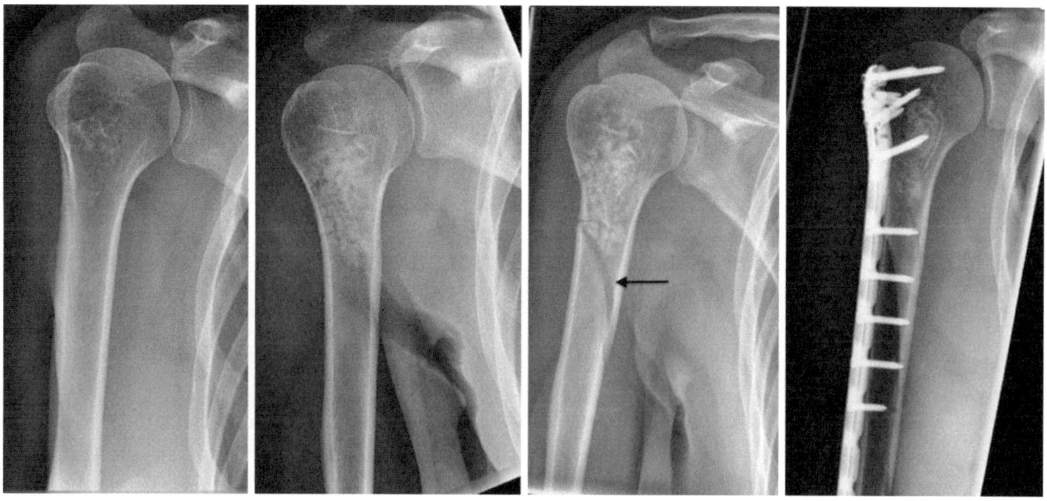

Fig. 19.2 Enchondroma of the proximal humeral metaphysis in a 49-year old female patient (*left picture*) and status after intralesional curettage and grafting with bone substitute (*second picture from left*). Pathological humerus fracture, originating from the caudal border of the bone window. The fracture occured 14 days after initial surgery, when the patient tried to open a water bottle (*third picture from left*). The *right picture* shows status after open anatomic reduction and stable fixation with a locking plate

healthy bones due to unphysiological loading (e.g. marching fracture) and is considered as chronic incident.

Epidemiology and Etiology

Compared to the total number of fractures excluding osteoporotic and insufficiency fractures pathological fractures are of rare occurence. In the current literature. Incidences between 0.5 and 5 % are given depending on author [3, 8]. Metastases are the most common malignant bone tumors and the most common cause of pathological fractures.

In contrast to the weight-bearing skeletal portions load-related pain, a common symptom of bone metastases, does usually not occur at the humerus. Thus quite often pathological fractures of the humerus are the first manifestation of a previously unknown underlying malignant disease [9].

Since the year 2000 in our University hospital, a total of 487 bone tumors of the upper extremity were treated surgically. Pathological fractures of the humerus occurred in 65 patients (13.3 %) whereas the most common benign cause of fractures was an enchondroma (n=9), followed by juvenile bone cysts (n=8). For metastases the renal cell carcinoma (n=10) and lung cancer (n=7) and in the primary malignant bone tumors, Ewing's sarcoma (n=5) followed by osteosarcoma (n=3) was present.

Diagnostics

An elaborate anamnesjs including fracture mechanism (traumatic vs. atraumatic), history (tumor history, endocrinological diseases, previous spontaneous fractures) and pre-existing complaints in the fractured area can help in diagnosing pathological fractures. After anamnesis the diagnosis of suspected pathological fractures relies primarily on performing radiographs in two planes so that the morphology of osseous lesions in general can be assessed. Lodwick et al. developed a classification system, which is helpful in correlating growth rate and radiographical morphology of a lesion [13]

The problem in definitely diagnosing pathological fractures is that the radiographichal morphology of tumorous lesions is often changed by fractures or tumor osteoid (e.g. in case of an osteosarcoma) might be misinterpreted as fracture callus [14].

For more detailed diagnostics both cross sectional imaging techniques in terms of Magnetic resonance imaging (MRI) and computed tomography (CT) are useful. MRI is usually performed to assess intra- and extraosseous tumor portions, the exact anatomical location of the tumor and its relation to other surrounding anatomical structures. CT allows for a three-dimensional visualization of the fracture and the extent of osseous destruction as well as the precise growth pattern of the lesion.

CT of thorax and abdomen using i.v. iodinated contrast media is recommended to search for primary tumors when osseous metastases have been found (e.g, carcinoma of the gastrointestinal tract) as well as to exclude or detect organ metastases.

Three-phase bone scintigraphy shows however information about the local bone metabolism of the lesion (osteoblastic activity) and also helps in detecting further metastases in the entire skeleton. However, it should be noted that scintigraphy might be disturbed by fractures as well as certain tumors, such as eosinophilic granuloma, simple bone cyst, multiple myeloma or aggressive osteolytic bone metastases may be silent on scintigrams (Fig. 19.3).

The diagnostic algorithm until the histopathological diagnosis is reached should always follow a strict pattern also in case of a pathological fracture: open or percutaneous image-guided biopsy of the suspicious lesion should thus be followed by immobilizing the injured limb by cast, occasionally even using external fixation. In order to avoid complication, biopsy should be performed at the same institution, which will be responsible for the final treatment. The technical performance of the biopsy should not limit the options of the definitive local treatment and should therefore be well planned in advance. The biopsy approach should be chosen in a way so that a tumor en bloc resection ultimately including the scar is still possibly achievable [15].

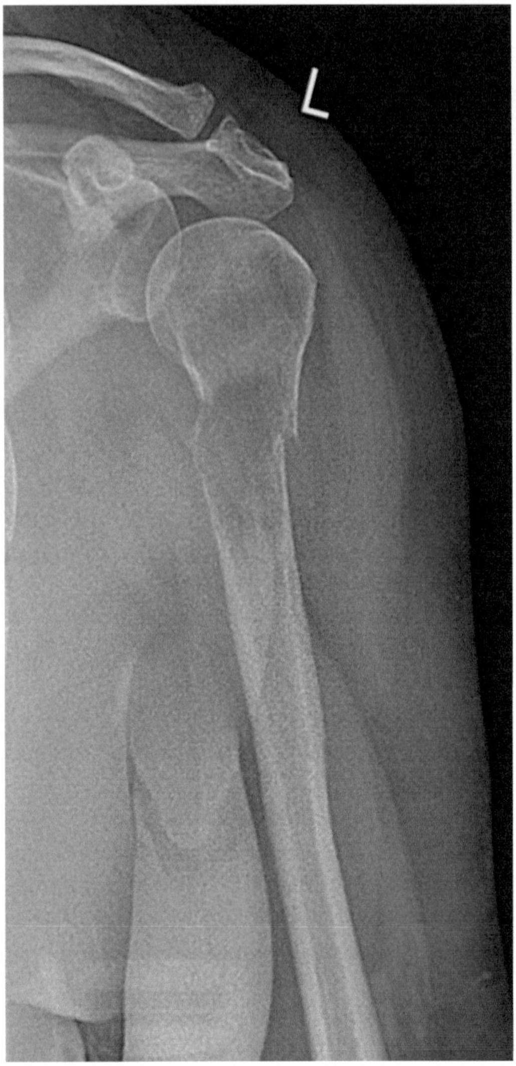

Fig. 19.3 Pathological proximal humerus fracture based on a osteolytic metastasis of a renal cell carcinoma in a 65-year old female patient

Benign Tumors

Benign bone tumors occur much more frequently than malignant ones. While the exact number of malignant bone disease is well documented in numerous national cancer indices, the majority of benign bone lesions remains undetected due to a lack of symptoms or are detected as incidental findings [16]. According to the classification of Enneking et al. benign tumors and so-called tumor-like lesions are divided in inactive, active and aggressive lesions [17].

Depending on the author and tumor center, the five most common benign bone tumors differ in their order of incidence. Cartilaginous exostosis (35 %) presents the most common benign bone tumor. However, the multiple manifestations forms in terms of pedunculated, sessile, solitary or multiple occurence does not predispose to pathological fractures.

Giant cell tumors (20 %) as well as enchondroma (10–25 %) and tumor-like lesions (current name: "Tumours of undefined neoplastic nature" [18]) such as juvenile bone cysts or aneurysmal bone cyst range among the most frequent benign bone lesions and regularly occur within the humerus. Since the biological behavior of these lesions ranges from active to aggressive it might be responsible for the occurence of pathological fractures.

Giant Cell Tumor

According to the current classification of musculoskeletal tumors of the World Health Organisation (WHO) giant cell tumors present as local aggressively growing benign tumors, also considered as tumors of intermediate malignancy by virtue of its biological behavior [18]. The relapse rate accounts for up to 25 % and lung metastases probably occur in 2 % of the cases. Pathological fractures occur in 5–10 % of all giant cell tumors. The radiograph shows an origin of the lesion at the bony epiphysis presenting as an eccentric osteolytic lesion characteristically with a destructive pattern type Lodwick 1c. MRI usually presents a low to intermediate signal intensity on T1-w images and intermediate to high signal intensity on T2-weighted images in contrast.

Open biopsy with subsequent immobilization of the limb is necessary to differentiate benign from malignant dedifferentiated giant cell tumors (<1). Only after the distinct diagnosis of a giant cell tumor is met and a malignancy is excluded a definitive surgical therapy with intralesional curettage, cement filling and osteosynthesis is to be performed. The initial reconstruction with autologous bone material is not indicated because of the high likelihood of recurrence. High primary stability, thermal adjuvant effects, the bone-saving approach and a good delineation of possible recurrence in imaging follow-up is in contrast to a revision including cement removal and biological reconstruction as well as a statistically increased risk of required endoprosthetical treatment of the adjacent joint [20, 21]. In very rare cases, it may be necessary in severe defect situations to use a primary endoprosthesis. Drug therapy with denosumab, an osteoclast-modifying human monoclonal antibody, shows promising results in several studies and becomes increasingly important in the treatment of unresectable or recurrent giant cell tumors [22–24] (Fig. 19.4).

Enchondroma

Due to its biological behavior the enchondroma, the second most common benign bone tumor, presents in several variants. All degrees reaching from asymptomatic incidental findings to sarcomatous degenerations including pathological fracture are possible. The proximal humerus presents the most commonly affected location following the small tubular bones of hands and feet (Fig. 19.5). Due to possible enossal erosion of the cortex (scalloping) and the resulting

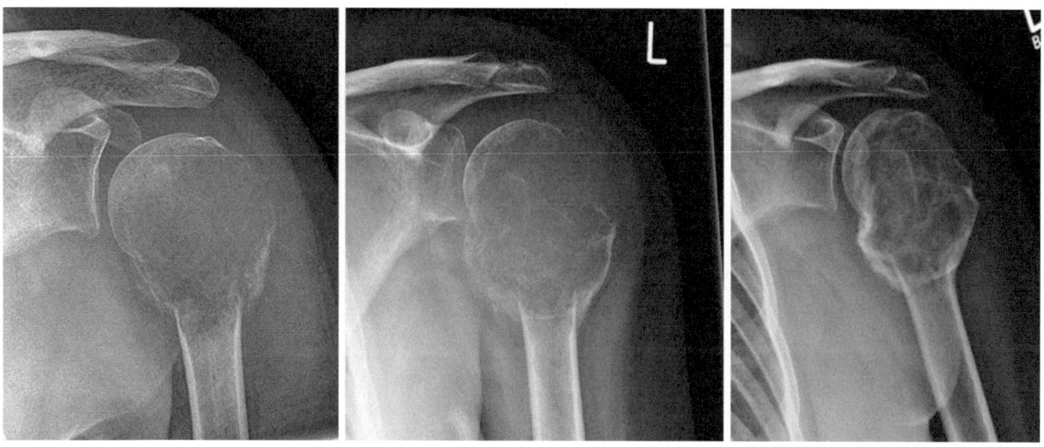

Fig. 19.4 Non-displaced, pathological humerus fracture in a 11-year old girl with histologically confirmed giant cell tumor. Surgical therapy was postponed due to initial egg-shell-like, thinned-out cortex and fear of loss of the proximal humerus. Within four month of s.c. therapy with Denosumab (Prolia©) bony concolidation is clearly visible

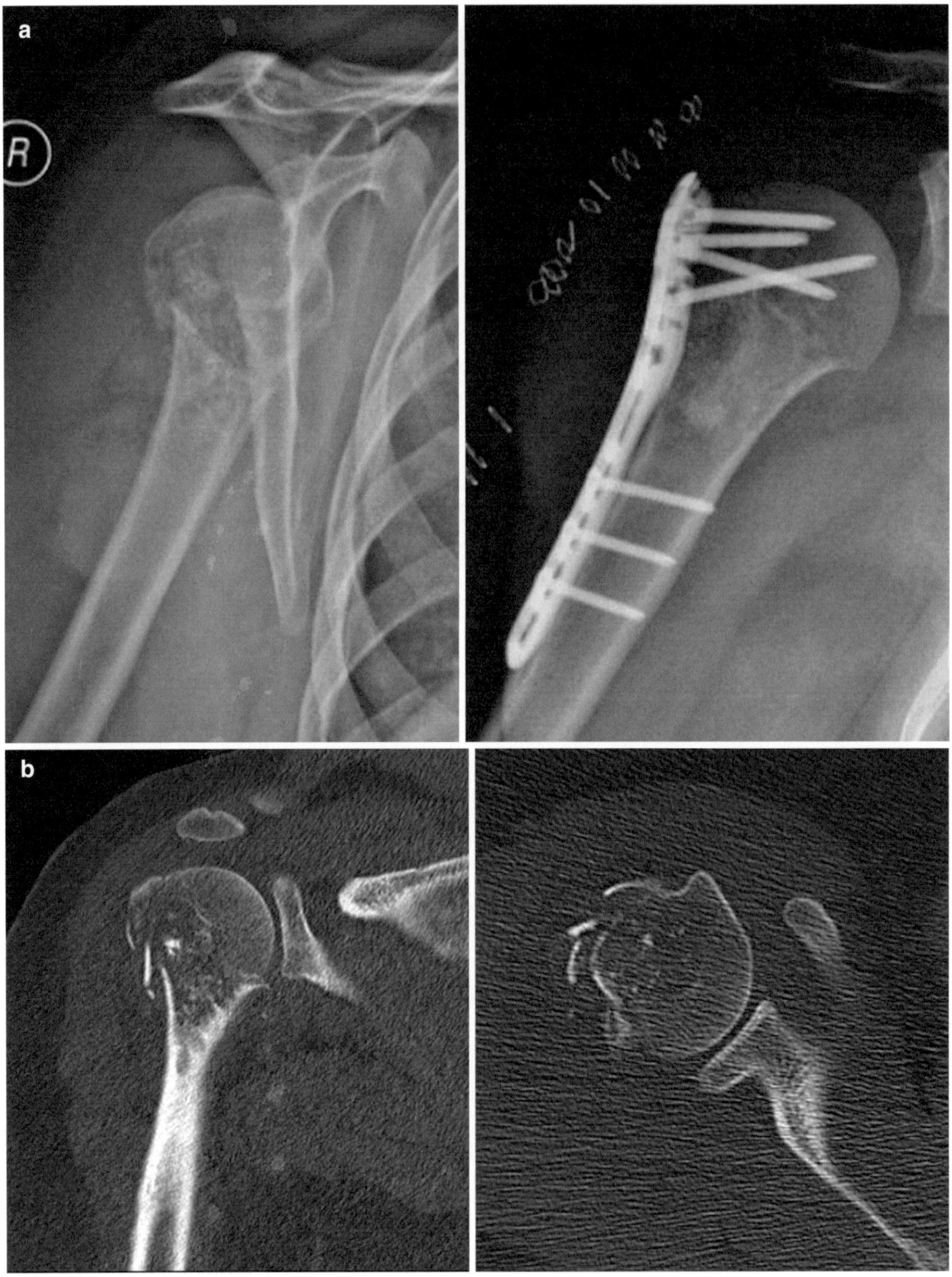

Fig. 19.5 Proximal humerus fracture based on an enchondroma in a 41-year old female patient. Conventional radiography, which was obtained after a fall on the right shoulder, clearly shows matrix mineralization, typically found in chondromatous bone tumours. Histopathological work-up of open biopsy confirmed diagnosis of enchondroma and allowed for a joint-preserving tumor resection. (**a**) Plain radiography pre- and postop; (**b**) preoperative coronal and axial CT-scans

reduced stability of the bone, pathologic fractures are also possible despite its benign dignity, but compared to metacarpals and phalanges of the hand of very rare occurence. A pathological fracture of the humerus in the presence of a chondromatous tumor should always remind the treating surgeon of a chondrosarcoma. A biopsy may not always lead the way despite a clinical and radiological suspected malignancy. The reason for this is that in practically all cases of low malignant highly differentiated chondrosarcoma histological malignancy criteria such as cellular atypia, pleomorphic stroma, increased mitotic activity are only focally and in many places the histological picture can not be distinguished from an enchondroma [25]. The reason for this is that in practically all cases of low grade, highly differentiated chondrosarcoma histological malignancy (cellular atypia, pleomorphic stroma, increased mitotic activity) are only focally and in many spots the histological picture can not be distinguished from an enchondroma [25]. Therefore, the diagnosis of low malignant chondrosarcoma G1 often derives besides the histopathological analysis from the combination of possible symptoms and findings and specific radiological criteria (see, chondrosarcoma).

Juvenile Bone Cyst

The juvenile bone cyst is a unilocular cavity lined with varying thick membrane filled with clear or sanguinary liquid [19]. In contrast to the aneurysmatic bone cyst (Abc), juvenile bone cysts do not present with any symptoms until a pathological fracture occurs due to its less aggressive behavior. On radiographs this type of cyst is usually located in the meta-diaphyseal junction, presents as a well-defined centric lesion with homogeneously decreased radioopacity (Fig. 19.6). In the location of the cyst the cortex is often thinned, on MR imaging a septation is either not or only sparsely present and the cyst appears to be filled with fluid isointense content without air-fluid levels. In general, there exists a grand variety of therapeutic options, including minimal invasive intralesional procedures [26], curettage with autologous bone grafting, implantation of cannulated screws or injection of autologous bone marrow aspirate or cortisone [27, 28]. In the presence of a pathological fracture the surgical treatment usually consists of an osteosynthetic stabilization by implanting an elastic stable intramedullary nail (ESIN), which also allows for an internal decompression of the cyst. In comparison to other therapeutical options if ESIN is

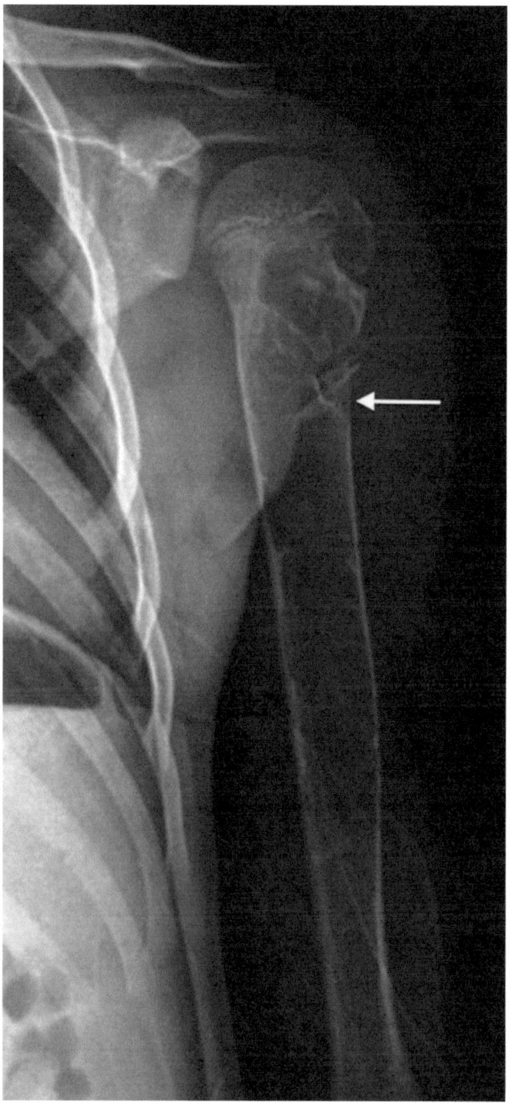

Fig. 19.6 Non-dispaced pathological humerus fracture in a 11-year old male patient with extensive unicameral bone cyst. *Arrow* shows the typical "fallen-leaf"-sign, representing a fragment of the thinned-out cortex in the cyst cavity

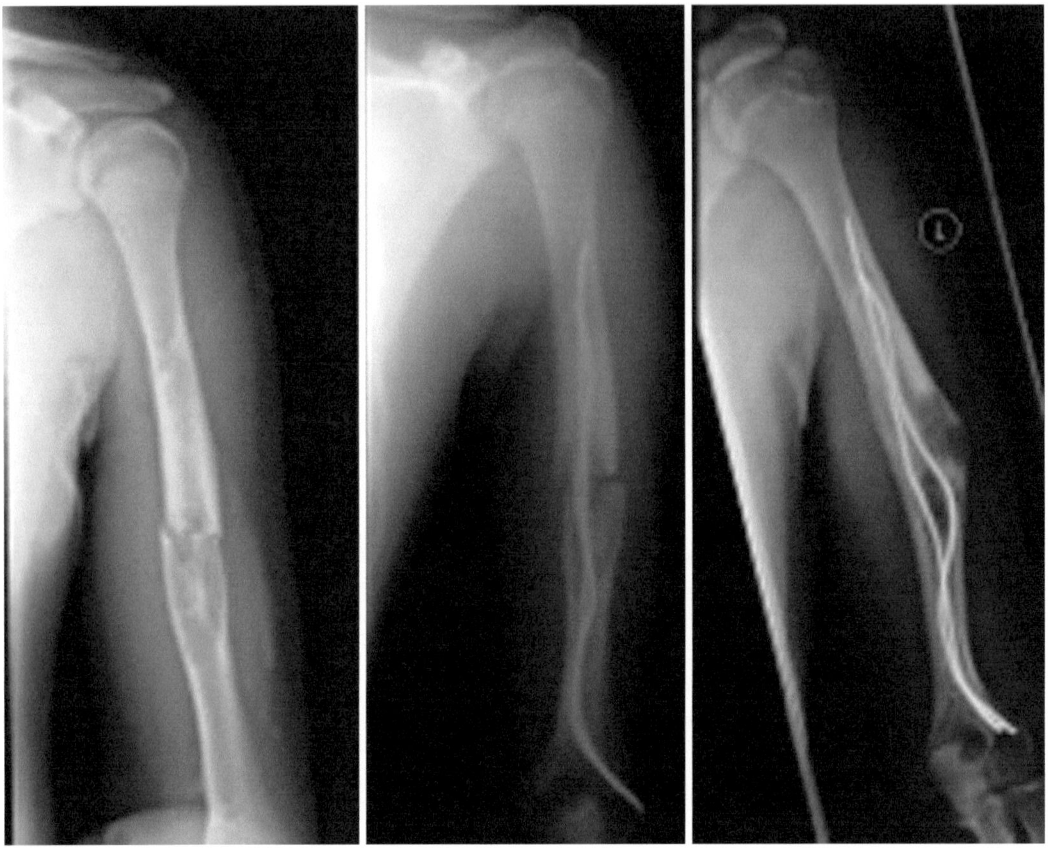

Fig. 19.7 Diaphyseal pathological humerus fracture based on a recurrent unicameral bone cyst in a 13-year old male patient (*left picture*), osteosynthesis with ESIN/Elastic Stable Intramedullary Nailing (*picture in the middle*) and bony consolidation of the fracture next to another recurrence/residuum with expansive cortical widening 7 month postop

performed there is no possibility to resect the cyst wall which can potentially increase the risk of recurrence (Fig. 19.7). However, in case a pathological fracture induces a decompression of the cyst so-called self-healing processes are initiated and thus, surgical treatment is in case of adequate immobilization not obligatory.

Primary Malignant Tumors

The 3 most common primary malignant tumors of the bone in terms of osteosarcoma, chondrosarcoma and Ewing's sarcoma show an annual incidence of approximately 10 per 1 million inhabitants. Whereas patients with osteo- and Ewing's sarcoma are mostly younger than 20 years old, the peak incidence of the primary (conventional) chondrosarcoma is in the fifth to seventh decade of life [16, 19]. Pathological fractures occur in patients suffering from osteo- and Ewing's sarcoma in 5–10 % of cases [10, 12, 29] and in patients with chondrosarcoma, depending on the degree of differentiation, in 2–25 % of the cases [37.1].

Diagnosis and treatment of osteo-, Ewing's sarcoma and chondrosarcoma may differ significantly, so that the major differences will be highlighted as follows:

Osteosarcoma

The "conventional" osteosarcoma can appear with a great variety on radiographs, but usually a mixed osteoblastic/osteolytic, eccentric-growing lesion is found in the metaphysis of the bone with concomitant cortical destruction, periosteal reaction and invasion of the surrounding soft tissue. If the osteosarcoma occurs in the diaphysis of the bone an increased risk for pathological fractures is present, but also in case of an osteolytic growth pattern and telangiectatic as well as fibroblastic osteosarcoma variants [30]. Compared to other anatomical locations, the osteosarcoma of the proximal humerus presents with a statistically higher incidence of pathological fractures (Fig. 19.8a, b) [31].

Ewing's Sarcoma

In case of manifestation of Ewing's sarcoma in long bones it is typically found in a diaphyseal location and characterized by a poorly definable, permeative or moth-damage like osteolytic osteodestruction along with onion peel-like periosteal reaction. Pathological fractures usually occur in association with neoadjuvant radiotherapy [30], but can also represent the first symptoms of a previously unknown tumor. While in osteosarcoma also low-malignant subtypes exist (e.g. paraosseal osteosarcoma G1) and local therapy may differ from a vast continuity interrupting resection, however, Ewing sarcoma, presents by definition always a low-differentiated, highly malignant tumor. After the diagnosis is confirmed by histology neoadjuvant therapy in terms of chemo- and/or radiotherapy should be initiated as soon as possible [16]. The definitive tumor resection and, if possible limb-preserving surgical reconstruction should consecutively be performed. Pathologic fractures due to underlying primary malignant bone tumors is not necessarily followed by ablative procedures along with amputation or exarticulation. In the current litera-

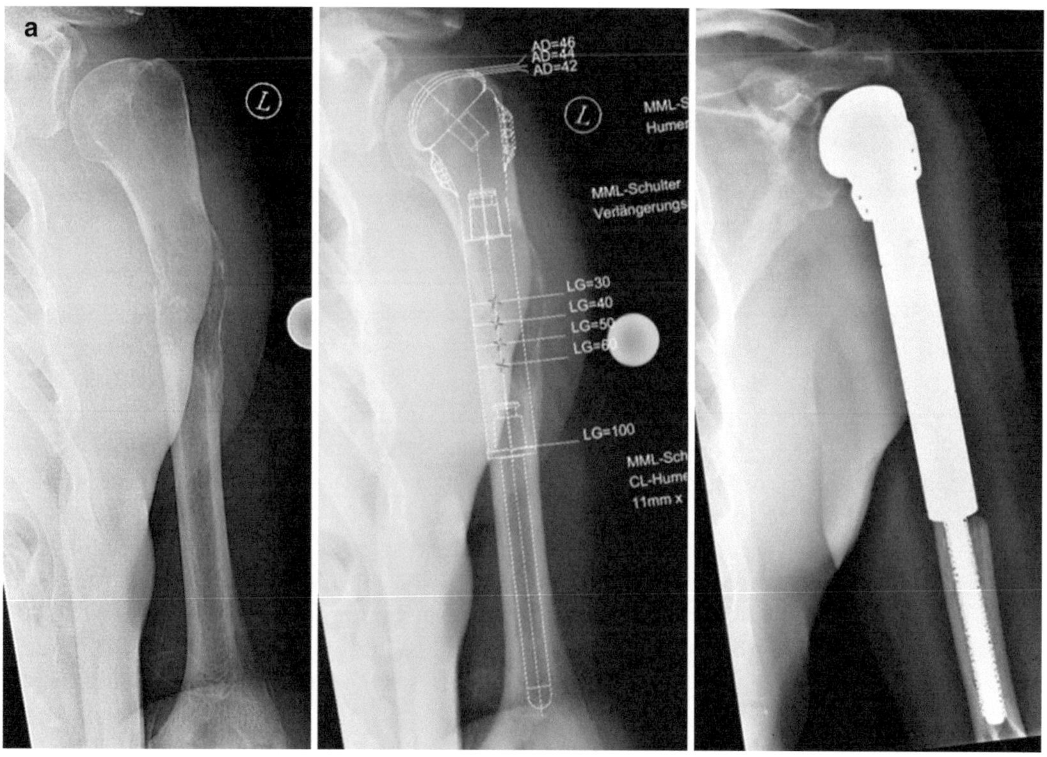

Fig. 19.8 (**a**) High-grade, giant-cell-rich osteosarcoma with pathological fracture of the left humerus in a 50-year old male patient (*left picture*). The picture in the *middle* shows preoperative planning including the level of resection and endoprosthetic reconstruction. Postoperative x-rays after wide tumor resection and implantation of a modular megaprosthesis (Orthodynamics, MML) in combination with a trevira tube for soft tissue reconstruction. (**b**) Local recurrence despite complete initial resection (R0) of the poorly differentiated giant-cell-rich osteosarcoma (G3) 27 month postop (*left picture*) and status after gleno-humeral disarticulation due to tumor-infiltration to the neuro-vascular bundle

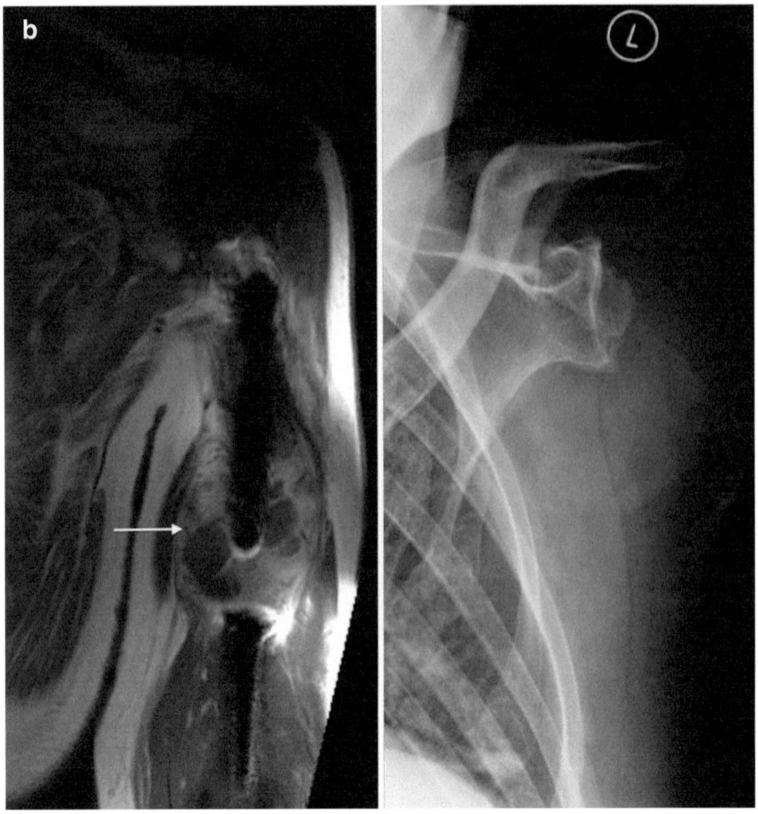

Fig. 19.8 (continued)

ture the risk of local recurrence is not described as increased if limb-preserving procedures are performed keeping tumor-free surgical margins and for pathological fractures including resection of the fracture hematoma [10, 12, 29, 32].

In the current literature risk factors for tumor-free survival are heterogeneously discussed. However, some authors do not see a negative influence of pathological fractures on the prognosis of Ewing's sarcoma, regardless of the time point when the fracture (before or during irradiation) occurs [10, 29]. However, in case of osteosarcoma the localization in the humerus as well as the presence of a pathological fracture seems to worsen the prognosis significantly [31, 33–35]. It needs to be stated that prognosis can not be improved by a more radical surgical therapy in terms of amputation. The reason why for Ewing's sarcoma the prognosis is not changing following a pathological fracture compared to osteosarcoma can be explained by the higher chemosensitivity of the tumor [29, 36].

Chondrosarcoma

In case of a pathological fracture due to underlying chondrosarcoma it stresses some exceptions regarding diagnosis and treatment of fractures. On the one hand the transition between enchondroma and low-grade chondrosarcoma is ambigous so that the histopathological analysis of a biopsy often does not allow for a definitive conclusion regarding dignity of the lesion. On the other hand no useful adjuvant therapy options exist since chondrosarcoma present as rather insensitive towards chemo- and radiotherapy. Chondrosarcoma in the humerus is found to be associated with a higher risk of pathologic fractures and of local recurrence respectively [37]. Pathological fractures, however, are not necessarily afflicted with higher rate of recurrence.

Pathological fractures due to chondrosarcoma seem also to negatively effect the mean survival rate as described for osteosarcoma but in contrast to Ewing's sarcoma [29]. In the literature some

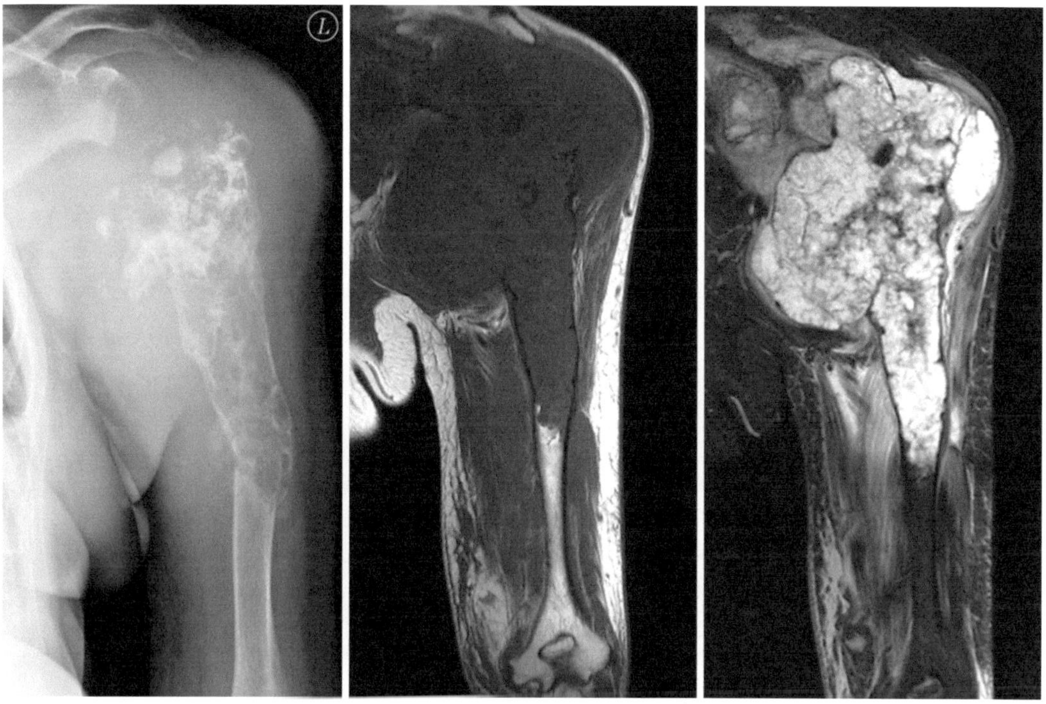

Fig. 19.9 Plain radiography and MRI with coronal T1- and T2- weighted cross sectional imaging of a dedifferentiated chondrosarcoma with pathological fracture in a 47-year old patient. Limb salvage was not viable and forquater amputation had to be performed

authors recommend more generous indications for ablative procedures [32, 37] due to the lack of chemo sensitivity of the tumor but sufficient studies of evidence are missing. The treatment recommendations should be based ultimately on the grading and the resectability of the tumor, since the prognosis of the primary (conventional) chondrosarcoma is directly correlated with the histological grade (Fig. 19.9). In case of low-grade chondrosarcoma (well differentiated, G1) of the extremities, followed by a pathological fracture, indication for intralesional currettage using chemical or thermal adjuvants has not changed. The difficulty is to distinguish well from a moderately or poorly differentiated tumors. Neither guide biopsy nor instantaneous section diagnostics can sometimes provide a clear graduation in case of insufficient representative tissue of a heterogeneous tumor. However, radiological criteria can help in decision making. As radiological criteria of aggressiveness an increase of the bony circumference and cortical thinning are considered as well as a deep scalloping (enosteal "nibbling" of the cortex) of the affected bone [38]. If these radiological criteria are present intralesional therapy should be refrained. Intramedullary tumor dimensions with a critical size of four to five cm as well as the presence, type and distribution of matrix calcification ("rings and arcs") are not any more considered as hard evidence of malignancy [38–42]. Permeative or moth-damage-related cortical destruction, perifocal edema and soft tissue component of the tumor are further suspicious changes suggesting a poor differentiated tumor presenting as argument against a primary surgical management of the pathological fracture with intralesional resection and also expressing the need of an extended biopsy or en bloc resection including tumor-free margins.

Multiple Myeloma

Multiple myeloma (MM) is different from all other tumors of the musculoskeletal system, since it presents a systemic disease with neoplastic proliferation of B lymphocytes [43]. Osteolytic lesions, which may result in pathological fractures, only represent a local osseous MM-manifestation and are caused by increased cytokine production of malignant plasma cells and the associated increased osteoclastic activity [44]. Therefore, diagnosistics and treatment of this disease also differs from the other previously described musculoskeletal tumors. Often MM-patients present with pain in the musculoskeletal system as initial symptom of a pathological fracture. On radiographs typically an increased radiolucency of the bone with focal lucency and enosseal cortical destruction is found [45] (Fig. 19.10). Further diagnostics consist of an extensive laboratory diagnostics. Serum- and 24-h urine electrophoresis are usually performed

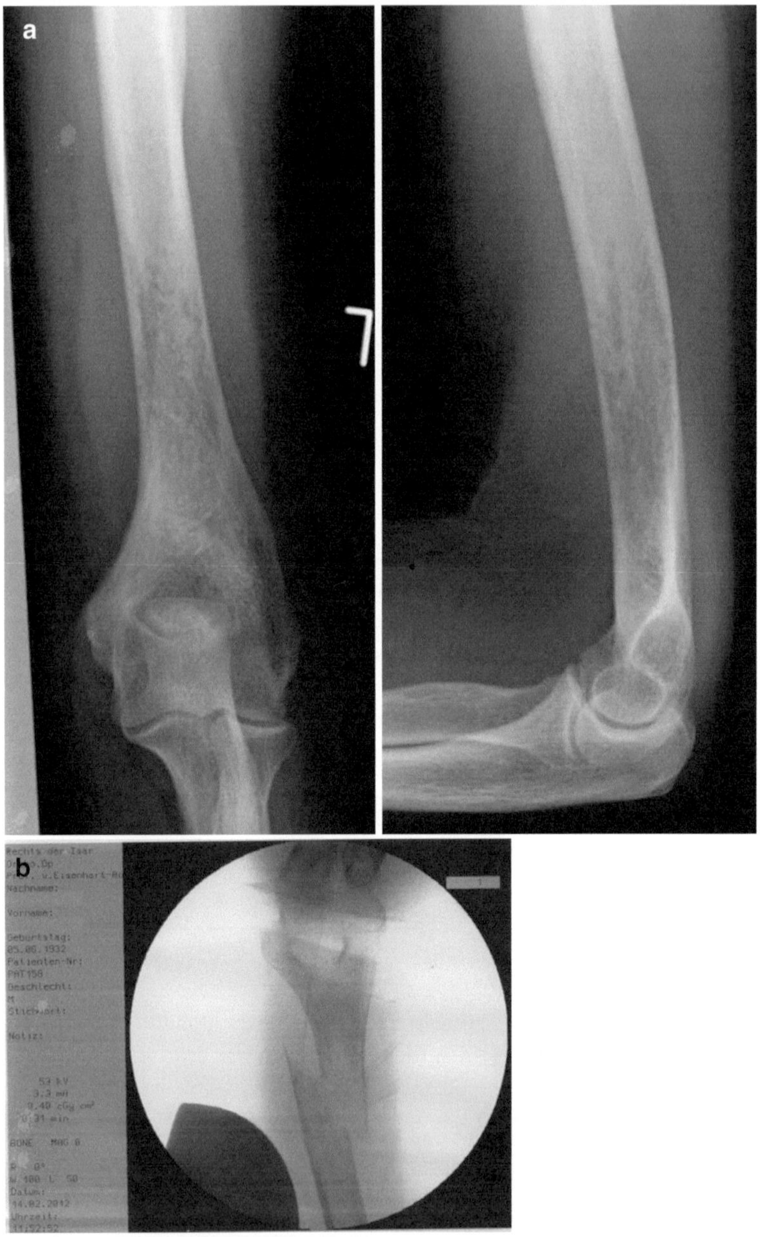

Fig. 19.10 Seventy-nine-year old male patient with a painful bone lesion of the distal diaphyseal humerus (**a**). Despite a Mirels-Score of <8p. a spontaneous pathological fracture occured (**b**). Surgery included intralesional tumor resection (curettage), open reduction and compound osteosynthesis with a locking compression plate (**c**)

Fig. 19.10 (continued)

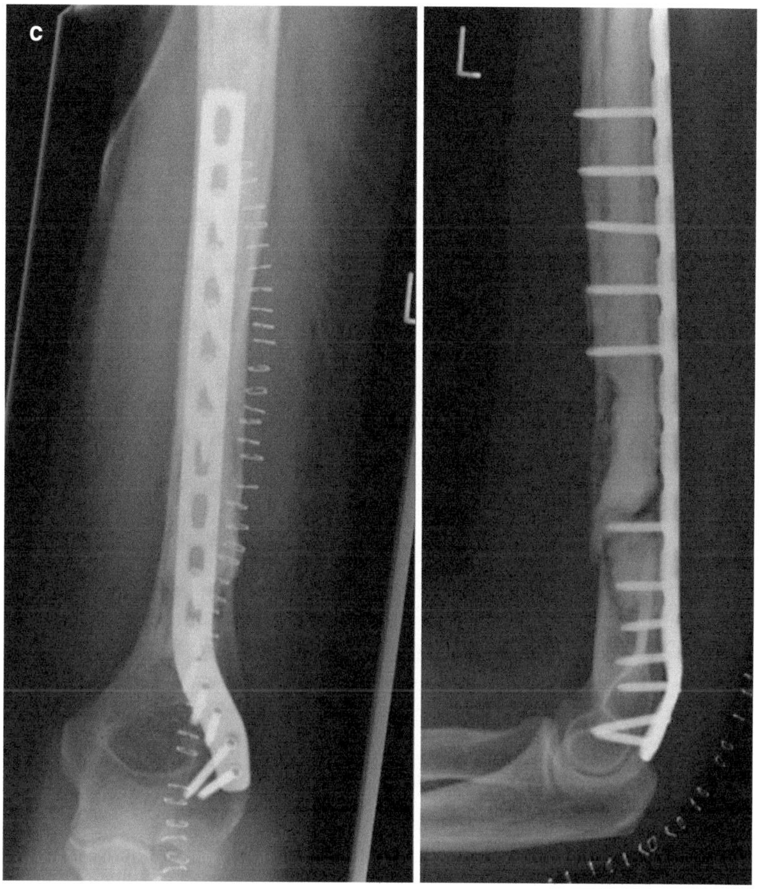

to detect the typically present monoclonal immunoglobulins. To confirm the diagnosis, however, a bone marrow biopsy is mandatory. The treatment of multiple myeloma primarily consists of systemic chemotherapy along with or without autologous stem cell transplantation (ASCT). However, in general multiple myeloma represents an incurable disease, which can be brought into remission. In the case of solitary focal plasmacytoma, radiation therapy can be performed as stand- alone therapy or as adjuvant therapy following surgery [44]. Osteolysis at risk for fracture or pathologic fractures, however, should always initially be treated surgically performing an intralesional resection and consecutive stabilization using osteosynthesis. At non-load-bearing bones such as the humerus a compound osteosynthesis is recommended by plate fixation and bone cement, since a high initial stability can be achieved with good function [46, 47]. In rare cases of severe bone destruction endoprothetic replacement may be indicated with additional adjuvant radiotherapy or combined radio/chemotherapy.

Metastases

Progress of the interdisciplinary treatment of malignant tumors lead and have lead to a permanent improvement in life expectancy, but also to an increasing incidence of bone metastases and pathological fractures. From the statistical point of view approximately 50 % of patients suffering from malignancies will develop metastases, whereas solitary metastases with a frequency of 5 % are of rare incidence [2, 48]. In a study already performed in the year 1950 on 1000 cancer patients undergoing autopsy 27 % of the cases presented already metastases [49]. The prevalence of secondary malignancies of the bone in terms of skeletal metastases, is compared to primary sarcomas of the bone at least 25 times higher [16]. Following lung and liver, most tumours then develop metastases in the skeleton whereas the spread consists of a hematogenious dissemination. Certain tumour entities such as prostate, breast, lung, renal and thyroid carcinoma have a designated affinity to bone accounting for up to 80 % until 93 % of all skeletal metastases [19, 50]. In principle, however, any malignant tumor may develop bone metastasis. Common sites for the occurrence of bone metastases are, in descending order, spine, ribs and pelvis as well as the proximal metaphyses of long bones femur and humerus. This can be explained by the mainly hematogenious spread in bone structures with a high proportion of hematopoetic bone marrow [51]. The incidence of pathological fracture of the humerus due to bone metastasis is between 10 and 29 % [2, 30, 52, 53], depending on the biological behavior of the primary tumour and its type of metastasis (osteolytic/osteoblastic/mixed, response to therapy, etc.). The surgical procedure in case of a metastasis induced pathological fracture of the humerus has the intention to enable the patient to improve quality of life and to recover as fast as possible to regain mobility and independence performing primary stable osteosynthetic or endoprosthetic treatment. However in most cases with multiple bone metastases the treatment plan is not of curative but rather of palliative character. In selected cases, however, the complete resection of a solitary metastasis may provide a significant increase of survival rate (Fig. 19.11a, b) although the average life expectancy is usually not determined by the treatment of bone metastases but by the nature of the primary tumor. Accordingly, the morbidity of the procedure and the prognosis of the underlying disease must always be taken into account. An exact estimation of life expectancy is essential. Miscalculation can lead to the problem that the selected operation method does not fulfill the increased survival regarding function and constancy. In general the presence of a solitary

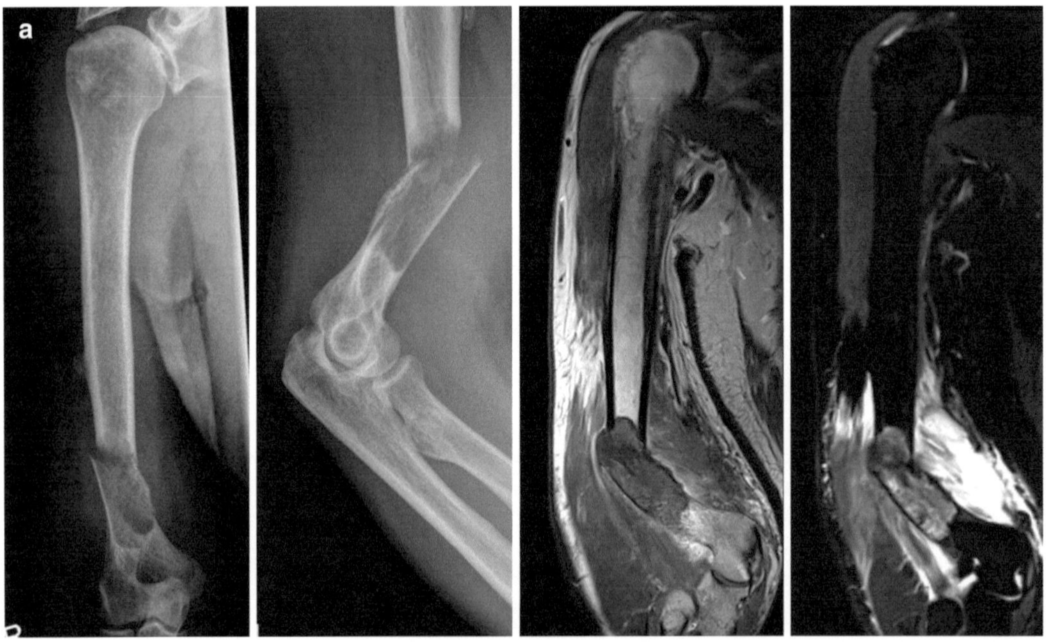

Fig. 19.11 (**a**) Plain radiography and MRI of a pathological distal humerus fracture in a 69-year old female patient without known tumor anamnesis. (**b**) Open biopsy and mounting of a external fixateur (*left picture*). After histopathological verification of the diagnosis, definite surgery consisting of wide tumor resection of a solitary metastasis of a renal cell cancer and reconstruction with a modular elbow prosthesis was carried out (*right picture*)

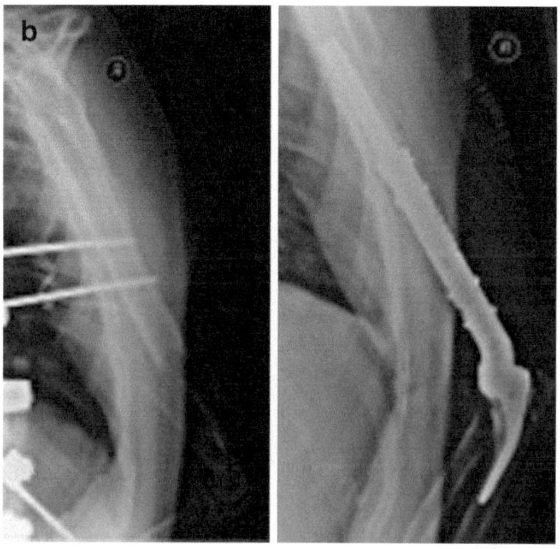

Fig. 19.11 (continued)

metastasis and the occurrence of bone metastases more than 3 years after the initial diagnosis of the primary tumour are considered as favorable prognosis [2]. Surgical treatment needs to be adapted accordingly. In these cases, not only a stabilization, but a tumor resection and, if necessary, reconstructive procedures should be performed. The reconstruction of epi-metaphyseal defects is performed by endoprosthetic joint replacement, diaphyseal defects by spacers, i.e. modular diaphyseal implant bridges.

Surgical Treatment

The treatment of pathological fractures of the humerus depends essentially on the dignity of the lesion and the prognosis of the underlying disease. Due to the numerous factors which have to be considered to come up with an individual treatment plan a general treatment recommendation is not possible, whereas the therapy spectrum ranges from conservative therapy with immobilization to amputation of the affected limb. The pathological fracture of the humerus represents an absolute indication for surgery. The only exception is in case such a fracture occurs in patients suffering from preterminal cancer who would not survive surgery or the remaining life expectancy accounts for only a few weeks. Here is a non-operative treatment indicated consisting of adequate sedation, analgesia and additional radiotherapy. The specific treatment of pathological fractures of the humerus on the basis of benign and malignant primary bone lesions has already been discussed. With the exception of a few, on imaging clearly identified benign lesion such as juvenile bone cyst, biopsy for histological verification of the lesion is primarily performed and followed by designated surgical treatment. Surgical treatment of bone metastases is in many cases subject to personal preferences of the surgeon or the philosophy of the treating hospital and department. An hieratic, or even to one singular surgical technique limited treatment strategy will not cope with the individual needs of each patient. Pathologic proximal humeral fractures based on metastasis require usually a treatment with an endoprosthesis because the bone quality is mostly reduced due to osteoporosis [2] (Fig. 19.12). Osteosynthetic attempts of reconstruction after intralesional resection of the metastasis are often associated with complications, especially if surgery should be followed by adjuvant therapy such as radiation or chemo therapy. Epiphyseal lesions should therefore be supplied with a cemented long-stem hemiarthroplasty, metaphyseal fractures with a modular tumor prosthesis. From the oncological point of view, a reattachment of the original insertion of the muscles of the rotator cuff especially should be performed. As luxation prophylaxis in case a modular mega prosthesis has been implanted, the use of a Trevira binding-tube is recommended [54], which is inserted between the glenoid and prosthesis. Meta-diaphyseal and diaphyseal pathologic fractures are usually treated with osteosynthesis. In patients in very poor general conditions, in addition with a poor prognosis, additionally increased risk for anesthesia and bone lesions with known adequate response to radiotherapy primary stabilization using an intramedullary nail without tumor resection is performed [2]. Benefits are, in comparison to open procedures, that the surgical procedure is shorter and less invasive, an immediate exercise stability is reached and the possibility

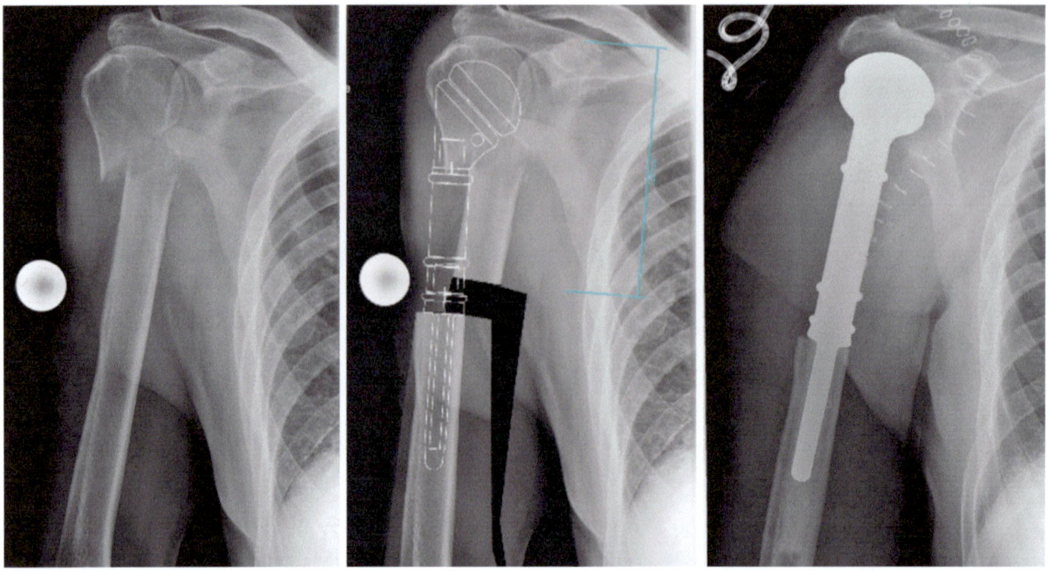

Fig. 19.12 Dislocated pathological humerus fracture based on a metastasis of an intermediate differentiated hepato-cellular carcinoma with multiple metastases in a 78-year old male patient (*left picture*). Preoperative planning (*middle*) and postop x-rays after marginal tumor resection and endoprosthetic reconstruction using a proximal humerus replacement (Implantcast, MUTARS)

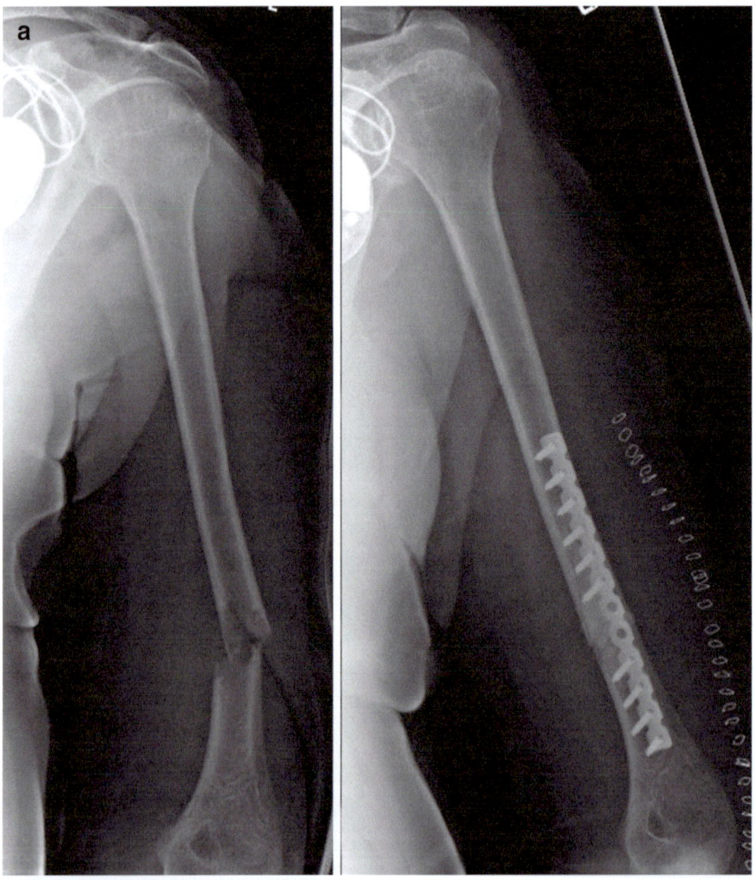

Fig. 19.13 (**a**) Multiple myeloma/plasmocytoma with pathological humerus fracture in a 84-year old male patient (*left picture*) and surgical therapy with compound ostesynthesis (*right picture*). (**b**) Implant failure of a 3.5 mm LCS plate

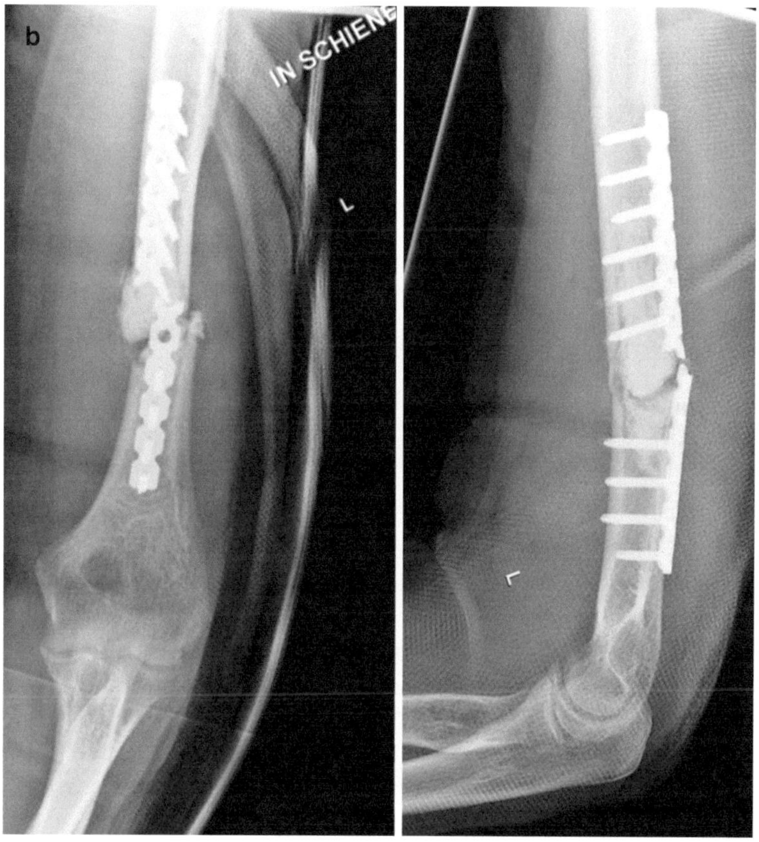

Fig. 19.13 (continued)

of early radiation therapy is given. Disadvantages are that there is no possibility of intralesional curettage and intraoperative application of chemical or thermal adjuvants as well as the dissemination of tumor material in the distal previously tumor free areas of the affected bone. A good prognosis requires a more sustainable operative care if adjuvant therapy is not performed or known to be ineffective. This sustainable operative care is usually done by an open, intralesional resection of metastases and the subsequently performed composite osteosynthesis. In this case the medullary canal is filled with bone cement across the osteolytic defect where also the fracture will be stabilized by one or two locking plates with regarding axis and rotation correct position (Fig. 19.13). Anderson et al. have shown that the two-plate technique is clearly superior to an intramedullary force carrier regarding torsional and flexing strength [67.2]. Adjuvant therapy possibly reducing the risk of local tumor recurrence or tumor progress include rinsing the already cleaned bone cavity with phenol, 95 % ethanol or H2O2 (chemical adjuvants) or cryotherapy with liquid nitrogen or electrocautery and PMMA plombage (thermal adjuvants) [55]. In a composite osteosynthesis using intramedullary nailing and bone cement without open reduction and tumor curettage it is recommended to use a pneumatic tourniquet at the level of the bone lesion to counteract an involuntary leakage of cement. With purely diaphyseal lesions in patients with good prognosis nowadays modular diaphyseal implants are available, which come from the development of modular mega prosthesis for reconstruction after resection of extended defect situations of aggressive bone tumors. These are anchored by cementable diaphyseal shafts while the point of the bony defect can be bridged by individual modules of different length. The use of bone cement for the fixation of the prosthetic stems is obligatory (Fig. 19.14) performing planned radiotherapy.

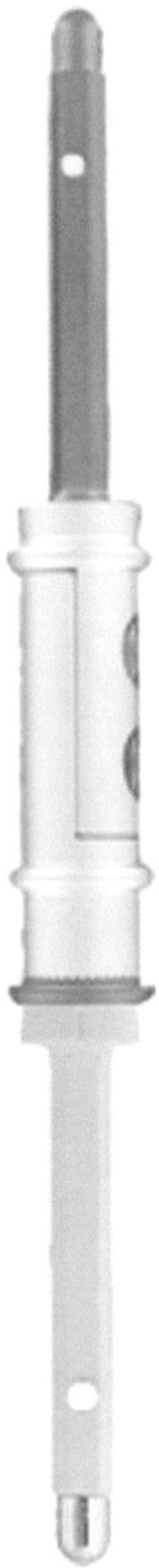

Fig. 19.14 Cemented modular diaphyseal tumor spacer prosthesis (Implantcast, MUTARS)

Conclusion

The humerus is one of the most common locations of pathological fractures. If osteoporotic and/or insufficiency fractures are excluded, most pathological fractures of the humerus occur due to bone metastases or similar aggressive neoplasia such as multiple myeloma. The remaining causes for pathological fractures are less common and significant, but are of multivarious character and require a profound background knowledge on the different therapeutic approaches regarding diagnostics and treatment of the relevant differential diagnoses. The biopsy remains the most important tool despite of modern diagnostic imaging to classify unclear bone lesions regarding dignity and entity clearly and to perform an adequate therapy. In general, an interdisciplinary therapeutic approach for the successful treatment of primary and secondary neoplasms of the bone is crucial.

References

1. Zeifang F, Sabo D, Ewerbeck V. Pathological fracture in primary malignant bone tumors. Chirurg. 2000;71(9):1121–5.
2. Capanna R, Campanacci DA. The treatment of metastases in the appendicular skeleton. J Bone Joint Surg Br. 2001;83(4):471–81.
3. Mutschler W, Wirbel R. Pathologische Frakturen. Unfallchirurg. 1997;100(6):410–29.
4. Maurer F, Ambacher T, Volkmann R, Weller S. Pathologic fractures: diagnostic and therapeutic considerations and results of treatment. Langenbecks Arch Chir. 1995;380(4):207–17.
5. Dietz P. Praxis der Kinder- und Jugentraumatologie. Berlin/Heidelberg: Springer; 2011.
6. Freyschmidt J. Pathological fractures from a pathological point of view. Trauma Berufskrankh. 2008;10 Suppl 2:165–6.
7. Krestan CR, Nemec U, Nemec S. Imaging of insufficiency fractures. Semin Musculoskelet Radiol. 2011;15(3):198–207. doi:10.1055/s-0031-1278420.
8. Kramer W, Gaebel G, Stuhldreyer G, Heitland W. Results of the treatment of pathologic fractures of long tubular bones. Unfallchirurgie. 1987;13(1):22–6.
9. Hardes J, Schultheiss M, Gosheger G, Schulte M. The juvenile bone cyst: treatment with continuous decompression using cannulated screws. Orthopade. 2009;38(3):256–62. doi:10.1007/s00132-009-1407-9.
10. Fuchs B, Valenzuela RG, Sim FH. Pathologic fracture as a complication in the treatment of Ewing's sarcoma. Clin Orthop Relat Res. 2003;415:25–30. doi:10.1097/01.blo.0000093893.12372.9d.
11. Jaffe N, Spears R, Eftekhari F, Robertson R, Cangir A, Takaue Y, Carrasco H, Wallace S, Ayala A, Raymond K, et al. Pathologic fracture in osteosarcoma. Impact of chemotherapy on primary tumor and survival. Cancer. 1987;59(4):701–9.
12. Natarajan MV, Govardhan RH, Williams S, Raja Gopal TS. Limb salvage surgery for pathological fractures in osteosarcoma. Int Orthop. 2000;24(3):170–2.
13. Lodwick G, Wilson A, Farrell C, Virtama P, Dittrich F. Determining growth rates of focal lesions of bone from radiographs. Radiology. 1980;134(3):577–83.
14. Freyschmidt J. Die pathologische Fraktur aus Sicht des Radiologen. Trauma Berufskrankh. 2008;10: 165–6.
15. Rechl H, Kirchhoff C, Wortler K, Lenze U, Toepfer A, von Eisenhart-Rothe R. Diagnosis of malignant

bone and soft tissue tumors. Orthopade. 2011;40(10):931–41. doi:10.1007/s00132-011-1821-7; quiz 933–42.
16. von Eisenhart-Rothe R, Toepfer A, Salzmann M, Schauwecker J, Gollwitzer H, Rechl H. Primary malignant bone tumors. Orthopade. 2011;40(12): 1121–42. doi:10.1007/s00132-011-1866-7.
17. Enneking WF. A system of staging musculoskeletal neoplasms. Clin Orthop Relat Res. 1986;204:9–24.
18. Grimer R. WHO classification of tumours of soft tissue and bone, vol. 5. 4th ed. Geneva: WHO Press; 2013.
19. Fletcher C, Unni K, Mertens F. World health organization classification of tumours: pathology and genetics of tumours of soft tissue and bone. Malignant fibrous histiocytoma of bone. Lyon: IARC Press; 2002.
20. Campanacci M, Baldini N, Boriani S, Sudanese A. Giant-cell tumor of bone. J Bone Joint Surg Am. 1987;69(1):106–14.
21. Gaston CL, Bhumbra R, Watanuki M, Abudu AT, Carter SR, Jeys LM, Tillman RM, Grimer RJ. Does the addition of cement improve the rate of local recurrence after curettage of giant cell tumours in bone? J Bone Joint Surg Br. 2011;93(12):1665–9. doi:10.1302/0301-620X.93B12.27663.
22. Branstetter DG, Nelson SD, Manivel JC, Blay JY, Chawla S, Thomas DM, Jun S, Jacobs I. Denosumab induces tumor reduction and bone formation in patients with giant-cell tumor of bone. Clin Cancer Res. 2012;18(16):4415–24. doi:10.1158/1078-0432.CCR-12-0578.
23. Chakarun CJ, Forrester DM, Gottsegen CJ, Patel DB, White EA, Matcuk Jr GR. Giant cell tumor of bone: review, mimics, and new developments in treatment. Radiographics. 2013;33(1):197–211. doi:10.1148/rg.331125089.
24. Thomas DM. RANKL, denosumab, and giant cell tumor of bone. Curr Opin Oncol. 2012;24(4):397–403. doi:10.1097/CCO.0b013e328354c129.
25. Freyschmidt JO, Ostertag H, Jundt G. Knochenutmoren mit Kiefertumoren: Klinik-Radiologie-Pathologie. Berlin/Heidelberg: Springer; 2010.
26. Hou HY, Wu K, Wang CT, Chang SM, Lin WH, Yang RS. Treatment of unicameral bone cyst: surgical technique. J Bone Joint Surg Am. 2011;93 Suppl 1:92–9. doi:10.2106/JBJS.J.01123.
27. Cho HS, Oh JH, Kim HS, Kang HG, Lee SH. Unicameral bone cysts: a comparison of injection of steroid and grafting with autologous bone marrow. J Bone Joint Surg Br. 2007;89(2):222–6. doi:10.1302/0301-620X.89B2.18116.
28. Donaldson S, Chundamala J, Yandow S, Wright JG. Treatment for unicameral bone cysts in long bones: an evidence based review. Orthop Rev (Pavia). 2010;2(1), e13. doi:10.4081/or.2010.e13.
29. Bramer JA, Abudu AA, Grimer RJ, Carter SR, Tillman RM. Do pathological fractures influence survival and local recurrence rate in bony sarcomas? Eur J Cancer. 2007;43(13):1944–51. doi:10.1016/j.ejca.2007.07.004.
30. Ruggieri P, Mavrogenis AF, Casadei R, Errani C, Angelini A, Calabro T, Pala E, Mercuri M. Protocol of surgical treatment of long bone pathological fractures. Injury. 2010;41(11):1161–7. doi:10.1016/j.injury.2010.09.018.
31. Cho WH, Song WS, Jeon DG, Kong CB, Kim MS, Lee JA, Yoo JY, Kim JD, Lee SY. Differential presentations, clinical courses, and survivals of osteosarcomas of the proximal humerus over other extremity locations. Ann Surg Oncol. 2010;17(3):702–8. doi:10.1245/s10434-009-0825-6.
32. Ebeid W, Amin S, Abdelmegid A. Limb salvage management of pathologic fractures of primary malignant bone tumors. Cancer Control. 2005;12(1):57–61.
33. Bramer JA, van Linge JH, Grimer RJ, Scholten RJ. Prognostic factors in localized extremity osteosarcoma: a systematic review. Eur J Surg Oncol. 2009;35(10):1030–6. doi:10.1016/j.ejso.2009.01.011.
34. Pakos EE, Nearchou AD, Grimer RJ, Koumoullis HD, Abudu A, Bramer JA, Jeys LM, Franchi A, Scoccianti G, Campanacci D, Capanna R, Aparicio J, Tabone MD, Holzer G, Abdolvahab F, Funovics P, Dominkus M, Ilhan I, Berrak SG, Patino-Garcia A, Sierrasesumaga L, San-Julian M, Garraus M, Petrilli AS, Filho RJ, Macedo CR, Alves MT, Seiwerth S, Nagarajan R, Cripe TP, Ioannidis JP. Prognostic factors and outcomes for osteosarcoma: an international collaboration. Eur J Cancer. 2009;45(13):2367–75. doi:10.1016/j.ejca.2009.03.005.
35. Bielack SS, Kempf-Bielack B, Delling G, Exner GU, Flege S, Helmke K, Kotz R, Salzer-Kuntschik M, Werner M, Winkelmann W, Zoubek A, Jurgens H, Winkler K. Prognostic factors in high-grade osteosarcoma of the extremities or trunk: an analysis of 1,702 patients treated on neoadjuvant cooperative osteosarcoma study group protocols. J Clin Oncol. 2002;20(3):776–90.
36. Wunder JS, Paulian G, Huvos AG, Heller G, Meyers PA, Healey JH. The histological response to chemotherapy as a predictor of the oncological outcome of operative treatment of Ewing sarcoma. J Bone Joint Surg Am. 1998;80(7):1020–33.
37. Puri A, Shah M, Agarwal MG, Jambhekar NA, Basappa P. Chondrosarcoma of bone: does the size of the tumor, the presence of a pathologic fracture, or prior intervention have an impact on local control and survival? J Cancer Res Ther. 2009;5(1):14–9.
38. Donati D, Colangeli S, Colangeli M, Di Bella C, Bertoni F. Surgical treatment of grade I central chondrosarcoma. Clin Orthop Relat Res. 2010;468(2):581–9. doi:10.1007/s11999-009-1056-7.
39. Parlier-Cuau C, Bousson V, Ogilvie CM, Lackman RD, Laredo JD. When should we biopsy a solitary central cartilaginous tumor of long bones? Literature review and management proposal. Eur J Radiol. 2011;77(1):6–12. doi:10.1016/j.ejrad.2010.06.051.
40. Kendell SD, Collins MS, Adkins MC, Sundaram M, Unni KK. Radiographic differentiation of enchondroma from low-grade chondrosarcoma in the fibula. Skeletal Radiol. 2004;33(8):458–66. doi:10.1007/s00256-004-0791-9.

41. Geirnaerdt MJ, Hermans J, Bloem JL, Kroon HM, Pope TL, Taminiau AH, Hogendoorn PC. Usefulness of radiography in differentiating enchondroma from central grade 1 chondrosarcoma. AJR Am J Roentgenol. 1997;169(4):1097–104. doi:10.2214/ajr.169.4.9308471.
42. Murphey MD, Flemming DJ, Boyea SR, Bojescul JA, Sweet DE, Temple HT. Enchondroma versus chondrosarcoma in the appendicular skeleton: differentiating features. Radiographics. 1998;18(5):1213–37; quiz 1215–44.
43. Hoffman R, Benz EJ, Furie B, Shattil SJ. Hematology: basic principles and practice. Philadelphia: Churchill Livingstone/Elsevier; 2009.
44. Pingali SR, Haddad RY, Saad A. Current concepts of clinical management of multiple myeloma. Dis Mon. 2012;58(4):195–207. doi:10.1016/j.disamonth.2012.01.006.
45. Greenspan A. Skelettradiologie: Orthop√§die, Traumatologie, Rheumatologie, Onkologie. München/Jena: Elsevier/Urban & Fischer; 2007.
46. Bohm P, Huber J. The surgical treatment of bony metastases of the spine and limbs. J Bone Joint Surg. 2002;84(4):521–9.
47. Kivioja AH, Karaharju EO, Elomaa I, Bohling TO. Surgical treatment of myeloma of bone. Eur J Cancer. 1992;28A(11):1865–9.
48. Katzer A, Meenen NM, Grabbe F, Rueger JM. Surgery of skeletal metastases. Arch Orthop Trauma Surg. 2002;122(5):251–8. doi:10.1007/s00402-001-0359-2.
49. Abrams HL. Skeletal metastases in carcinoma. Radiology. 1950;55(4):534–8.
50. Braun S. Operative Therapie und Prognose bei Patienten mit skelettären Karzinommetastasen. München: Ludwig-Maximilians-Universität München; 2004.
51. Layer G. Skelettmetastasen. In: Stäbler AF, Freyschmidt J, editors. Handbuch diagnostische Radiologie, Muskuloskelettales System 2. Berlin: Springer; 2005. p. 329.
52. Piccioli A, Maccauro G, Rossi B, Scaramuzzo L, Frenos F, Capanna R. Surgical treatment of pathologic fractures of humerus. Injury. 2010;41(11):1112–6. doi:10.1016/j.injury.2010.08.015.
53. Hardes JG, Gosheger G. The pathologic fracture from the viewpoint of the orthopaedic specialist and trauma surgeon. Trauma Berufskrankh. 2008;10 Suppl 2:167–74.
54. Gosheger G, Hillmann A, Lindner N, Rodl R, Hoffmann C, Burger H, Winkelmann W. Soft tissue reconstruction of megaprostheses using a trevira tube. Clin Orthop Relat Res. 2001;393:264–71.
55. Gollwitzer H, Toepfer A, Gerdesmeyer L, Gradinger R. Tumors and tumor-like lesions of the foot and ankle: diagnosis and treatment. In: Saxena A, editor. Special procedures in foot and ankle surgery. New York: Springer; 2013. doi:10.1007/978-1-4471-4103-7.

Further Reading

Schulz T, Prietzel T, Kluge R, Schneider JP, Tannapfel A, Kahn T. Efficient diagnosis of pathological fractures. Rontgenpraxis. 2006;56(3):75–92.

Goudarzi YM, Sautmann F. Pathological fractures in childhood and adolescence in benign and semi-malignant bone tumors and tumorous and inflammatory bone changes. Aktuelle Traumatol. 1987;17(2):73–9.

Jacofsky DJ, Haidukewych GJ. Management of pathologic fractures of the proximal femur: state of the art. J Orthop Trauma. 2004;18(7):459–69.

Mirels H. Metastatic disease in long bones. A proposed scoring system for diagnosing impending pathologic fractures. Clinical Orthop Relat Res. (249):256–64.

Franzius C, Daldrup-Link HE, Sciuk J, Rummeny EJ, Bielack S, Jurgens H, Schober O. FDG-PET for detection of pulmonary metastases from malignant primary bone tumors: comparison with spiral CT. Ann Oncol. 2001;12(4):479–86.

Franzius C, Sciuk J, Daldrup-Link HE, Jurgens H, Schober O. FDG-PET for detection of osseous metastases from malignant primary bone tumours: comparison with bone scintigraphy. Eur J Nucl Med. 2000;27(9):1305–11.

Yanagawa T, Shinozaki T, Iizuka Y, Takagishi K, Watanabe H. Role of 2-deoxy-2-[F-18] fluoro-D-glucose positron emission tomography in the management of bone and soft-tissue metastases. J Bone Joint Surg Br. 2010;92(3):419–23. doi:10.1302/0301-620x.92b3.23131.

Campanacci M. Bone and soft tissue tumors: clinical features, imaging, pathology and treatment. 2nd ed. Wien: Springer; 1999.

Campanacci DA, Scoccianti G, Franchi A, Roselli G, Beltrami G, Ippolito M, Caff G, Frenos F, Capanna R. Surgical treatment of central grade 1 chondrosarcoma of the appendicular skeleton. J Orthop Traumatol. 2013;14(2):101–7. doi:10.1007/s10195-013-0230-6.

Evans HL, Ayala AG, Romsdahl MM. Prognostic factors in chondrosarcoma of bone: a clinicopathologic analysis with emphasis on histologic grading. Cancer. 1977;40(2):818–31.

Lee FY, Mankin HJ, Fondren G, Gebhardt MC, Springfield DS, Rosenberg AE, Jennings LC. Chondrosarcoma of bone: an assessment of outcome. J Bone Joint Surg Am. 1999;81(3):326–38.

Harousseau JL. Ten years of improvement in the management of multiple myeloma: 2000-2010. Clin Lymphoma Myeloma Leuk. 2010;10(6):424–42. doi:10.3816/CLML.2010.n.076.

Anderson JT, Erickson JM, Thompson Jr RC, Chao EY. Pathologic femoral shaft fractures comparing fixation techniques using cement. Clin Orthop Relat Res. 1978;131:273–8.

Physical Therapy and Rehabilitation 20

Marcus Schmitt-Sody

Physiotherapy After Surgical Treatment of Proximal Humerus Fractures

Functionality of the Shoulder Joint

The aim of rehabilitation after humerus fractures is the restoration of muscle power and the functionality of the joint. The shoulder joint is the most flexible joint in the human body. The articulation surface is incongruent and is composed of the glenohumeral joint and the subacromial space. Because of these circumstances, the shoulder joint is not as stable as other joints. In everyday life, it is mostly affected by tensile loading. Stabilization of the joint is primarily facilitated by musculature and the capsule-ligament apparatus. The most important ligaments are the glenohumeral ligament and the coracohumeral ligament, the so-called cruciate ligaments of the shoulder joint.

In the neutral position of the arm, two muscle groups work together: the stabilizators and the muscles which cranialize the humerus head.

The following muscles belong to the first group:

- Supra- and infraspinatus
- Teres minor and major
- Subscapularis
- Latissimus dorsi
- Biceps brachii (caput longum)

The following muscles belong to the second, cranializing and dynamic group:

- Deltoideus
- Pectoralis
- Triceps caput longum
- Coracobrachialis
- Biceps caput breve

As the upper arm is not fixed to the trunk, but to the scapula, and is located in some kind of a suspension, a frictionless motion sequence is facilitated not only by the muscular stabilization, but above all by the location of the scapula and the scapulothoracic plain bearing. Therefore, the setting and stability of the scapula are decisive for the correct motion sequence of the shoulder joint.

The scapula is mainly stabilized and actuated by the Serratus anterior muscle (external rotation) together with the Rhomboideus muscle and the Levator scapulae muscle (internal rotation). If the Serratus anterior is overbalanced, the scapula is rotated internally and clings to the Levator scapulae muscles and the Trapezius pars descendens muscle, which can cause afflictions of the cervical spine.

M. Schmitt-Sody
Orthopaedic Department, Medical Park Chiemsee, Bavaria, Germany
e-mail: M.Schmitt-Sody@medicalpark.de

P. Biberthaler et al. (eds.), *Fractures of the Proximal Humerus*, Strategies in Fracture Treatments,
DOI 10.1007/978-3-319-20300-3_20

The humerus head has the physiologic tendency to decenter. In most cases, this is caused by a muscular disequilibrium and a misaligned scapula towards cranial and ventral.

A movement of the arm in the shoulder joint is possible in all three planes and axes. The normal range of motion is: anteversion/retroversion 90/0/50; abduction/adduction 90/0/45; external rotation/internal rotation 40–60/0/95. Elevation up to 170° (in case of anteversion) or 180° (in case of abduction) only works when the shoulder girdle is involved and the spine is stretched.

Recording of Findings and Documentation

Inspection

Before starting physical therapy in an in- or outpatient department, the current (postoperative) findings have to be recorded and documented. Therefore, it is necessary that recent X-ray images are available for assessment.

For a rapid assessment of the shoulder joint, shoulder stand (hanging, pulled upwards, asymmetry), contours of the joint and changes of clavicle and sternoclavicular acromioclavicular joint have to be inspected first. Also, muscle atrophies and position of the scapula have to be taken into account.

The inspection of the surgical wound for a regular healing process is obligatory. Care must be taken of edema and soft tissue swelling, warmth or local signs of inflammation. In case of critical findings, photographic documentation is recommended as a follow-up. The perifocal and peripheral circulatory conditions should also be examined. Type and location of pain have to be inquired from the patients.

Assessment of the Range of Motion

Neutral Zero Method

For objective comparison purposes, the current range of motion has to be measured by the neutral zero method as far as the actual condition allows it.

The normal or neutral position is the position taken by the joints during upright stance with the arms hanging down and keeping the feet together. The ranges of motion are determined from this normal position as the zero point, starting in both directions and recorded one by one. The value for flexion is usually listed first, followed by the neutral position denoted as zero, and finally the range of motion for extension is noted. See Chap. 1 for the normal values of motion in the shoulder joint. A complete restoration of range of motion is often not achieved after surgical treatment of humeral fractures.

Palpation

The main palpable findings at the shoulder joint are:

- Stability in the SC joint: examination of the relocatability of the clavicle
- Checking the AC joint: in adduction of the arm with flexed elbow
- Palpate joint space: in elevation and extension
- Palpate long biceps tendon: between the tuberculum majus and minus
- Palpate infraspinatus insertion: at the tuberculum majus
- Palpate supraspinatus tendon: in extension of the arm below the acromion
- Palpate subscapularis tendon: with external rotation at tuberculum minor

Assessment of Instabilities

In the acute postoperative stage, no clinical assessment for instability can be performed. After the consolidation of fractures or healing of ligament reconstructions, capsule stability tests can be performed. Usually, a distinction is made in unidirectional or multidirectional instability.

Muscle Function Test

Assessment of Muscle Strength

Muscle strength grades are assessed according to Vladimir Janda and divided into five stages. Full strength corresponds to 5/5. Here, further

Table 20.1 Muscle function grades according to Vladimir Janda

Level 5: N	Normal	100 %	Full, normal muscle strength
Level 4: G	Good	Approx. 75 %	Medium resistance can be overcome in full range of motion
Level 3: F	Fair	Approx. 50 %	Movement against gravity can be performed in full range of motion
Level 2: P	Poor	Approx. 25 %	Full range of motion possible with exclusion of gravity
Level 1: T	Trace	Approx. 10 %	Trace of tension in the muscle
Level 0: Z	Zero	0 %	No muscle contraction possible
Addition	S		Spasticity
Addition	K		Contracture

distinctions such as fatigability of a muscle are not detected. This assessment is also helpful for communicating with the physiotherapist for the description of existing or permitted load capacity and objectification of improvements in the findings of patients. Partial pareses, which are imposed during the neurological examination are furthermore quantified (Table 20.1).

Functional Testing

For the function of each muscle see Table 20.2:

Anteversion is also denoted flexion, while retroversion can also be called extension. The resistance test is usually done in sitting position. Immediately after surgery, it should be avoided. Isometric strength tests are to be omitted after surgery. In addition to the shoulder joint, flexion and extension and pronation and supination in the elbow joint should always be tested.

To assess the shoulder joint function and document the subjective history of patients, questionnaires can be used:

- Constant score: Summarizes subjective (35 %) and objective (65 %) parameters to a total of 100 points; it covers e.g. pain, strength, agility and everyday functionality; it is recommended by the SECEC (European Society of Shoulder and Elbow Surgery) as well as the DVSE (German Society of Shoulder and Elbow Surgery) as a standard tool for the assessment of shoulder function
- Oxford Score: Captures the results of shoulder surgery and the influence of shoulder injuries on daily activities and quality of living in 12 points
- DASH (Disabilities of Arm, Shoulder and Hand): A subjective score, which measures the ability to carry out everyday activities; the way in which these activities are carried out is not recorded.
- SPADI (Shoulder Pain and Disability Index): Subjective score, pain and impairment in activities of daily living are recorded

Table 20.2 Characteristic muscles and their functions at the shoulder joint

Muscle	Function
M. supraspinatus	Initiates abduction
M. infraspinatus	External rotation, adduction
M. subscapularis	Internal rotation, adduction
M. deltoideus	Abduction from about 30°
M. teres minor	External rotation, adduction
M. biceps	Caput longum: abduction
	Caput breve: adduction
M. pectoralis major	Adduction
M. coracobrachialis	Adduction, internal rotation, anteversion
M. trapezius pars deszendens and aszendens	Elevation beyond horizontal
M. serratus anterior	Connects shoulder joint and trunk; pulls the scapula in ventral direction and allows rotation
M. latissimus dorsi	Adduction

Neurological Status

A complete examination includes the orientational neurological status of the relevant nerves in the shoulder joint. Indications of motor deficits are already obtained in parallel to the muscle function test. Basically, the innervation is realized via the brachial plexus (segment C4–C6). An overview of the innervation of each muscle is provided in Table 20.3.

Table 20.3 Shoulder muscles and their innervation

Muscle	Innervation
M. supraspinatus	N. suprascapularis
M. infraspinatus	N. suprascapularis
M. subscapularis	Nn. subscapulares (from the fasciculus post. of the Plexus brachialis)
M. deltoideus	N. axillaris
M. teres minor	N. axillaris
M. biceps (caput longum and caput breve)	N. musculocutaneus
M. pectoralis major	N. pectoralis (from N. suprascapularis)
M. coracobrachialis	N. musculocutaneus
M. trapezius pars deszendens and aszendens	N. accessorius and branches of the cervical plexus
M. serratus anterior	N. thoracicus longus
M. latissimus dorsi	N. thoracodorsalis

Due to its location close to the humerus, the radial nerve is often affected in addition to the mentioned muscles in fractures or storage damages. Nerves that are also frequently lesioned are: the axillary nerve, the musculocutaneous nerve and the median nerve.

Radial Nerve

If there is a lesion of the radial nerve in the front third region of the proximal humerus, there will be a paralysis of the triceps (not in case of a lesion at the level of the mid upper arm!), brachialis and all wrist extensors. An extension of the elbow joint is no longer possible, as well as there is a weakness in flexion of the elbow in the middle position. The symptom of the typical "drop hand" occurs, as the active extension of the hand is paralyzed. In addition, no active abduction of the thumb is possible due to the failure of the M. abductor pollicis. The hand is pronated.

Axillary Nerve

The axillary nerve contains fibers from the spinal cord segments C5 and C6. It runs very close to the humerus in the quadrangular space. A lesion of the axillary nerve occurs very frequently in shoulder dislocations, but also in humerus fractures. As a result of a lesion, a functional failure of the deltoid and teres minor will occur, so that the arm can not be lifted up to the horizontal plane. In case of hypo- or atrophy of the deltoid muscle, the symptom of "acute shoulder" will result.

Sensory disturbances will occur at the outside of the proximal shoulder joint.

Musculocutaneous Nerve

The n. musculocutaneus provides motoric innervation to the coracobrachialis, the biceps and the brachialis. In case of lesions, atrophies of the anterior upper arm muscles occur accordingly. This leads to loss of function of flexion and supination of the forearm, which can be compensated by other muscle groups. The failures of the coracobrachialis can also be compensated in case of an isolated lesion. Nevertheless, a misalignment of the humerus head occurs in any type of lesion.

Median Nerve

In case of irritations of the median nerve, the known "monkey hand" occurs when the patient is asked to close his hand to a fist. Fingers I–III remain stretched, while only fingers IV and V can be bent as they are supplied by the ulnar nerve. As the M. opponens pollicis malfunctions, only an incomplete closure of the fist is possible. Typically, a bottle cannot be held anymore. This condition is termed as "positive bottle sign". Sensory disturbances occur in case of median nerve lesions of the thumb, forefinger and middle finger and partially on the ring finger.

Therapeutic Regimens Overview

A surgeon acting responsibly should also set the guidelines for the treatment, because he knows the intraoperative findings best. Here, he has to predetermine the actually permitted ranges of motion and define details for the load in each case, as well as to define the further increase over time in a regular healing process. The earliest possible mobilization under sufficient analgesia and the degrees of movement and exercise levels set by the surgeon are important in any case. The partially necessary immobilization of 3–4 weeks is already leading to contractures in the capsular-ligament system, whereby the subsequent mobilization is considerably more difficult and delayed. The availability of studies regarding the optimum time interval of immobilization is not satisfactory [1].

General Therapeutic Measures

Positioning and Splint Supply

Postoperative positioning should preferably be comfortable and painless for the patient, as far as possible under the permitted ranges of motion.

The shoulder joint should be stored in a slight internal rotation and abduction. A functionally correct positioning of the elbow joint is flexion of 90–100° and a slight pronation. Pillows, wedge pillows, blankets, foam, roll pillows, sand bags and splints can be used to position the patients.

Congenital or acquired functional limitations must be considered. With the patient lying in an acute stage, slight elevation above heart level is recommended to favor the decongestion. Possible nerve pressure points and exposed wound or scar areas must be padded well.

Depending on the type of surgery and intraoperative situation, the surgeon prescribes 3–6 weeks of immobilization of the shoulder joint. The existing auxiliary devices for this are:

- Desault dressing: maximum immobilization, therefore used for no longer than 2–3 weeks; shoulder joint in neutral position and maximum internal rotation, elbow in 90° flexion
- Gilchrist dressing: zero position and maximum internal rotation of the shoulder joint, elbow joint in 90° flexion; the hand can and may be moved and used; in case of stable osteosyntheses only necessary for a few days (Fig. 20.1a)
- Abduction pillow: relieves capsular ligaments by 40–60° – abduction position and internally rotated arm; elbow joint in 90° flexion; applied postoperatively usually for 4–6 weeks, especially in case of prosthetic treatment (Fig. 20.1b)
- Arm sling/Bronner sling: sometimes used as a transition to relief at the stage of active training or exercise-stable osteosyntheses; rotation of the shoulder joint possible

a b

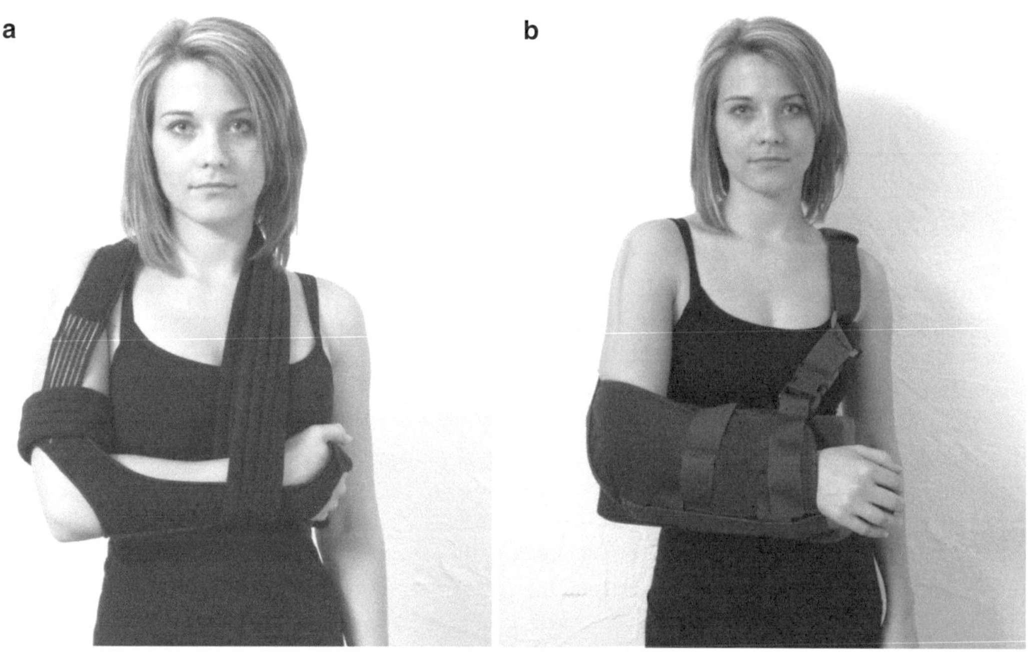

Fig. 20.1 Examples of shoulder ortheses (**a**) gilchrist, (**b**) abduction pillow

Analgesia

Modern pain management should be sufficient to counteract peri- and postoperative chronic pain and to allow early mobilization. Through a proactive basic analgesia, better pain relief is achieved at a lower total dose. Centrally, regionally and locally acting analgesics are used. Centrally acting opioids are mainly applied intraoperatively and in the early postoperative phase. The patients have to be monitored sufficiently (respiratory depression). In outpatient surgery, usually no centrally acting substances are used.

In case of very painful procedures (e.g. arthrolysis), the installation of a pain catheter in the supraclavicular plexus or patient-controlled analgesia (PCA) is useful with computer-controlled, need-based administration of opioids. Only in this way, an adequate analgesia for earliest possible mobilization can be achieved. It is important to check the involved nerves for their regular functioning before installing the catheter.

The use of nonsteroidal anti-inflammatory drugs (NSAIDs) is well-established in the further course of treatment because of the additional decongestant and anti-inflammatory compounds of these substances in the first 10–14 postoperative days. Additionally, Novaminsulfon or Tramal can be administered. In principle, treatment is conducted according to the WHO staging system. If pain is occurring during rehabilitation treatment with intensive exercising, a local steroid infiltration therapy can be successful in addition to a reduction of the intensity.

Cooling Applications

To reduce swelling and hyperthermia, cooling applications in the form of ice, cooling pads, quark compresses or alcohol covers etc. are suitable. In addition, cryotherapy is one of the preparatory and accompanying measures of motor-functional treatment methods. Short-term measures of 5–15 s have a rather superficial effect on the sympathetic nervous system. Heat dissipation is accelerated, the tissue tone decreases, the pain is muted and the motor system is activated. Fast rubbing with ice promotes the disposition of a weakened muscle to contract.

Long-term applications of 10–30 min, act further in depth in the sense of a dampening, depending on the fat layer. The pain relief outlasts the time of application about two to three -times. Cold water covers promote the absorption of edema. Cryotherapy can therefore on the one hand reduce pain, on the other hand stimulate muscles. It should be noted that the pain threshold is increased by the application of ice so that pain as a protective function is partially disabled. Patients sometimes allow too intense exercise and in some cases develop increased pain symptoms only hours after treatment. During the first 2 postoperative weeks, only dry ice packs with textile cover should be used for cooling at the surgical site until removal of the suture.

The cooling system should be rather mild and carried out in an interval principle. The ice-swab technique is also proven. Ice compression bandages should only be applied in exceptional circumstances and under supervision. If cold pain occurs, the patient must have an opportunity to remove the cooling cover immediately, otherwise there is a risk of ice burns. Injuries associated with sensory loss are particularly at risk.

Heat Applications

In the **acute state**, the application of heat in the injured shoulder is absolutely contraindicated because it intensifies the stimulus sensitivity and inflammatory responses and leads to increased edema. Under certain circumstances, even bleeding or rebleeding can be triggered or at least strengthened.

It makes sense, however, to use the heat in some remote regions as relaxing and circulation-enhancing measure, for example, to the strained neck muscles. Typical application forms are the classic mud pack and hay flower sachets and the so-called “hot roll”. In this case, a rolled up hand towel is soaked with boiling water. The towel roll is just as hot as tolerated by the patient (approximately 45 to a maximum of 65 °C) and is repeatedly pressed and unrolled at different points in the treatment area. After cooling, the procedure is repeated. The treatment takes 10–20 min. Advantage over the Fango treatment is the individualized dose of warmth and prevent heat build-up.

In the **chronic stage**, heat is well-suited for the treatment of contractures. Under heat used therapeutically in the range of 40–45 °C, collagen fibers do not completely reverse back to their original length after increasing strain. A partial extension remains even after the stretching stimulus is removed. The treatment is less strength-consuming for the therapist, because the resistance to movement is reduced by the application of heat and the maximum passive movement speed increases.

Massages

Manual Lymphatic Drainage

Manual lymph drainage is a special form of massage. By particularly soft, tissue-sparing techniques, intra- and extravascular tissue fluid is tried to be mobilized and drained to relieve the accumulated body region. Depending on the surgical incision, small lymphatic vessels will be interrupted so that there are perifocal lymphedema. Through the lymph drainage, the own motor function of the wall muscle is stimulated in the transport vessels and promotes the formation of new lymphatic vessels.

The treatment is based on the anatomical course of the lymphatic tracks. In contrast to stroking, it is used for the lymphatic drainage from proximal to distal direction. It starts with a light pressure massage in the armpit area to initially promote the drainage from the local lymph nodes. With different techniques, such as rotating, cupping and transverse techniques according to Dr. Vodder or the edema technique according to Dr. Asdonk is subsequently worked gradually in distal direction. Each technique is repeated six to seven times. Finally, the limb should be wrapped with elastic bandages over a soft cotton padding. If this is not possible due to the injury pattern, the arm at least elevated [2].

Scar Massage

For mobilization of the connective tissue, a so-called scar massage can also be performed after adequate tissue consolidation in the scar area. In contrast to classical massage, the strongest possible tightening of the muscles is aimed at to get the clearest possible distinction between contractile structures and scar tissue during treatment. Techniques which stress the scar on traction are called shifting techniques. In addition, the scar tissue can be mobilized by transverse and lateral distortion as well as lifting of the skin.

In order to achieve a better depth effect, a scar stick can be used. The pressure response and the stroke pattern depend on age, condition and location of the scar. It starts with edging lines in rhombic shape. Then, diagonal lines (5–10 repetitions) are stroked over the scar tissue, and finally the scar and the surrounding tissue must be stroked manually from distal to proximal direction. Strongly touch-sensitive scars can be treated with local anesthetics. Alternatively, a strained nociceptive-vegetative pain blockade can be accomplished by inhibiting the sympathetic nervous system with strokes of the scar stick before starting the treatment [2].

Traditional Massage

In the acute state, traditional massage is not performed directly in the operated area. However, a massage over the entire area of the often muscularly tense shoulder girdle, the cervical and thoracic spine can have a great effect. As a result, a dampening of sympathetic nervous system can be achieved, which leads to a reduction of the entire muscle tone. In addition, segments relevant to the innervation of the arm (C5-Th1) are relieved. Overall, it also achieves improvement in posture through the harmonization of muscle tone and reduces tension pain. Through **stroking**, the venous and lymphatic flow and the removal of metabolic waste products are stimulated. In addition, the muscular defense tension is reduced. By **transverse friction** corresponding to the soft tissue technique according to Cyriax, the deeper tissue layers can be reached. In this method, "friction" for muscle and tendon insertion is applied transversely, for example with small surfaces (thumb, palm, finger pad) pressure is exerted on the tissue in straight, circular or spiral movements. The circulation is stimulated. The elasticity and intrinsic mobility of the tissue is improved, individual muscle fibers or scar strands are dissolved and the healing process is stimulated. In order to solve adhesions of the subcutaneous fat tissue, **kneading** is performed. In this case, the muscle is targeted across the grain, and slightly lifted off the pad and the tissue is stretched maximally by intermittent traction.

Electrotherapy

In electrotherapy, various therapeutic current forms are used to influence disease processes with general and specific effects. The current modes can be selected according to the respective disease. Effects are achieved at the site of electrode placement, but also within the central nervous system, autonomic nervous system and via reflex arcs in internal organs. It is necessary to distinguish between pain relief, regeneration-promoting electrotherapy, and electrical muscle stimulation to improve motor skills.

In the following, some frequently used forms of therapy are explained in more detail (Table 20.4).

TENS

Transcutaneous electrical nerve stimulation, shortly called TENS, is a method of counter-irritation. Electrodes are glued to the skin through which electrical stimuli are set to cover the pain sensation. The electrical stimulus parameters, such as amplitude, pulse duration, frequency, and the proper placement of the electrodes must be developed individually for each patient.

For example, with which electric current can nociceptive forwarding of information be inhibited at the level of the dorsal horn? This is done by the excitation of fast-conducting fibers of the peripheral nerves. TENS also promotes the formation of endorphins which also contribute to pain relief.

Table 20.4 Overview: forms and effects of electrotherapy

Pain relief	
Local:	**Central**:
Diadynamic currents	TENS
Ultra Stimulation according to "Träbert"	High-voltage currents
Galvanization	Diadynamic currents
APL-Tens	Galvanization
Regeneration/Circulation support	
Local:	**Central**:
Diadynamic currents	TENS
Ultra Stimulation according to "Träbert"	High-voltage currents
Galvanization	Diadynamic currents
	Galvanization
Muscle stimulation	
Neofaradic threshold currents	
AMF currents	
Exponential current	
And other types of electricity depending on the frequency range	

Iontophoresis

Iontophoresis is used for the targeted introduction of analgesic and/or anti-inflammatory substances in the depth of the tissue to produce an amplified local effect. There are two electrodes applied, for which the correct positioning of the electrodes is essential for the production of the desired effect. Depending on the charge of the substance particles in the galvanic field, movement will be towards the cathode (positive) or anode (negative) instead. Negatively charged substances such as salicylic acid, hydroxyethyl salicylate (e.g. Mobilat), diclofenac, dipyrone and heparin (minus) are applied under the anode and are attracted by the cathode (plus) across the tissue. Conversely, positively charged substances such as local anesthetics, histamine, acetylcholine or hyaluronidase are placed under the anode (negative) and move to the cathode (positive). Metal implants are a contraindication for iontophoresis!

Ultrasound

Ultrasound is considered an in-depth heating method with a penetration depth of up to 7 cm, by which also near bone structures and muscle insertions can be reached. The effect is like a kind of micro-massage, with the help of which swelling and pollutants can be more effectively removed and the metabolism in the application area can be excited by means of activation at cell level [4]. With the help of an ultrasonic device, medication can also be "sounded in". Ultrasound is also used in combination with iontophoresis.

Structure of Joint Mobilization

After determining the current function and stability of the shoulder joint from biomechanical point of view, the short- and long-term aim of the treatment should be discussed with the patient and communicated as detailed as possible to the therapist (therapy map, feedback about the progression). The crucial factor primarily is the assessment of the surgeon, only he knows the intraoperative findings.

The precise control of the course of treatment and the exchange between patient, doctor and therapist are important. The findings should be checked regularly and adapted to treatment duration and intensity if necessary. Overall, beginning of the exercise treatment as early as possible is desirable to avoid adhesions and contractures. On the other hand, the extremely gentle treatment dosage is crucial, because too rigorous physical therapy is associated with the formation of calcifications and can cause severe pain and irritation in the subacromial space.

The restoration of **functionality**, **stability and analgesia** of the shoulder is the overall target. Late effects such as muscle insufficiency, capsular shrinkage, motor impairment and poor posture should be avoided. The three main pillars of physiotherapy are:

- **Centering of the humeral head:**
- Centering of the humeral head (see Fig. 20.2) is on the one hand facilitated by passive techniques such as manual therapy, on the other hand by **strengthening the stabilizing muscles** that oppose a decentering of the humeral head in a cranial direction and thus expand the subacromial space. These muscles include: M. supra- and infraspinatus, Teres minor and major, subscapularis, latissimus dorsi and biceps brachii caput longum.
- **The cranial muscles** are gently stretched and relaxed by physical applications: including the deltoid, pectoralis, triceps caput longum, coracobrachialis and biceps caput breve muscles.
- **Scapula setting**:
- To guarantee a biomechanically correct movement in the shoulder joint, the scapula must be fixed properly to the thorax and be able to slide and rotate undisturbedly. The serratus anterior, the rhomboid muscles and the trapezius with his transverse and ascending part provide sufficient retraction of the shoulder and fixation of the scapula to the thorax and an erection of the thorax, whereby the rotator cuff muscles are activated. These functional conditions can be restored by manual therapy, physiotherapy and home exercises, so that a smooth scapulo-thoracic rhythm is given (see Figs. 20.3 and 20.4)
- **Core stability**:
- An incorrect posture or insufficiency of the ESPE leads to shortening and weakening of the trapezius muscle. Thereby, the ventral parts of the deltoid muscle are activated and the humerus moves cranially. On the other hand, the scapula fixation onto the thorax is deteriorated. In addition, there is often a shortened pectoralis, resulting in an anterior instability of the glenohumeral joint.
- Therefore, posture training and strengthening of the core stability is a critical cornerstone for a regular shoulder function (see Fig. 20.5).

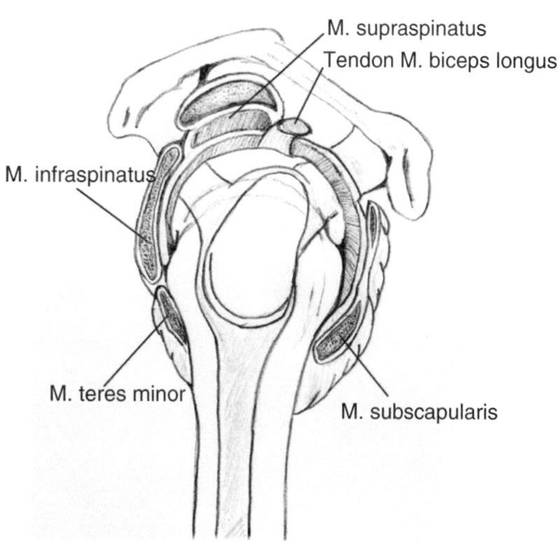

Fig. 20.2 Regular, centered position of the humeral head

The rehabilitation treatment can be divided into four phases:

- Acute phase/immobilization
- Exercise stability
- Rehabilitation training
- Load stability

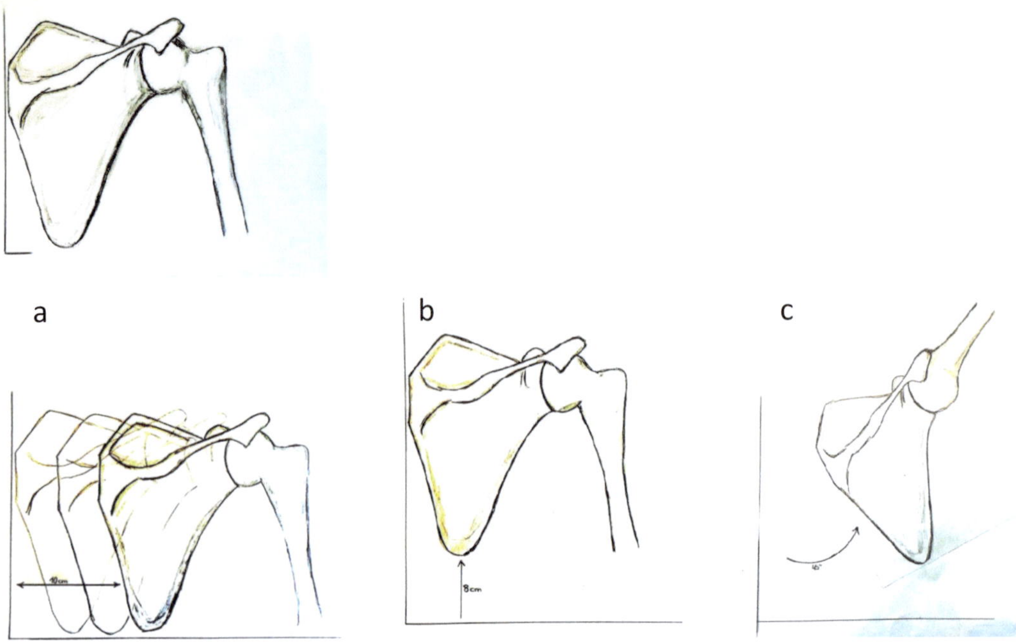

Fig. 20.3 Scapulo-thoracic rhythm, (**a**) medio-lateral shift, (**b**) cranialisation, (**c**) abduction

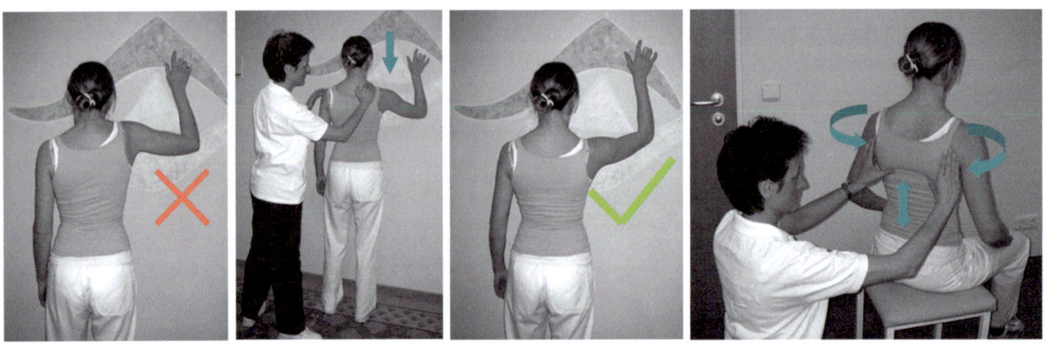

Fig. 20.4 Dynamic scapula stabilization and scapular setting

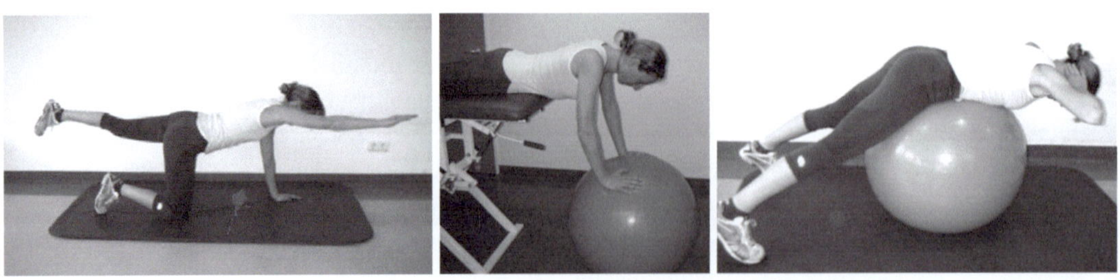

Fig. 20.5 Exercises for trunk stabilization

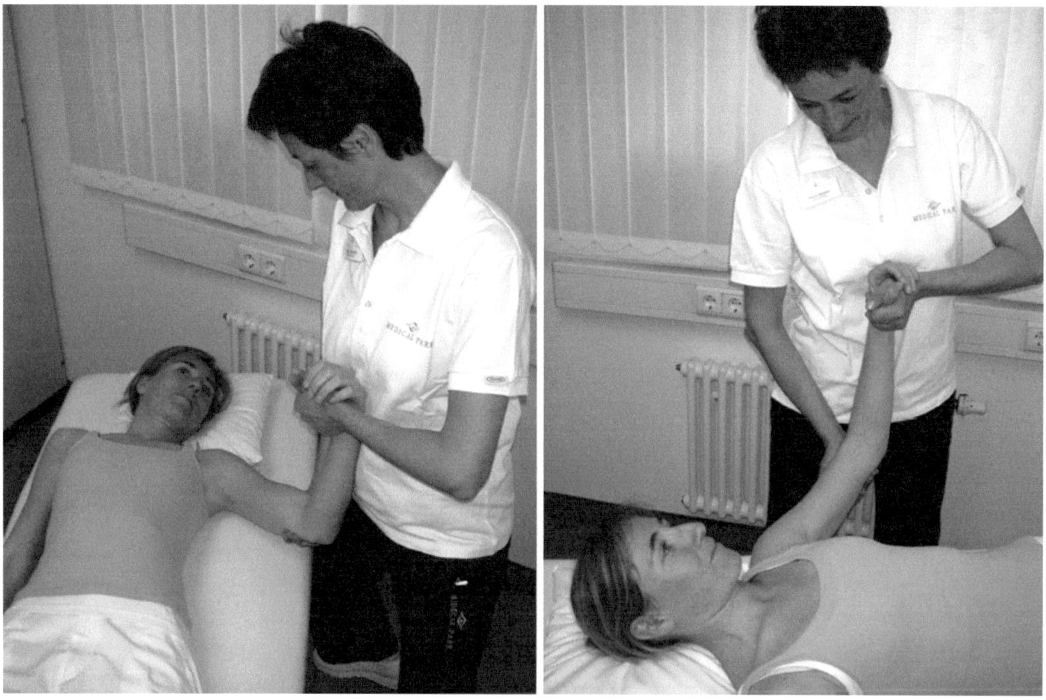

Fig. 20.6 Passive abduction and elevation of the shoulder joint

Acute and Early Stage

As long as the Redon drains are placed in the muscle compartment or joint, only **passive exercising** is allowed. The limb remains in the prescribed postoperative position. Required sterile dressings are generally kept during the exercise treatment.

The first aim of physiotherapy is to center the humeral head. In the first stage, this centering can be done mostly passive. To avoid reflectory tension of the muscles, ice compresses and relaxation techniques can be used in addition. First, gentle isometric tensing of the centering muscle groups can take place in the splint. These are mainly the adductors and external rotators, which center the humeral head caudally and dorsally.

The tension change is repeated as often as possible, finally muscle relaxation follows. Conscious relaxing and aware recreation of the comfortably resting arm can also help. In addition, cold applications are recommended. The patient himself can do finger exercises that stimulate blood circulation and the lymphatic drainage at this stage. Letting the arm limp prevents contractures of the elbow. The cervical spine can be exercised to avoid tension and poor posture. The exercises have to be dosed carefully. In case of increasing swelling and hyperthermia, the intensity should be reduced.

Passive Mobilization (Exercise Stability)

Once **stability during exercise** is reached, **passive motion exercises** with correct axis alignment can be performed without the splint and with a decreased body gravity, ideally as terminal as possible (see Fig. 20.6). The lesion-specifically defined amounts of movement must be respected and the pain threshold considered.

Furthermore, isometric exercises that center the humeral head should be performed. Centering can also be realized by manual translation from the glenoid and active re-tensioning.

By means of posture correction, trunk control, scapula mobilization and respiratory therapy, the scapula setting can be initiated, which

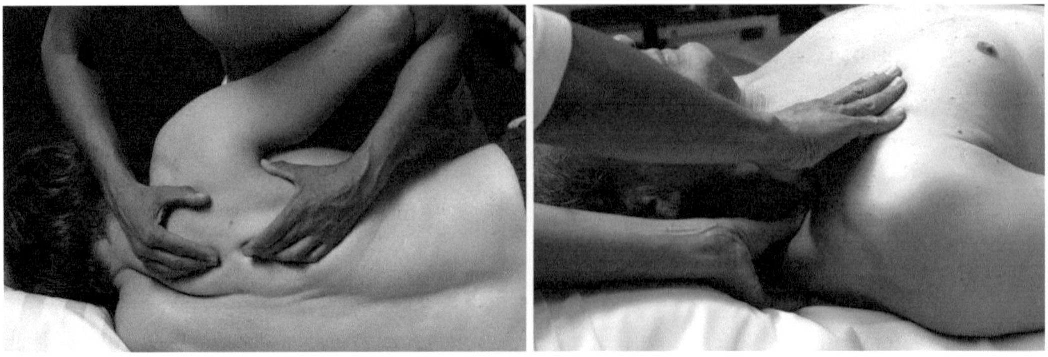

Fig. 20.7 Manual scapula mobilization

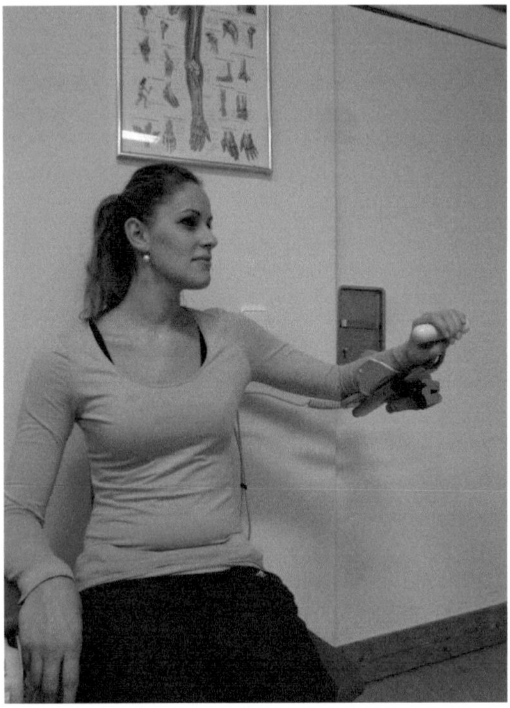

Fig. 20.8 Treatment with the CPM splint

is indispensable for movements in the shoulder joint (see Fig. 20.7).

Motorized Exercise Splint

Passive movement therapy can be supported in the early phase of rehabilitation depending on the type of the injury and a permitted range of motion by motorized exercise splints. These are also known as **CPM (continuous passive motion) rails**. According to the catalogue of therapeutic appliances, CPM therapy is indicated at the shoulder joint after surgically treated fractures of the humerus. The positive effect on the mobility of the shoulder is proven [5].

If possible, it is used several times a day with short treatment times. In the course, treatments can be reduced to one to two times per day for a treatment period of 20–30 min each. Before first use, the current range of motion should be determined manually in compliance with the pain threshold according to the parameters of the splint (Fig. 20.8).

Load Stability

Transition to Active Movement

As progression after purely passive movements, the patient now increasingly supports the same motion control of the correct axial flexion/extension with the same technique as the therapist with his own muscle activity. This stage is called **active-assistive movement** with a decrease of gravity. The allowed amounts of movement and the pain threshold must still be observed. The active support of the therapist is slowly reduced to a purely guiding contact. This ensures a correct axial movement and prevents evasive movements. In this phase, the patient may begin active-assistive home exercises (see Fig. 20.9).

The patient gradually adopts more muscle activity against gravity. Now we speak of **active motion exercise against gravity**. Also the initiation of therapy in a exercise pool has proven to be successful in this phase, if wound healing is completed (see Fig. 20.10). The buoyancy of the

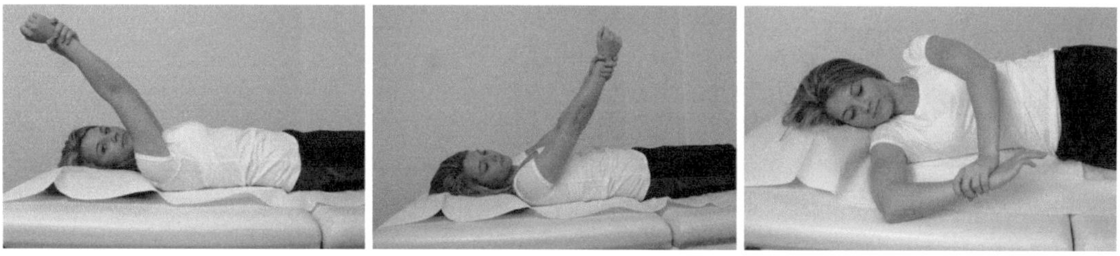

Fig. 20.9 Active-assistive home exercises

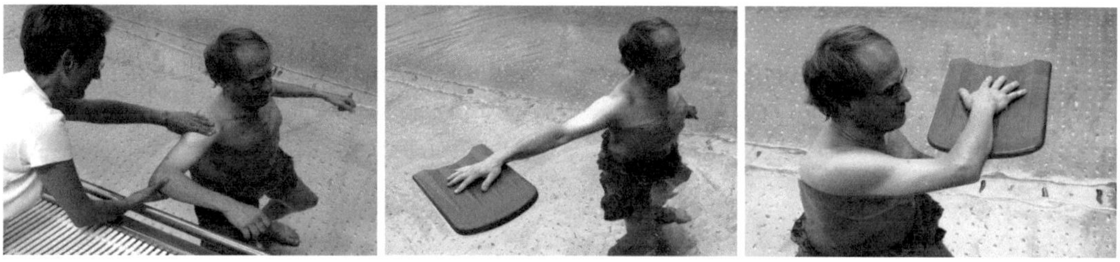

Fig. 20.10 Therapy in an exercise pool

water allows exercises with seeming weightlessness with low muscle strength and coordination. The elevation and abduction in the often strained shoulder area is encouraged. The exercise resistance of a movement can be smoothly dispensed. Warm water has a generally relaxing effect on the muscles and therefore has a very beneficial impact in the treatment of contractures.

Cervical spine and distal joints must be kept free. This means with shoulder lesions, elbow and wrist are also included in the exercise therapy to avoid stiffness by false posture.

Exercise Against Resistance (Load Stability)

Prior to further load increase, **X-ray checks** should be performed. With these, it is determined whether the achieved consolidation allows a permission for load stability. If this is the case, practicing against resistance can be started as the next level. In addition to the increase of load, the movement amounts are extended gradually. From this stage on, exercises in the form of PNF patterns are especially recommended. **PNF** means proprioceptive neuromuscular facilitation. The PNF method decomposes complex movements in a variety of basic patterns of muscle (group) movements. These are unconscious components of everyday movements and extend three-dimensionally and diagonally across the body, because the muscles are set up spirally. Each of these individual patterns can now be trained separately with the patient. In this process, the musculoskeletal system is stimulated by elongation, as well as tension and pressure on the joints or the skin by touching, the eye by eye contact or the ears by hearing commandos. The PNF method takes advantage of the fact that the brain is reminiscent of complex movements, although the body cannot perform them at the moment.

PNF exercises can be performed as active physiological movement patterns

- against manual contact
- against matched manual resistance
- against maximum resistance
- against device resistance or body weight (closed chain)
- against fixed resistors such as walls or door frame.

By gradually increasing the exercise resistance, the improvement of muscle strength and endurance is trained in parallel to mobilization. In an affection-free joint, the resistance can be increased.

Implementation and dosage of PNF exercises have to be adjusted individually to current stability, mobility and resilience of the lesion (fracture, soft tissue, ligament injury, surgery).

Orthopedic Manipulative Therapy (OMT)

Manual therapy according to the concepts of Maitland and Kaltenborn-Evjenth are physiotherapeutic procedures acknowledged by the WHO.

There is a focus on the mobilization of joints by traction and purely translational sliding movements within a joint with small amounts of movement according to fixed rules and definitions.

The application of techniques from manual therapy is recommended for shoulder lesions to solve agglutination and adhesion in the joint area and thus resolve malfunctions.

Ergotherapy to Recover the Functionality

The already discussed mobilization is aimed at functional improvements. In particular, the complex motion patterns that are practiced in the context of PNF patterns are already preparing the necessary **everyday movements**. A variety of devices can also be incorporated into the training program such as staves, ropes or dumbbells. It is favorable to practice in front of a mirror for self-control. It is also possible to form groups, if there are several patients with equivalent load status. In contrast to physical therapy, the focus of ergotherapy is focused on the functionality in everyday life from the beginning on. Especially with rehabilitation needs in the arm/hand area, it is important to integrate ergotherapy from the start of the exercise therapy. It is seen as a useful addition to physiotherapy.

The main goal of ergotherapy is to make the patient independent in activities of daily living. Therefore, supporting patients with relevant **adjuvants** is also a responsibility of the therapist, such as combs or cutlery with long handles in case of impossible elevation of the shoulder joint. The ergonomically correct use of prescribed items will be practiced with the patient in order to avoid the creation of motion deficits by relieving posture and evasive movements. In the ward, this part of therapy is called ADL training (Activities of Daily Living). The task of the therapist is a detailed diagnostic assessment in relation to the current situation of the patient in home care, work and leisure. Initial training will be fitted to the individual patient. He practices what he needs most and what corresponds to his previous habits and requirements (athletes, seniors, craftsmen, etc.) Family members who participate in the daily life of the patient should be included in the ADL training. When it can be assumed that a complete cure will be possible, ergo therapy is a temporary support and complement of physiotherapy.

In the context of the actual postoperative functional exercise, it is important to note the general joint protection rules. All planned measures should then be examined critically.

It is important to avoid axial deviations of the joint in the required movements. Pain and stress thresholds must be strictly observed to be stopped instantly in doubt. Therefore, timely and adequate breaks should be included in the training program. To avoid muscle tension, an optimal seating and working posture should be ensured. The activities should be designed as dynamic as possible, which means that the required range of motion should be as large as possible.

So-called functional games are applied. These are usually simple board games that meet the timeframe of a therapy unit. Through various oversized pieces, specifically selected movements can be improved. In the horizontal plane there is e.g. an oversized "Solitaire". For vertical exercising the "clothespin tree" is used (see Fig. 20.11).

(a) "Clothespin Tree": Clothespins are pegged to exercise the vertical movement (can be performed without pronation and supination)
(b) Oversized "Solitaire" to exercise the horizontal movement (with and without pronation and supination feasible)

Building Phase

Medical Training Therapy/ Physiotherapy with Devices

Medical training therapy or MTT already represents the transition to independent practice of

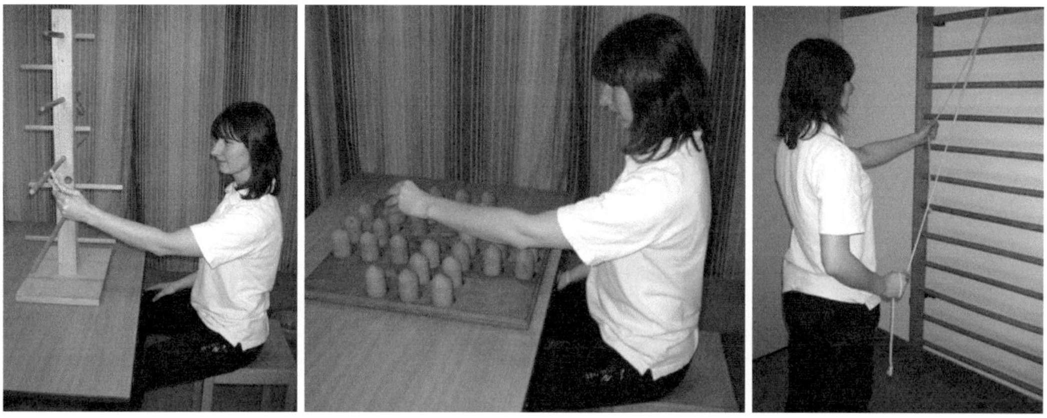

Fig. 20.11 Examples of ergotherapeutic games

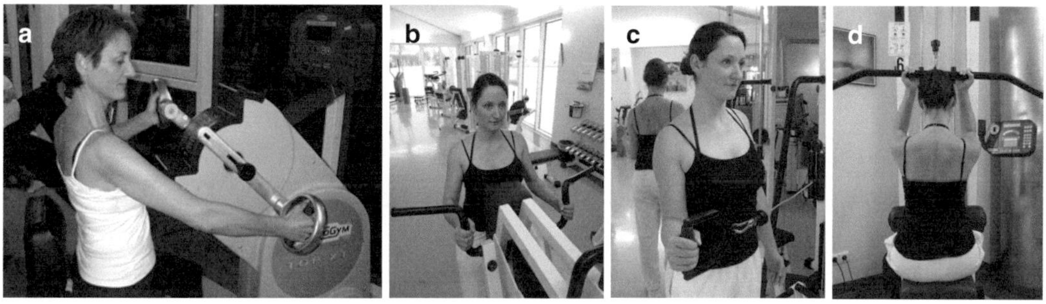

Fig. 20.12 MTT training. (**a**) Hand crank (**b**) rhomboids trainer (**c**) external rotators (**d**) latissimus dorsi

patients, but is also available in the field of inpatient rehabilitation. The term medical training is defined as a specific muscle training with light weight, with the aim to train joint flexibility and endurance. The shoulder joint must already be sufficiently resilient. Equipment and assistive devices which fit the specific rehabilitation needs are applied. The use of these devices facilitates a more accurate exposure dose during the exercises. Stimulus density, intensity and duration can be accurately measured during MTT and adapted according to the individual needs by means of scientific criteria of training theory. MTT should always be conducted by experienced coaches who at the beginning guide the implementation of the exercises in detail and supervise the training process continuously. The training staff should be able to recognize symptoms during or after therapy such as excessive strains in the form of pain, redness and warmth and if necessary adjust or stop the training program in consultation with the attending physician.

In case of full resilience and sufficient mobility of the shoulder joint, the program may proceed to the training phase. This is characterized by

- Plyometric training
- Increased neuromuscular training
- Progressive cardio and strength training of the entire shoulder and trunk muscles
- Whole-body workout

The muscles centering the humerus head and those stabilizing the scapula rotation and fixation to the trunk are particularly trained (see Chap. 1). The scapulo-thoracic rhythm should be exercised extensively to train a physiologically functional movement pattern in the shoulder joint (see Figs. 20.12 and 20.13).

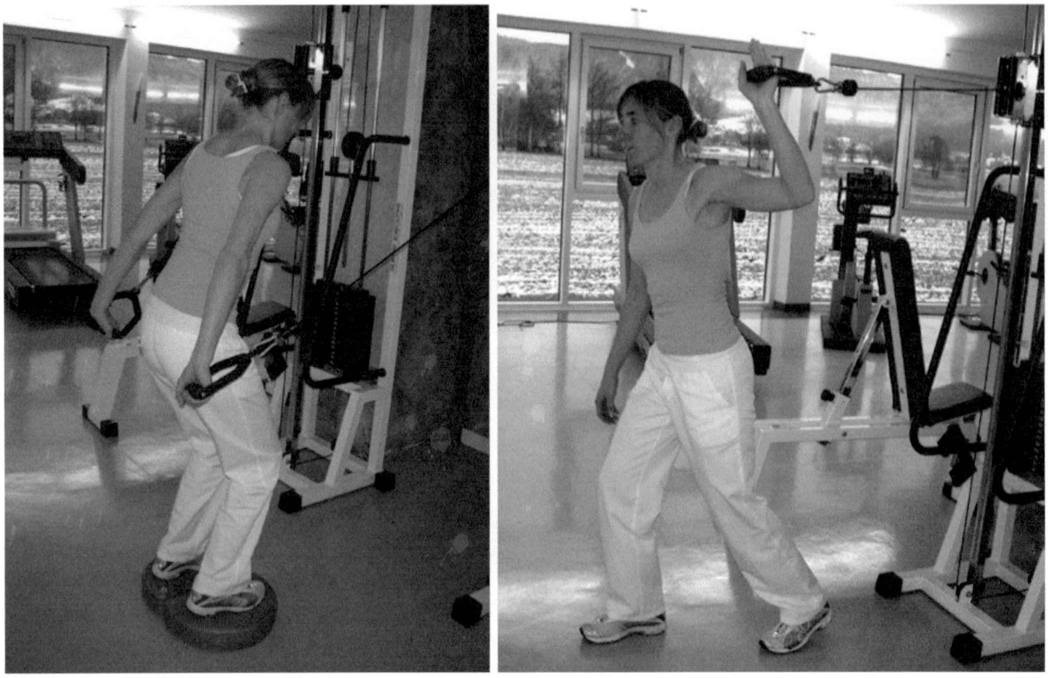

Fig. 20.13 Training with a winch

Gyrotonic (Neurophysiological Complex Therapy)

Gyrotonic training can incorporate movements of entire chains of muscles and can be trained holistically and in three-dimensional sequences against even gliding resistance. The joints are subject to a minimum axial load (see Fig. 20.14), simultaneously developing of strength, coordination and agility. This requires adequate joint and muscle stability.

The Way to Everyday Life

For the period after the acute inpatient or outpatient rehabilitation, the patient should receive guidance on **behavior in everyday life**.

After an inpatient rehabilitation measure, the continuation of outpatient physical therapy is usually recommended. Thus, the learned functions will further be strengthened and setbacks are avoided. Hence, the patient continuously proceeds from the consolidation phase, which may take up to a year, to the prevention phase.

In outpatient surgery, the patient must receive exact behavior rules and get instructions for home exercises immediately after surgery. The patient needs to know what he has to practice and what he ought to avoid, how much and for how long he should load and move. Warning signs have to be pointed out, such as perifocal pain, swelling, redness and/or warmth that make an immediate visit to the doctor necessary.

Homework for Patients

To expand the daily practice time, the patient should also get some "homework" to practice for himself already during the hospital stay or rehabilitation. The exercises must be adapted to the individual patient, depending on the type of lesion or surgical intervention, the further postoperative course and the basic performance. The patient receives correct instructions of the exercise and training sheets for the correct execution only under follow-up of the attending doctor and therapist.

Examples for Exercises in the Acute Phase

In the acute phase, the home exercises may just be performed to a very limited extent. The following **finger and hand exercises** are recommended for correctly positioned extremities:

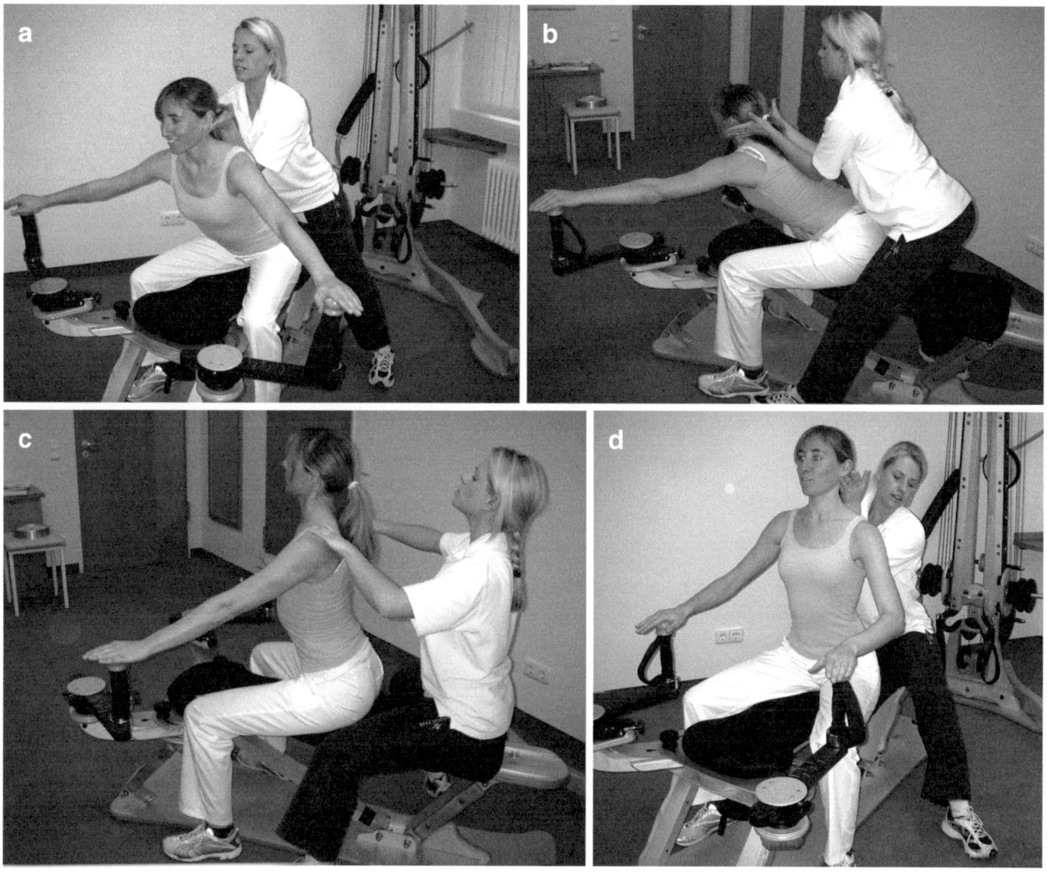

Fig. 20.14 Gyrotonic

- Finger: spread and close fingers on a flat surface repeatedly
- Thumb: repeated abduction, adduction, circles and opposition of the thumb to each finger
- "Small fist": repeated finger flexion and extension in the middle and end joints
- "Large fist": normal fist closure, finger flexion in the base, middle and end joints; fist closure with small soft ball
- Hand: extension and flexion at the base joint
- Hand: radial ulnar abduction

The number of repetitions should be increased stepwise. In the beginning, it is preferable to exercise multiple times per day, but only for a few minutes.

Examples and Exercise Stability

- "Wipe": The patient performs "wiping exercises" on the table. Here, the elbow is mobilized in addition. It should be practiced on slippery surfaces with low frictional resistance.
- "Swing": The patient is in walking stance and is holding on to secure support, bends the upper body forward and swings the arm hanging loosely in front of the body left/right and next to the body back and forth. This exercise should be done several times a day for a few minutes.
- "Creaming": In this exercise, the hand is moved as if creaming with lotion in a circular motion loosely along the body, to the extent permitted by the range of motion without pain. The advantage of this exercise is that the hand

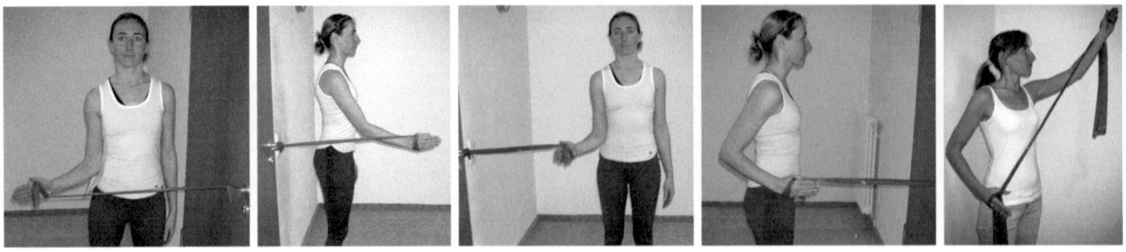

Fig. 20.15 Exercises with Thera-Bands. From *left* to *right*: external rotation, anteversion, internal rotation, retroversion, complex therapy

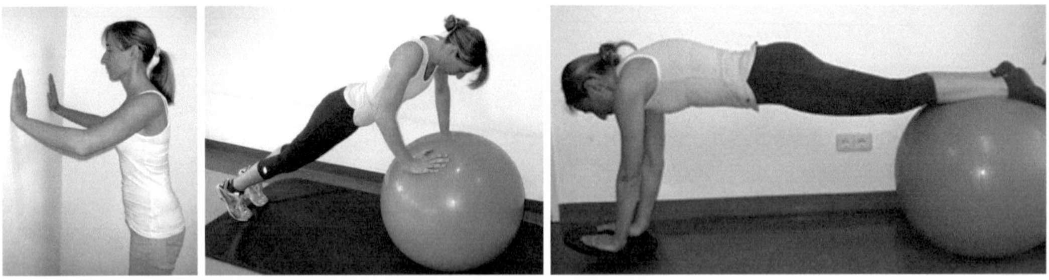

Fig. 20.16 Self-exercise for setting the scapula

is guided through physical contact and rapid uncontrolled movements are avoided.

Examples and Load Stability

Under load stability, the patient can practice independently without orthosis. The variation of the exercises is diverse. The use of **Thera-Bands** is convenient, because they can be used for multiple PNF-like complex movements (Figs. 20.15 and 20.16).

Rehabilitation Training

The rehabilitation training in the context of MTT is performed with variable exercises depending on the function deficit. If no postoperative motion or load limits are noted, the patient increases his exercises pain-adaptedly.

Important Questions and Issues for Everyday Life

- What may I lift and carry?
- Application of additional pain medication
- When should I see a doctor (pain, inflammation, functional impairment)?
- Follow-up at the surgeon
- Regular muscle training, physiotherapy if necessary

References

1. Hodgson S. Proximal humerus fracture rehabilitation. Clin Orthop Relat Res. 2006;442:131–8.
2. Heisel J. Physikalische Medizin. Stuttgart: Thieme; 2005.
3. Ergotherapie Zeitschrift für angewandte Wissenschaft Jg.5(2). November/Dezember 2004.
4. Ebenbichler GR, et al. Ultrasound therapy for calcific tendinitis of the shoulder. N Engl J Med. 1999;340(20):1533–8.
5. Michael JW, et al. Efficiency of a postoperative treatment after rotator cuff repair with a continuous passive motion device (CPM). Z Orthop Ihre Grenzgeb. 2005;143(4):438–45.

Scoring

21

Marc Beirer

Introduction

In shoulder surgery scoring instruments are well-established to evaluate functional outcome and patient satisfaction. A distinction is made between self-assessment questionnaires allowing for long-term follow-up examination of large patient collectives despite of long distances to the clinic without requiring face-to-face contact and physician-based scoring systems mostly used in the clinical setting. In general Patient-Reported Outcome (PRO) questionnaires showed to be more suitable for outcome research due to their superior validity in comparison to clinician assessed parameters [1]. Furthermore self-assessment eliminates selection or examiner observation bias of physicians rating the patients they treated before much better than other physicians or patients themselves [2]. Since subjective patient-satisfaction is not necessarily directly linked to physician-based objective examination [3], numerous scoring tools have been developed in the recent years. As most studies use different scoring systems, comparison of treatment results with literature, with the aim to improve therapeutic strategies, is limited. Consequently, the risk of maintaining inadequate treatment concepts is increased leading to reduced treatment quality and decreased patient satisfaction. Recently a new PRO shoulder questionnaire, the Munich Shoulder Questionnaire, was developed to calculate already well-established shoulder scores out of one single questionnaire [4] to compare the results of different therapeutic approaches with the objective on selecting the most effective treatment strategies and quitting obsolete therapy regimes.

The Munich Shoulder Questionnaire (MSQ) [4]

The MSQ is a universally applicable patient reported outcome (PRO) questionnaire which has been developed for an effective follow-up of shoulder patients. Analysing the items of already existing and well established shoulder scores (Shoulder Pain and Disability Index (SPADI), Disability of the Arm, Shoulder and Hand (DASH) and the Constant Score) for congruency in measurement and subsequent condensing of numerous items into one single question led to a 30 items containing tool. Typical shoulder movements are depicted as photographs to assess the range of motion. The MSQ has been demonstrated as a valid questionnaire allowing for reliable calculation of the SPADI, the DASH and the Constant Score and is currently in use in outcome research [5]. The Munich Shoulder Questionnaire

M. Beirer
Department of Trauma Surgery, Klinikum rechts der Isar, Technical University of Munich, Munich, Germany
e-mail: marc.beirer@mri.tum.de

P. Biberthaler et al. (eds.), *Fractures of the Proximal Humerus*, Strategies in Fracture Treatments,
DOI 10.1007/978-3-319-20300-3_21

is available at http://www.chirurgische-klinik.de/download/inhalt/fachgebiete/unfallchirurgie/MSQENG.pdf

The Shoulder Pain and Disability Index (SPADI) [6]

Roach et al. [6] developed a self-administered questionnaire consisting of 13 equally weighted items divided in two subscales to measure pain (see Table 21.1) and disability (Table 21.2) in shoulder diseases. The 5 items for pain and the 8 items for disability are visualized as visual analog scales ranging from 0 to 10 (0=no pain/no difficulty; 10=worst pain imaginable/so difficult required help).

The Disability of the Arm, Shoulder and Hand (DASH) [7]

The DASH is a 30-item self-administrated measurement tool to assess physical function and symptoms in patients with musculoskeletal disorders of the upper extremity. It was developed by the American Academy of Orthopedic Surgeons (AAOS), the Council of Musculoskeletal Specialty Societies (COMSS) and the Institute for Work and Health (Toronto, Ontario) to be used by physicians in daily practice and as a research tool. Two optional modules for work and sports or performing arts provide an amendment to measure symptoms and function in athletes, artists and other workers whose jobs require a high degree of physical performance. The DASH has been translated in numerous languages and is available under http://dash.iwh.on.ca free of charge.

Table 21.1 Pain subscale of the SPADI

How severe is your pain?
At its worst?
When lying on the envolved side?
Reaching for something on a high shelf?
Touching the back of your neck?
Pushing with the involved arm?

Reprinted with permission from Roach et al. [6]

Table 21.2 Disability subscale of the SPADI

How much difficulty do you have?
Washing your hair?
Washing your back?
Putting on an undershirt or jumper?
Putting on a shirt that buttons down the front?
Putting on your pants?
Placing an object on a high shelf?
Carrying a heavy object of 10 lb?
Removing something from your back pocket?

Reprinted with permission from Roach et al. [6]

The Constant Score [8]

The Constant Score was developed as a physician-based measurement tool to provide an overall clinical functional assessment [8]. It is a 100 point scaling system divided into four subscales: pain (15 points; Table 21.3), activities of daily living (20 points; Table 21.4), strength measurement (25 points) and range of motion (40 points; Table 21.5a, b). Shoulder strength is measured as abduction power at 90° with the wrist as point of loading [9].

Table 21.3 Pain subscale of the Constant Score

Pain	None	15
	Mild	10
	Moderate	5
	Severe	0

Reprinted with permission from Constant and Murley [8]

Table 21.4 Activities of daily living subscale of the Constant Score

Activities of daily living	Full work	4
	Full recreation/sport	4
	Unaffected sleep	2
Positioning	Up to waist	2
	Up to xiphoid	4
	Up to neck	6
	Up to top of head	8
	Above head	10

Reprinted with permission from Constant and Murley [8]

The Relative Constant Score (Age- and Sex-Related) according to Gerber et al. [10]

The strength subscale of the Constant Score constitutes a potential source of error due to gender-related differences in absolute lean body mass resulting in an average lower muscular force in women compared to men [11]. Brinker et al. [12] reported a relevant bias of both age and gender on the total Constant Score in favour of young men. Therefore Yian et al. [10] developed normative age- and sex-specific Constant Scores and strength values in a large population sample (Table 21.6).

Table 21.5 Range of motion subscale of the Constant Score

(a) Flexion/abduction		
Flexion	0–30°	0
	31–60°	2
	61–90°	4
	91–120°	6
	121–150°	8
	151–180°	10
Abduction	0–30°	0
	31–60°	2
	61–90°	4
	91–120°	6
	121–150°	8
	151–180°	10
(b) External/internal rotation		
External	Hand behind head with elbow held forward	2
	Hand behind head with elbow held back	2
	Hand on top of head with elbow held forward	2
	Hand on top of head with elbow held back	2
	Full elevation from on top of head	2
Internal rotation	Dorsum of hand to lateral thigh	0
	Dorsum of hand to buttock	2
	Dorsum of hand to lumbosacral junction	4
	Dorsum of hand to waist (3rd lumbar vertebra)	6
	Dorsum of hand to 12th dorsal vertebra	8
	Dorsum of hand to interscapular region	10

Reprinted with permission from Constant and Murley [8]

The American Shoulder and Elbow Surgeons Standardized Shoulder Assessment Form [13]

This shoulder score was developed by the Research Committee of the American Shoulder and Elbow Surgeons (ASES) as a standardized method of assessing musculoskeletal function to facilitate the communication between investigators [13]. It constitutes a baseline measurement tool applicable to all shoulder patients regardless of diagnosis. The form consists of demographic information (Fig. 21.1), a patient self-evaluation section and a physician assessment section. The patient self-evaluation form is divided into three subscales (Fig. 21.2a–c): pain, instability and activities of daily living. The physician assessment portion of the form consists of a range of motion (Fig. 21.3a), a clinical signs (Fig. 21.3b), a strength (Fig. 21.3c) and an instability section (Fig. 21.3d).

Summary

In general scoring instruments are widely used to assess the preoperative and postoperative status of patients with shoulder diseases. Besides already existing physician-based scores

Table 21.6 Normative age- and sex-specific Constant Score

	Constant score	
Age (years)	Male	Female
21–30	94	86
31–40	94	86
41–50	93	85
51–60	91	83
61–70	90	82
71–80	86	81

Reprinted with permission from Yian et al. [10]

Shoulder assessment form Americam shoulder and elbow surgeons		
Name:		Date
Age:	Hand dominance: R L Ambi	Sex: M F
Diagnosis:		Initial Assess? Y N
Procedure/Date:		Follow-up: M; Y

Fig. 21.1 Demographic information of the ASES standardized shoulder assessment form (Reprinted with permission from Richards et al. [13])

numerous self-evaluation questionnaires have been developed to eliminate observer bias of physicians rating the patients they treated before. The Munich Shoulder Questionnaire, a patient-reported measurement tool, was especially developed for an effective self-evaluation of shoulder patients and allows for a quantitative assessment of the Constant, Shoulder Pain and Disability Index (SPADI) and Disabilities of the Arm, Shoulder and Hand (DASH) score. It presents a universally applicable baseline measurement tool to select the most effective treatment strategy and to facilitate communication of investigators.

a

Patient self-evaluation		
Are you having pain in your shoulder? (circle correct answer)	Yes	No
Mark where your pain is		

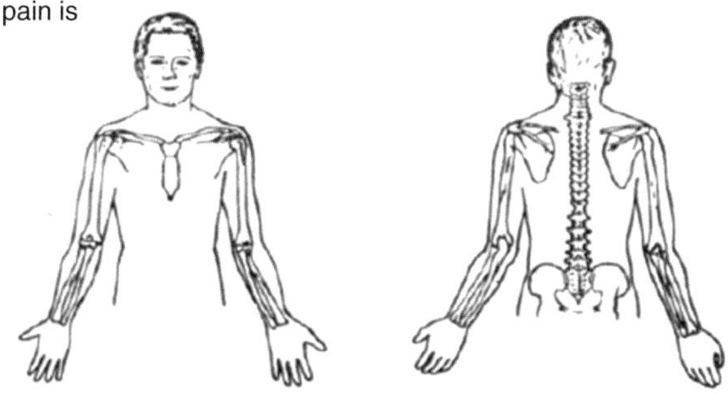

Do you have pain in your shoulder at night?	Yes	No
Do you take pain medication (aspirin, Advil, Tylenol etc.)?	Yes	No
Do you take narcotic pain medication (codeine or stronger)?	Yes	No
How many pills do you take each day (average)?	pills	
How bad is your pain today (mark line)? 0 – 10 No pain at all ... Pain as bad as it can be		

b

Does your shoulder feel unstable (as if it is going to dislocate?)	Yes	No
How unstable is your shoulder (mark line)? 0 – 10 Very stsble ... Very unstsble		

c

Circle the number in the box that indicates your ability to do the following activities:
0= Unable to do; 1 = Very difficult to do; 2 = Somewhat difficult; 3 = Not difflcult

Activity		Right arm	Left arm
1. Put on a coat		0 1 2 3	0 1 2 3
2. Sleep on your painful or affected side		0 1 2 3	0 1 2 3
3. Wash back/do up bra in back		0 1 2 3	0 1 2 3
4. Manage toiletting		0 1 2 3	0 1 2 3
5. Comb hair		0 1 2 3	0 1 2 3
6. Reach a high shelf		0 1 2 3	0 1 2 3
7. Lift 10 lbs. above shoulder		0 1 2 3	0 1 2 3
8. Throw a ball overhand		0 1 2 3	0 1 2 3
9. Do usual work - List		0 1 2 3	0 1 2 3
10. Do usual sport - List		0 1 2 3	0 1 2 3

Fig. 21.2 (**a**) Self-evaluation: pain section of the ASES standardized shoulder assessment form (Reprinted with permission from [13]). (**b**) Self-evaluation: Instability section of the ASES standardized shoulder assessment form (Reprinted with permission from Richards et al. [13]). (**c**) Self-evaluation: Activities of daily living section of the ASES standardized shoulder assessment form (Reprinted with permission from Richards et al. [13])

a

Physician assessment				
Range of motion Total shoulder motion Goniometer preferred	Right		Left	
	Active	Passive	Active	Passive
Forward elevation (Maximum arm-trunk angle)				
External rotation (Arm comfortably at side)				
External rotation (Arm at 90° abduction)				
Internal rotation (Highest posterior anatomy reached with thumb)				
Cross-body adduction (Antecubital fossa to opposite acromion)				

b

Signs 0 = none; 1 = mild; 2 = moderate; 3 = severe			
Sign		Right	Left
Supraspinatus/greater tuberosity tenderness		0 1 2 3	0 1 2 3
AC joint tenderness		0 1 2 3	0 1 2 3
Biceps tendon tenderness (or rupture)		0 1 2 3	0 1 2 3
Other tenderness - List:		0 1 2 3	0 1 2 3
Impingement I (Passive forward elevation in slight internal rotation)		Y N	Y N
Impingement II (Passive internal rotation with 90° flexion)		Y N	Y N
Impingement III (90° active abduction - classic painful arc)		Y N	Y N
Subacromial crepitus		Y N	Y N
Scars - location		Y N	Y N
Atrophy - location:		Y N	Y N
Deformity : describe		Y N	Y N

c

Strength (record MRC grade) 0 = no contraction; 1 = flicker; 2 = movement with gravity eliminated 3 = movement aganist gravity; 4 = movement aganist some resistance; 5 = normal power.		
	Right	Left
Testing affected by pain?	Y N	Y N
Forward elevation	0 1 2 3 4 5	0 1 2 3 4 5
Abduction	0 1 2 3 4 5	0 1 2 3 4 5
External rotation (Arm comfortably at side)	0 1 2 3 4 5	0 1 2 3 4 5
Internal rotation (Arm comfortably at side)	0 1 2 3 4 5	0 1 2 3 4 5

Fig. 21.3 (**a**) Physician assessment: range of motion section of the ASES standardized shoulder assessment form (Reprinted with permission from Richards et al. [13]). (**b**) Physician assessment: Clinical signs section of the ASES standardized shoulder assessment form (Reprinted with permission from Richards et al. [13]). (**c**) Physician assessment: Strength section of the ASES standardized shoulder assessment form (Reprinted with permission from Richards et al. [13]). (**d**) Physician assessment: Instability section of the ASES standardized shoulder assessment form (Reprinted with permission from Richards et al. [13])

d

Instability

0 = none; 1 = mild (0 - 1 cm translation)
2 = moderate (1 - 2 cm translation or translates to glenoid rim)
3 = severe (> 2 cm translation or over rim of glenoid)

Anterior translation	0 1 2 3	0 1 2 3
Posterior translation	0 1 2 3	0 1 2 3
Inferior translation (sulcus sign)	0 1 2 3	0 1 2 3
Anterior apprehension	0 1 2 3	0 1 2 3
Reproduces symptoms?	Y N	Y N
Voluntary instability?	Y N	Y N
Relocation test positive?	Y N	Y N
Generalized ligamentous laxity?	Y N	

Other physical findings:

Examiner's name:

____________________________ ________________ Date

Fig. 21.3 (continued)

References

1. Kosinski M, Zhao SZ, Dedhiya S, Osterhaus JT, Ware Jr JE. Determining minimally important changes in generic and disease-specific health-related quality of life questionnaires in clinical trials of rheumatoid arthritis. Arthritis Rheum. 2000;43(7):1478–87.
2. Boehm D, Wollmerstedt N, Doesch M, Handwerker M, Mehling E, Gohlke F. Development of a questionnaire based on the Constant-Murley-Score for self-evaluation of shoulder function by patients. Unfallchirurg. 2004;107(5):397–402.
3. Hollinshead RM, Mohtadi NG, Vande Guchte RA, Wadey VM. Two 6-year follow-up studies of large and massive rotator cuff tears: comparison of outcome measures. J Shoulder Elbow Surg. 2000;9(5):373–81.
4. Schmidutz F, Beirer M, Braunstein V, Bogner V, Wiedemann E, Biberthaler P. The Munich Shoulder Questionnaire (MSQ): development and validation of an effective patient-reported tool for outcome measurement and patient safety in shoulder surgery. Patient Saf Surg. 2012;6(1):9.
5. Biberthaler P, Beirer M, Kirchhoff S, Braunstein V, Wiedemann E, Kirchhoff C. Significant benefit for older patients after arthroscopic subacromial decompression: a long-term follow-up study. Int Orthop. 2013;37(3):457–62.
6. Roach KE, Budiman-Mak E, Songsiridej N, Lertratanakul Y. Development of a shoulder pain and disability index. Arthritis Care Res. 1991;4(4):143–9.
7. Hudak PL, Amadio PC, Bombardier C. Development of an upper extremity outcome measure: the DASH (disabilities of the arm, shoulder and hand) [corrected]. The Upper Extremity Collaborative Group (UECG). Am J Ind Med. 1996;29(6):602–8.
8. Constant CR, Murley AH. A clinical method of functional assessment of the shoulder. Clin Orthop Relat Res. 1987;214:160–4.
9. Constant CR, Gerber C, Emery RJ, Sojbjerg JO, Gohlke F, Boileau P. A review of the Constant score: modifications and guidelines for its use. J Shoulder Elbow Surg. 2008;17(2):355–61.
10. Yian EH, Ramappa AJ, Arneberg O, Gerber C. The Constant score in normal shoulders. J Shoulder Elbow Surg. 2005;14(2):128–33.
11. Katch MK. Measuring and improving muscular strength. In: Exercise physiology energy, nutrition, and human performance. Philadelphia: Lippincott Williams and Wilkins; 1991.
12. Brinker MR, Cuomo JS, Popham GJ, O'Connor DP, Barrack RL. An examination of bias in shoulder scoring instruments among healthy collegiate and recreational athletes. J Shoulder Elbow Surg. 2002;11(5):463–9.
13. Richards RR, An KN, Bigliani LU, Friedman RJ, Gartsman GM, Gristina AG, Iannotti JP, Mow VC, Sidles JA, Zuckerman JD. A standardized method for the assessment of shoulder function. J Shoulder Elbow Surg. 1994;3(6):347–52.

Assessment of Functional Deficits Caused by Fracture of the Proximal Humerus

22

Gertrud Kirchhoff, Chlodwig Kirchhoff, and Rainer Kirchhoff

An injury of the upper extremity by a proximal humerus fracture is connected to an immobilization of the extremity, what concerns size and period are dependent on the applied surgical method. It is to start out from an accident by definition if the person insured or not insured suffers a health damage involuntarily by an event suddenly having an effect on his body from outside [8].

The assessment of the respective damage compensation is dependent on several factors if there is such a claim.

It can be an accident which has to be compensated in the context of the statutory accident insurance. Possibly it could be a domestic accident or a sporting accident for which a personal accident insurance is responsible possible as cost carrier. It can be an accident in the context of a road accident or other accident [2, 7, 10]. It can be an event in the context of any illness process the private or legal health insurance has to compensate and an assessment in the context of legal claims according to seriously handicapped persons.

It can be the determination of efficiency in the context of an application for inability to work for a private pension fund or also for the legal social insurance [2].

There is the determination of ability for professional rehabilitation by legal social insurance and also the determination of housekeeping damage [9].

In principle the impairment of professional efficiency has to be checked in certain professions, on the general labor market as well as also with public employers for a limited time or for duration [6].

The statutory accident insurance covers damages which have resulted from a work accident, way to work accident or an occupational disease [4, 6]. Unlike the assessment in health insurance or the pension insurance which is based on the principles of finality, the base of decision is the principle of causality in legal work insurance, in which a causality which is justifying liability and filling out liability. This means that the respective decision of probability is based on full proof and not on the basis of probability [2, 3, 5].

Decisive basis in legal work insurance(GUV) is, that the assessment is not carried out for a profession determined or practiced last but as an

G. Kirchhoff (✉)
Institute for Assessment and Occupational Medicine, Munich, Germany
e-mail: info@zemba.de

C. Kirchhoff
Unfallchirurgische Klinik des Klinikums R.d.Isar der Technischen Universität München, Klinikum rechts der Isar, Technical University, Ismaninger Str. 22, 81675 Munich, Germany
e-mail: Chlodwig.kirchhoff@mri.tum.de

R. Kirchhoff
DEZEMBA-Deutsches Zentralinstitut für Begutachtungs- und Arbeitsmedizin, Institute for Assessment and Occupational Medicine, Munich, Germany

MEDEX Plus, Diessen-Riederau, Germany
e-mail: info@zemba.de

P. Biberthaler et al. (eds.), *Fractures of the Proximal Humerus*, Strategies in Fracture Treatments,
DOI 10.1007/978-3-319-20300-3_22

abstract decline in performance for the general labor market [6]. This is particularly often difficult to understand since one certain damage possibly represents an impairment influencing more strongly a profession practiced at the time of the event than in the general labor market. The professional impairment is discontinued and only the abstract damage has to be compensated. This is expressed with a MdE-value, i.e. a number which is used only at the assessment in the context of the statutory work insurance [6, 8].

Ludolph has built a MdE-table for damages of the upper extremities which counts on empirical values. You assume that the use-arm is rated just the same as the con-arm [5] (Table 22.1).

For determination of MdE-value clinical examination is required with determination of movement measures as well as motoric and neurological failures. A evaluation of specific professional conditions is not interesting [4, 5, 8].

Analogous to assessment of the results of a proximal humerus fracture in context of determination of the degree of handicap according to the seriously handicapped person law it is just usual to fix function deficits. Handicap is a condition against the rules differing from the norm which lasts more than 6 months and exceeds age corresponding measure. Therefore the anyway existing age corresponding changes cannot be evaluated in the form of arthrotic and degenerative changes in the shoulder [1, 2].

The tables to the assessment of the degree of handicap therefore contain an estimation space in which the function deficits are contained as a rule [1] (Table 22.2).

The sensibility failures and neurological deficits are not so precisely determined like in the case of the GUV-evaluation since they are not so important in everyday life [5].

The complete damage is not compensated in the personal accident insurance which is interpreted as a sum insurance. The sum insured at the time of conclusion of a contract is authoritative for the amount of compensation. Basis of the determination is the idea of the disability, namely the economic consequences as a result of the accident by a ever lasting impairment. The results of an accident must be asserted and proved at least within a year plus 3 months [2, 3]. Thus it can be avoided that that calculable long-term damages are excluded. The assessment is aligned with the provable function damages. One assumes in the schedule of compensation that shaft injuries can cause permanent consequences for example axis deviation, rotation, malpositions, varus and valgus position, shortening, prolongation as well as stable or unstable pseudarthrosis [3]. Scars, joint injuries with participation of the bones, ribbons and cartilage also have to be decided besides neurological and motorical deficits. The assessment is carried out as fractions of amount of the

Table 22.1 Malfunction of the upper extremity [4] modified by Kirchhoff R

Malfunction	MdE in %
Stiffening of a shoulder joint and bandolier in function position (30° forward-and side lifting and 30° inner rotation free	40
Stiffening of a shoulder joint in function position	30
Concentric movement restriction in a shoulder joint around the half	25
Movement restriction in a shoulder joint: Forward free-/side lifting of the arm to 90°, rotation free	20
Movement restriction in a shoulder joint: Forward free-/side lifting on the arm to 120°, rotation free	10
Total or part prosthetic substitute one or both shoulder joints with a free function	10
Movement restriction in an elbow joint (stretching/diffraction 0/30/90)	20
Movement restriction in an elbow joint (stretching/diffraction 0/30/120)	10
Abolition of the forearm turn into neutral 0-position	30
Abolition of the forearm turn in inwards turn as of 20°	25
Concentric movement restriction in the wrist around the half	15
Complete failure of the N. axillaris	30
Complete failure of an N. radialis in proximal section	30
Complete failure of an N. radialis in middle section	25
Complete failure of an N. radialis in distal section	20
Complete failure of an N. radialis and N. axillaris (the same appendage)	60

Table 22.2 GdB tables [1] modified by Kirchhoff R

Function deficit	GdB degree
Stiffening of the shoulder joint in a favorable position	30
Stiffening of the shoulder joint in an unfavorable position	40–50
Movement restriction of the shoulder joint, raise arm only around 120° in a corresponding qualified sense of the trick and spreading ability	10
Movement restriction of the shoulder joint, raise arm only around 90° in a corresponding qualified sense of the trick and spreading ability	20
Upper arm pseudarthrosis tight	20
Upper arm pseudarthrosis limp	40
Movement restriction of the elbow joint of stronger degree	20–30
Abolition of the forearm trick movability isolated in a middle pronation position	10
Abolition of the forearm trick movability isolated in an unfavorable position	20
Abolition of the forearm trick movability isolated in an extreme supination	30

Table 22.3 Fraction amount of moving deficits of the upper extremity – schedule of compensation [4–6] modified by Kirchhoff R

Movement size	Assessment
Arm increase to 120°	2/20 arm value
Arm increase to 90°	4/20 A
Arm increase to 60°	6/20 A
Shoulder joint ruin after head necrosis	5/10 A
Elbow joint stretching/diffraction 0-30-120 with forearm turn 45-0-45	5/20 A
Elbow joint stretching/diffraction 0-30-90 with forearm turn 45-0-45	7/20 A
Loss of the forearm turn	6/20 hand value
Upper arm pseudarthrosis tight	1/10 A
Upper arm pseudarthrosis unstable	3/10 A

determined extremity. This method makes the calculation of the compensation possible. So for example a loss 1/1 of a hand values 55 % of the sum insured or 1/1 loss of a leg values 40 % of the sum insured. So results of a proximal humerus fracture can be assessed following depending on the schedule of compensation [3, 4] (Table 22.3).

Table 22.4 Malfunction of the upper extremity and performance exclusions [2]

Malfunction	Performance exclusion
Arm increase to 120°	Over-brain-work
Arm increase to 90°	Work pre-holds into arm
Arm increase to 60°	Work about table standard
Forearm streching/-diffraction	Heavy lift/handbarrows of medium difficulty, constant load, Assembly work
Forearm turn	Manual activities
Sensitive failures	Injury danger

Furthermore compensation is also possible besides schedule of compensation in per cent in the private accident insurance (PUV) also for internal and psychic damages [3].

There are damage compensations at which it furthermore depends alone on the ability of function and capacity of an organ in an occupational activity. Inability to work has in the statutory pension insurance the same importance as discussed for the general labor market. Normally if a proximal humerus fracture is healed without complications, no relevant restriction has to be derived for activities on the general labor market. For the general labor market the original use arm also can be used as con-arm if there is made no particular requirement on skill and movability. This will never result to a full or partial pension in the statutory pension insurance [8, 10].

The relevance is quite different to the private occupational disablement insurance. The inability to work has to be examined in the learned profession here and for the BUZ insurance it particularly depends on the specific activity performed especially last. The relegation to other activities still has to be checked if necessary. The assessments like in the pension scheme also be applied to the determination of the inability to work. If healing with functional deficits resulted decision whether it is the use-arm or the con-arm is necessary. So performance exclusions result [2, 7, 8] (Table 22.4).

The determination is different to the inability to work. It has to be decided how far the resulting damage effects the specific professional workload.

It has to be checked which individual performances of the occupational activity can be performed no more or only limited. This determination requires an exact knowledge of the special job and the specific and individual activities carried out. This mostly can only be fixed out by an analysis of the workplace and analysis of the workflow. There are different degrees of the inability to work now in which these also can be insured. The most usual one is the inability to work of more than 50 % [2, 7, 8]. In this determination the restriction both the qualitative and the quantitative efficiency flow must be considered. In administrational professions it can be considered as rule that all functional deficits following proximal humerus fracture do not cause any restriction of more than 50 %. Also in all intellectual professions assumed that written work is still possible with the damaged extremity as well as the operation of a keyboard. A split-up of the individual performances is required into manual, organizational, logistical, communicative and educational segments as well as an separation of all other works to time approaches. The determination of the inability to work is problematic at employers, which are working alone in the enterprise. Here the case could occur that inability to work happens at a inability degree of below 50 % if by failure of essential segments which characterize the occupational activity, this job then can no longer be performed competitively [2].

In case of an accident and the resultant damage has happened in the traffic, sports or in the private area and for which a liability carrier exists, the acute consequences of the proximal humerus fracture on the one hand have to be considered and on the other hand all long term consequences. The acute consequences appear in the necessity of operative or conservative, stationary or outpatient treatment. The immobilization of a shoulder often leads to a stiffness up to frozen shoulder. This requires an intensive physiotherapy. Regularly it can be assumed, that at an uncomplicated healing course an inability to work time commercially lasts at least 3 months and this time period can itself be prolong at mobilization due to a stiffness also for 6–9 months at working persons especially if a chronic pain syndrome develops under circumstances in connection with a M. Sudeck [3, 4, 7, 8]. A tendency toward expansion of the inability to work times can be recognized with workers unlike employees educated academically. The time period of 100 % of disability to work is not defined legally in the health insurance. It is different at the private health insurance and the determination of the sickness daily allowance. It is demanded that the injured must be unable not to any part of the activity executed before the accident. This will have to be particularly negatively determined, when the damaged extremity for the mastering of the work does not have any outstanding function. The permanent consequences have to be assessed as well as in the case of the statutory pension insurance, the work inability insurance or the PUV in case of working persons [3, 5].

If permanent injuries have to be determined at persons no more working or pensioners, it depends on the restriction in the daily lifestyle. This contains the functional deficits which arise a practiced sporting activity, practiced secondary occupation or honorary activity from restrictions till now. This only can be concluded by an exact analysis of the individual segments. However, daily lifestyle contains the household of the damaged both among working persons as well as among pensioners so that a socalled housekeeping damage must be estimated [9].

Schulz-Borck/Pardey [9] say, that such damages of the housekeeping have to be included about a time factor. Basis is the recording of a socalled household type which includes how many persons the household contains, as how many children live in the household in which age and who from the parents is working. One assumes unlike earlier assessments of it that the activities contain not only the partners in the household but this also has to be applied to life partnerships. It is practice today at the same time that the household activities do not confine themselves to the female person in the household but also the companion or the other part at life partnerships of the same sex is tied into the household activity as well. This can cause that a damage decreases depending on the share of performance which is expected by the other companion. At the specification of the household

Table 22.5 Malfunction of the upper extremity [9] modified by Kirchhoff R

Activity	Shoulder stiffening (%)	Movement deficit arm up to the horizontal position (%)	Radial paralysis (%)
Obtaining	15	10	20
Diet Supply inventory	15	10	20
Washing the dishes	15	10	30
Cleaning	25	20	20
Laundry	20	20	25
Gardening	20	15	25
Housekeeping	0	0	0
Support of children	15	20	25
Detailed work	10	5	15
Complete handicap depending on household type in %	17–18	13–14	20

type also individual factors have to be taken into considering like this one whether it is an average household or a simple or elevated with broad eating supply, high cultural standard or also around one in which older people are looked after. All this requires an exact analysis of the circumstances which must cover the apartment/house, the facilities, the technical equipment, structural unusual features, care of plants and animals, garden, motor vehicles and tools as well as also the purchase, cleaning and the complete food supply. It has been successful to split the household activity up into some segments and to put the damages in order as well. However, an addition of the failures must not be carried out at multiple damages but only functional assignment. The functional deficits are taken more easy since more compensation possibilities consist in the household like in the acquisition economy [2, 9] (Table 22.5).

A week load in hours which refers to the handicap arises from the household type. The determined complete handicap can be determined and identified as a cash value in per cent value of the hour load.

The assessment of the acute damage has to be formed besides the determination of the permanent consequences if differently it is a no longer improvable condition. The time of the admission of the damage until the completion of the immobilization after a proximal humerus fracture has to be practically equated to an arm loss by Schulz-Borck/Pardey tables. This causes a housekeeping damage of 80–82 % depending on household type [9].

References

1. Federal Ministry of a health and social safeguarding supply medicine ordinance with the supply medical principles. Berlin. 2009.
2. Kirchhoff R, Kirchhoff G, Nguyen T, Kirchhoff Ch Insurance medicine. Stuttgart-NewYork: Thieme Publishing House; 2013 (submitted).
3. Lehmann R. Private casualty insurance bases. In: Ludolph E, editor. The accident man. Berlin/Heidelberg: Springer; 2013.
4. Ludolph E. Bemessungsempfehlungen for the private casualty insurance. In: Ludolph E, editor. The accident man. Berlin/Heidelberg: Springer; 2013.
5. Ludolph E. Proof demands and burden of proof. In: Ludolph E, editor. The accident man. Berlin/Heidelberg: Springer; 2013.
6. Ludolph E. Statutory accident insurance. In: Ludolph E, editor. The accident man. Berlin/Heidelberg: Springer; 2013.
7. Mehrhoff E, Fritze E. The statutory accident insurance. In: Fritze E, editor. The medical assessment. Darmstadt: Steinkop; 2001.
8. Mehrtens G, Valentin H, Schönberger A. Work accident and occupational disease. Berlin: Erich Schmid; 1993.
9. Schulz-Borck H, Pardey F. Der haushaltsführungsschaden. 7. Auflage. Karlsruhe: Versicherungswirtschaft GmbH; 2009.
10. Triebig G, Kentner MR. Arbeitsmedizin. Stuttgart: Gentner Publishing House; 2008.

Part VII

Complication Management

23 Complication Management Malunion/Non-union Proximal Humeral Fractures

Thomas R. Duquin and John W. Sperling

Introduction

Proximal humeral fractures are common injuries, especially in elderly and osteoporotic patients. The initial management can be operative or non-operative, depending on the fracture pattern and patient factors. The development of symptomatic non-union or malunion of proximal humeral fractures is rare, and can occur with both operative and non-operative treatment of the acute fracture. The non-union rate following proximal humeral fractures has been reported to be from 1 to 20 % in the literature [1–3]. A recent systematic review of non-operative management of proximal humerus fractures revealed a radiographic union rate of 98 % [1]. Malunions are much more common with a 13 % rate of varus malunion reported in the same study. However, malunions are frequently asymptomatic or well-tolerated especially in the elderly, a low demand population that typically suffers from these injuries. Similar rates of non-union and malunion have been reported with operative management of proximal humerus fractures [4]

T.R. Duquin, MD (✉)
Department of Orthopaedic Surgery, University at Buffalo, 462 Grider Street, Buffalo, NY 14215, USA
e-mail: tduquin@ecmc.edu

J.W. Sperling, MD
Department of Orthopaedic Surgery, Mayo Clinic, Rochester, MN, USA
e-mail: sperling.john@mayo.edu

A non-union of the proximal humerus is defined as a lack of healing after nine months of non-operative management or a lack of radiograph progression of healing over 3 months. Non-union most frequently occurs at the surgical neck, but can involve the greater or lesser tuberosity as well. The development of a non-union can be associated with patient factors such as poor bone quality, medical comorbidities, smoking or noncompliance with treatment. The fracture pattern and management can also result in impaired healing potential. Metaphyseal comminution and greater than 33 % translation of the surgical neck fracture have been shown to significantly increase rates of non-union [2]. Treatment modalities, such as hanging casts, early mobilization and devascularization due to soft tissue stripping in open reduction and internal fixation, have been identified as contributors to non-union of the proximal humerus.

Proximal humeral malunions are defined as greater than 45° of angulation or 1 cm of displacement according to the Neer classification. The importance of the greater tuberosity alignment in rotator cuff function and avoiding impingement on the acromion has led most to use a more stringent 5 mm of displacement when treating the greater tuberosity fracture. The management of complex proximal humeral fractures in the elderly often involves benign neglect resulting in the development of malunion. In these patients there is often a functional loss of

P. Biberthaler et al. (eds.), *Fractures of the Proximal Humerus*, Strategies in Fracture Treatments,
DOI 10.1007/978-3-319-20300-3_23

overhead activity and strength that is generally well-tolerated in the low demand population. In younger and more active patients the functional limitations and pain can be debilitating. The development of the initial treatment plan for a proximal humeral fracture should include a detailed discussion with the patient and family regarding the daily activities and functional goals of the patient.

Clinical Presentation/Evaluation

Patients with proximal humeral non-union or malunion present with complaints of both pain and limited function. They often report minimal or no improvement from the time of the initial injury, and can often be frustrated with the prolonged course of treatment without success. Due to the significant morbidity we recommend close evaluation and early intervention if patients demonstrate signs of a non-union or malunion.

Non-union of the proximal humerus results in limited range of motion, pain and weakness that is frequently debilitating and not generally well-tolerated. A detailed history is important in the assessment of patients with non-union. Identifying risk factors that contributed to the non-union can be important in preventing further treatment failures. The initial fracture type and treatment, as well as medical comorbidities, medications and social history, are important to investigate. The presence of an undiagnosed infection or metabolic disorder should be suspected in every patient who presents with a non-union. Often these conditions can be identified following a detailed history and confirmed using laboratory tests.

Malunions often are not associated with medical comorbidities, but can be the result of inappropriate initial fracture management, insufficient strength of fixation or patient non-compliance. A detailed history is important to clearly identify the patient's limitations and complaints to determine if the malunion is the source of the problem. The most common complaint following a malunion is limited range of motion and pain due to impingement of the displaced tuberosity on the acromion or glenoid depending on the direction of the displacement. Some patients with symptomatic malunions may have relatively well-preserved range of motion, but weakness associated with the disadvantaged pull of the rotator cuff muscles.

Physical Examination

The initial examination should involve simple observation of the patient's general health, function and ability to ambulate with or without the need for upper extremity assistance. Inspection of the shoulder includes assessment for deformity, muscle atrophy, skin break down and signs of infection. The determination of active and passive range of shoulder motion is important in determining the etiology of the patient's complaints. Patients with a non-union will frequently have very limited active range of motion with painful, but relatively well-preserved passive range. Those with malunions often have limitations and pain with both active and passive range of motion. A detailed assessment of the upper extremity muscle strength, as well as a thorough neurologic examination, is an essential part of the physical examination. Deltoid and rotator cuff function can often be difficult to assess due to pain and limited function, and in circumstances where there is suspected nerve injury electromyography and nerve conduction, studies are helpful diagnostic tools.

Radiographic Studies

The initial assessment should include AP, axillary and scapular-y radiographs of the shoulder. In certain circumstances the use of internal or external rotation views may add additional information regarding the presence of a malunion or non-union. A CT scan is helpful if there is a question as to the presence of healing or bridging callous in a suspected non-union. CT scans are also important in the characterization of a malunion which is essential prior to proceeding with surgical intervention. An MRI is often of limited value

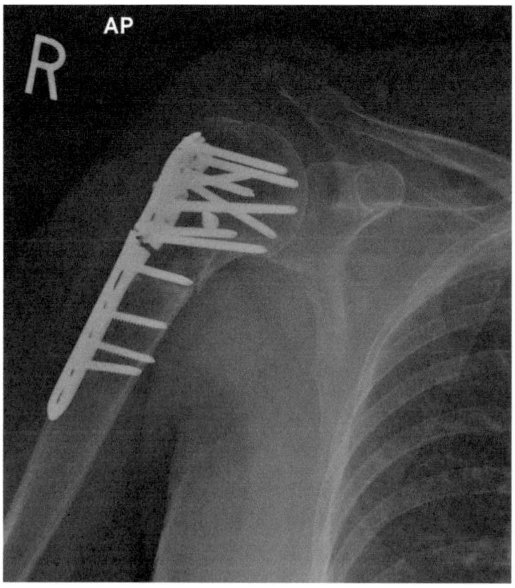

Fig. 23.1 Radiograph of 56 year-old female 1 year after open reduction and internal fixation of proximal humerus fracture with a surgical neck nonunion and a broken proximal humeral locking plate

in the assessment of a non-union or malunion unless there is a suspected pathologic fracture or associated soft tissue pathology such as rotator cuff or labral tears. In a recent study of MRI findings at the time of injury and at one year follow up after proximal humerus fractures, there were full thickness rotator cuff tears in 5 and 11 % of patients respectively [5]. Other studies such as bone scans or tagged white blood cell scans can be useful in rare occasions (Fig. 23.1).

Laboratory Studies

It has been well-documented that metabolic or endocrine disorders can contribute to fracture non-union. The rate of metabolic or endocrine abnormalities in patients with non-union and without inappropriate management or technical error has been reported to be nearly 85 % [6]. Blood and urine tests to identify abnormalities in vitamin, mineral or hormonal levels should be performed in patients with suspected metabolic disorders. The most common problems encountered are vitamin D deficiency and abnormal thyroid function. Often referral to an endocrinologist is employed if any abnormalities are suspected.

In patients with prior surgery an infection should always be suspected as the etiology of the non-union. Laboratory values have shown variable ability to detect infections in shoulder surgery [7]. However, basic screening blood work including a CBC with differential, ESR and C-reactive protein should be performed. Aspiration and culture is the gold standard for patients with a suspected infected non-union. Proprionbacterium acnes has been identified as a common pathogen in shoulder surgery, which requires cultures to be held for extended periods of time (2–3 weeks) to rule out infection.

Treatment

The treatment of proximal humeral non-union or malunion can vary depending on multiple factors, including degree of deformity, bone quality and patient comorbidities. In young, active patients with good bone stock options that reconstruct, the native articulation, such as open reduction and internal fixation or osteotomy, is preferred. However, these options in the elderly low-demand patient with poor bone quality are less appealing, and typically joint replacement options have more reliable outcomes.

Non-union

The management of a non-union depends on the quality of the available bone and the type of non-union. Classification of the non-union as atrophic or hypertrophic can help identify the factors that contributed to the failure to heal, and therefore suggest how to treat the cause of the non-union. In atrophic non-unions the etiology is a lack of biologic response to generate a fracture callous, and most commonly, is due to poor blood supply. In contrast, the hypertrophic non-union has all the biology needed to heal the fracture, but inadequate stability to allow for solid union. The treatment of an atrophic nonunion should include attempts at improving the biologic healing capacity of the fracture or joint arthroplasty options. Hypertrophic non-unions require rigid fixation, and often will have adequate bone stock that makes joint replacement less likely.

In cases where there is adequate bone stock in the humeral head and no evidence of arthritic changes, open reduction and internal fixation has historically had variable results. Multiple techniques have been employed, including conventional plate and screw fixation, intramedullary rods and fixed angle devices. The use of intramedullary fixation with a tension band construct originally showed high rates of healing in a small series by Neer [8]. However, all of the patients required reoperation due to stiffness and painful hardware, and subsequent attempts to reproduce the results in the original series by Neer have been met with high rates of failure [9]. Recent series using fixed-angle plate constructs with structural bone grafting using a fibular allograft or iliac crest have demonstrated healing rates of 90–95 % and improved clinical outcome scores [10, 11]. The author's preferred treatment for non-unions with good bone stock and no evidence of avascular necrosis or arthritis is open reduction and internal fixation with a proximal humeral locking plate with an intramedullary fibular allograft strut (Fig. 23.2a, b).

Non-unions that have severe cavitation of the humeral head, advanced osteoporosis, avascular necrosis or glenohumeral arthritic changes are contraindications to attempted fixation and bone grafting. In these instances joint replacement, consisting of hemiarthroplasty, total shoulder arthroplasty or reverse shoulder arthroplasty, is the preferred treatment. Traditionally hemiarthroplasty has been the most common joint replacement for the treatment of proximal humeral non-unions. Hemiarthroplasty for proximal humeral non-union is a very challenging procedure due to both bone and soft tissue compromise. Multiple studies have demonstrated improvement in pain scores, but limitation in function outcomes with high rates of

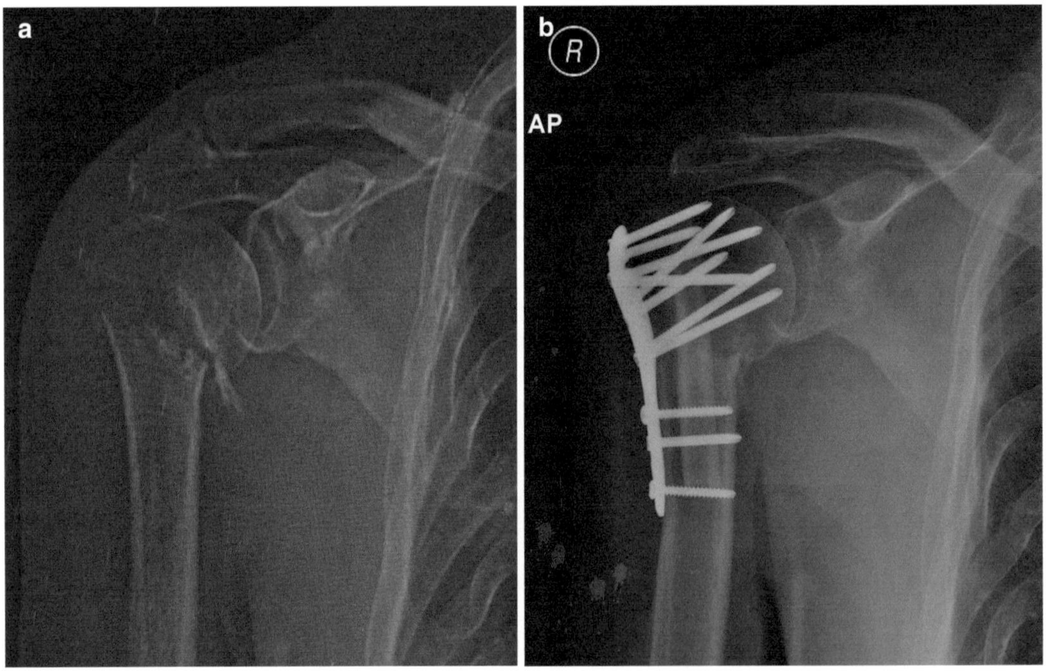

Fig. 23.2 (**a**) Radiograph of a 60 year-old male with non-union of a surgical neck fracture of the proximal humerus with no evidence of glenohumeral arthritic changes or rotator cuff pathology. (**b**) Radiograph 6 months following open reduction and internal fixation with fibular allograft strut and proximal humeral locking plate. Radiographs demonstrate healing of the proximal humeral fracture non-union and no evidence of avascular necrosis or arthritic changes

component malposition and tuberosity malunion, non-union or resorption [12, 13]. Despite improved implant design, fixation techniques and bone grafting, the rates of tuberosity complications are still high. As a result of the difficulties with tuberosity healing, interest has developed in the use of reverse total shoulder arthroplasty for the treatment of proximal humeral nonunions [14]. There are still only small series and limited evidence to support the use of the reverse, and further study is still needed to determine if the results are superior to hemiarthroplasty. The author's preferred treatment currently is to use hemiarthroplasty for patients who are young or active, or who are not amenable to open reduction and internal fixation techniques. However, in the elderly or lower demand patient, we do use the reverse total shoulder replacement for proximal humeral non-unions (Figs. 23.3a, b and 23.4a, b).

Non-union treatment flow chart

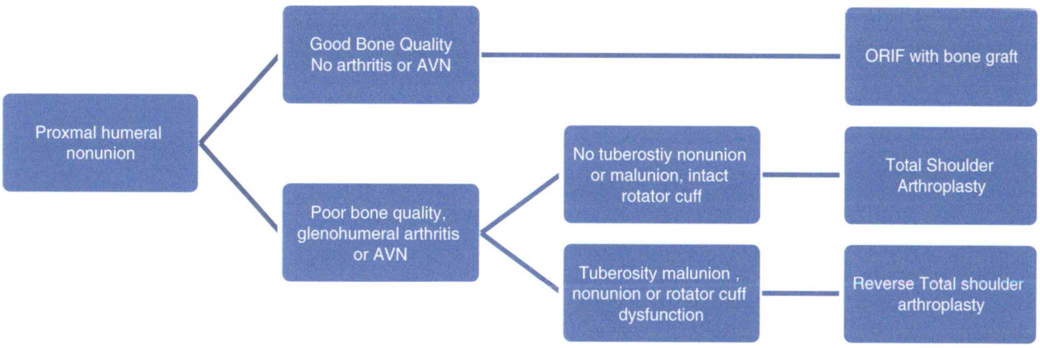

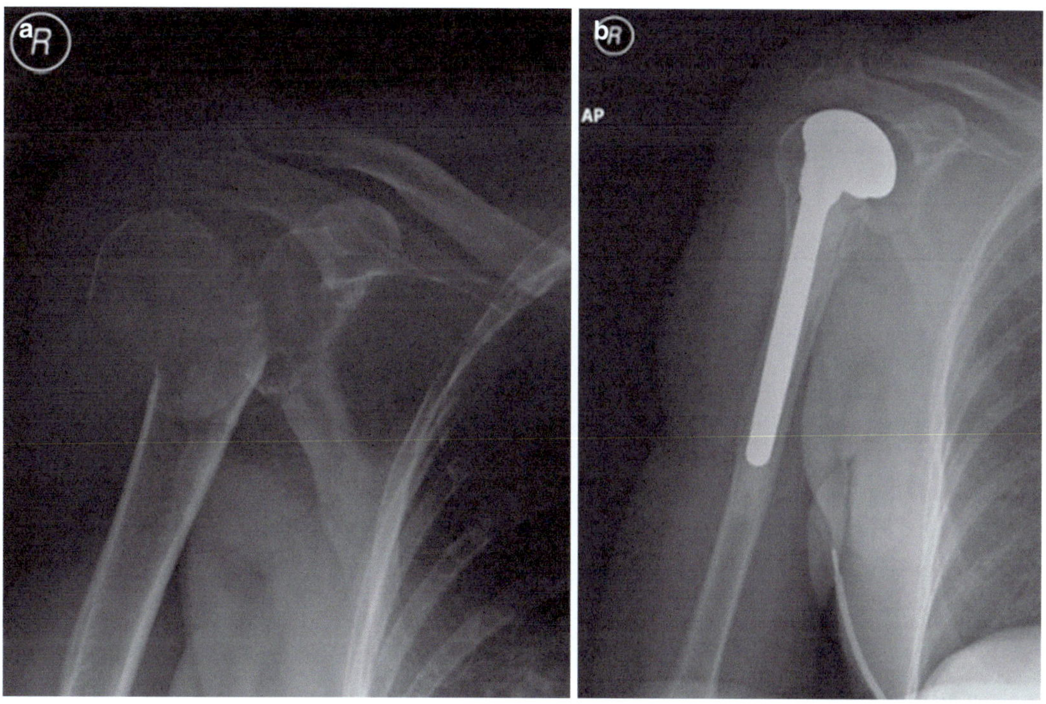

Fig. 23.3 (**a**) Radiograph of 65 year old female 4 months after 3 part proximal humerus fracture with nonunion of the surgical neck and tuberosity fractures. The patient had good bone stock and intact rotator cuff at time of surgery. (**b**) Radiograph 9 months after treatment with hemiarthroplasty demonstrating anatomic healing of the tuberosity fragment

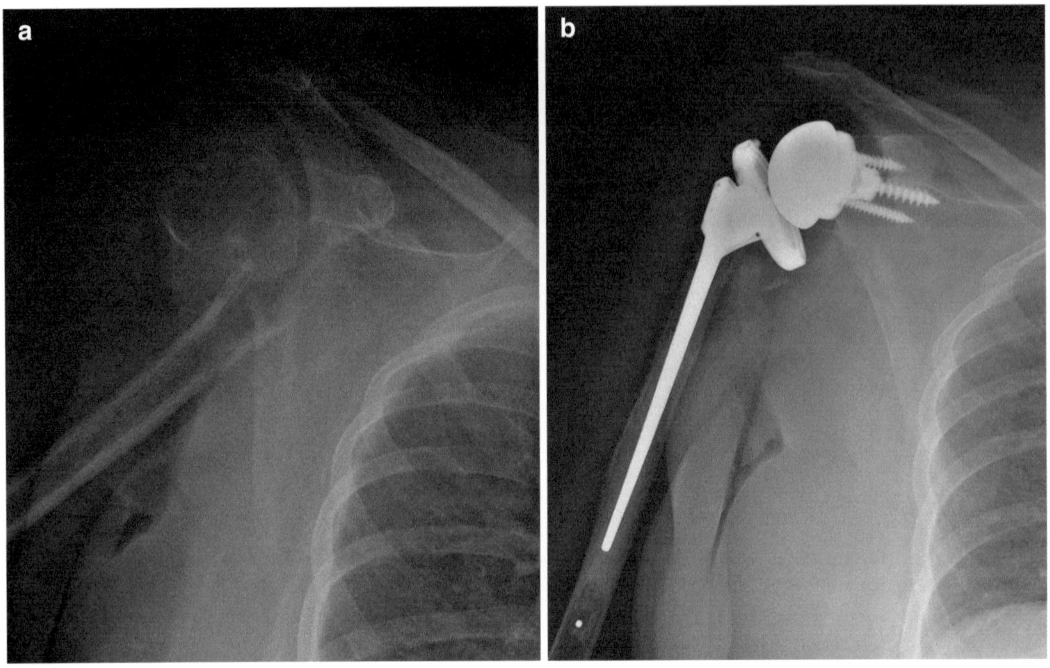

Fig. 23.4 (**a**) Pre-operative radiograph of a 64 year old female 1 year after proximal humeral fracture treated non-operatively. Patient had cavitation of humeral head with significant bone loss and osteoporosis at the time of surgery. (**b**) Radiograph on year after reverse total shoulder

Malunion

The treatment of proximal humeral malunions depends on multiple factors, including the type of deformity, as well as patient factors, such as bone quality and the presence of associated arthritic changes [15]. Procedures that preserve the native glenohumeral articulation including osteotomy, ostectomy, tuberoplasty or acromioplasty are preferred in the young and active population. Arthroscopic treatment of impingement or contractures that result from proximal humeral malunions has shown good results in small clinical series [16, 17]. A recent study by Ladermann et al. reported improved function and pain scores with good and excellent results in six of nine patients treated with arthroscopic tuberoplasty with detachment, and advancement, and repair of the rotator cuff [16]. In cases of varus malunions with more severe deformity, a valgus osteotomy of the proximal humerus is a treatment option. Benegas et al. demonstrated improvement in pain and functional range of motion with union in 5 of 5 patients treated with a valgus producing osteotomy of the proximal humerus [18]. Due to the small sample sizes and lack of controlled trials, there is no clear superiority of one technique over another, and each surgeon should use clinical judgment to determine the best treatment option for patients with milder deformity and no glenohumeral joint incongruence or arthritis (Fig. 23.5a, b).

In patients with advanced deformity, avascular necrosis or arthritic changes, joint replacement options are indicated. Arthroplasty for proximal humeral malunions can be challenging due to bone deformity and soft tissue contractures. The presence of soft tissue contractures, including the joint capsule and rotator cuff, result in significant difficulty with exposure and balancing of the joint. Mobilization of the rotator cuff, utilizing both articular and bursal releases, in addition to extensive capsular excision is often required to regain range of motion. In cases with signifi-

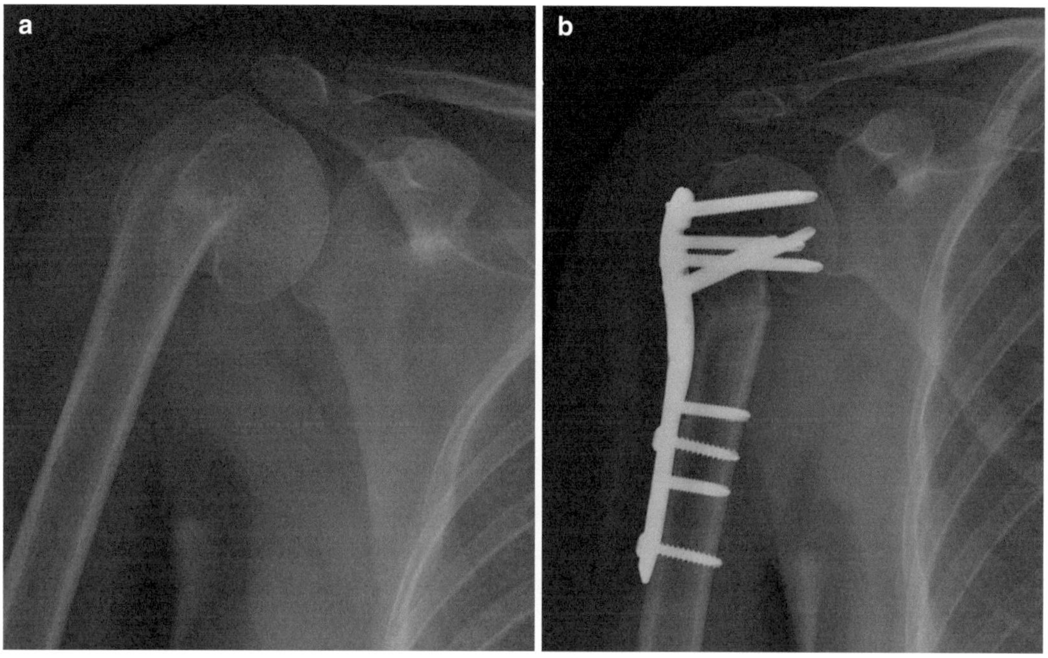

Fig. 23.5 (**a**) Radiograph of a 18 year-old female 6 months after proximal humerus fracture with varus malunion resulting in limited range of motion and pain. (**b**) Radiograph following valgus osteotomy of the proximal humerus resulting in improved range of motion and no pain

cant bone deformity that results in impingement or weakening of the rotator cuff leaver arm, an osteotomy may be needed to allow for implantation of a prosthesis. However, multiple studies have shown poor outcomes when an osteotomy is performed in conjunction with an anatomic unconstrained arthroplasty for proximal humeral malunion [19–22]. Every effort should be made to avoid tuberosity osteotomy, including modification of the humeral prosthesis to accommodate for deformity. The advent of new technology, including small humeral stems or resurfacing implants, has made this easier to accomplish (Fig. 23.6a, b).

Reported outcomes following anatomic shoulder arthroplasty for proximal humeral malunions have been variable in the literature. Most series have demonstrated improvement in pain and function, compared to the preoperative state, with high rates continued unsatisfactory outcome scores due to persistent limitation in function [19–22]. Better outcomes have been demonstrated in patients without distortion of the tuberosities and those with an acromiohumeral distance greater than 8 mm at follow up [22]. Poor prognostic fac tors include advanced age, prolonged duration of symptoms, rotator cuff pathology and severe tuberosity malunion requiring osteotomy [19–22]. In instances where there is no glenoid wear with intact cartilage, the use of hemiarthroplasty may be a reasonable option. However, total shoulder arthroplasty has been shown to have less pain and lower reoperation rates than hemiarthroplasty for patients with degenerative arthritis, and similar results would be expected in the case of humeral malunions [23].

The role of reverse total shoulder arthroplasty is still unclear. In circumstances where there is associated rotator cuff pathology or severe deformity that would require tuberosity osteotomy, the reverse total shoulder may provide a more reliable result. Additional study is still needed to determine if reverse total shoulder designs outperform standard anatomic arthroplasty for the treatment of proximal humeral malunions.

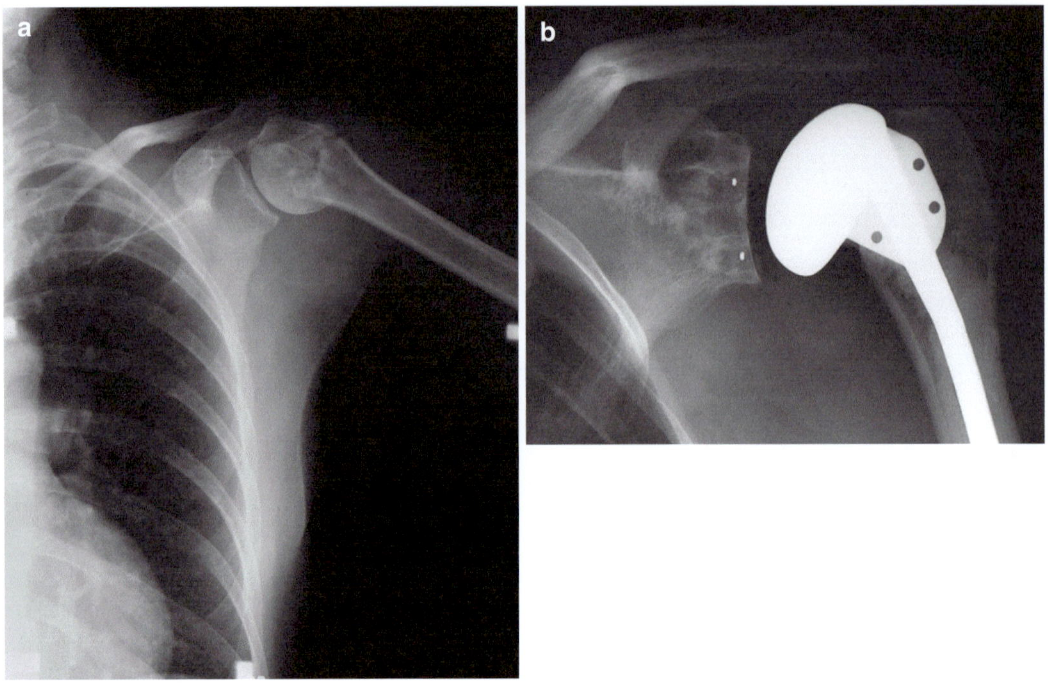

Fig. 23.6 (**a**) Radiograph of a 58 year-old woman, 6 months following a three part proximal humerus fracture treated non-operatively with a nonunion of the surgical neck and malunion of the greater tuberosity. (**b**) Two-year follow-up radiograph showing a total shoulder replacement with bending of the humeral stem to accommodate the tuberosity malunion at the time of surgery. The surgical neck nonunion has gone on to union and there is no evidence of loosening or displacement of the humeral or glenoid components

Malunion treatment flow chart

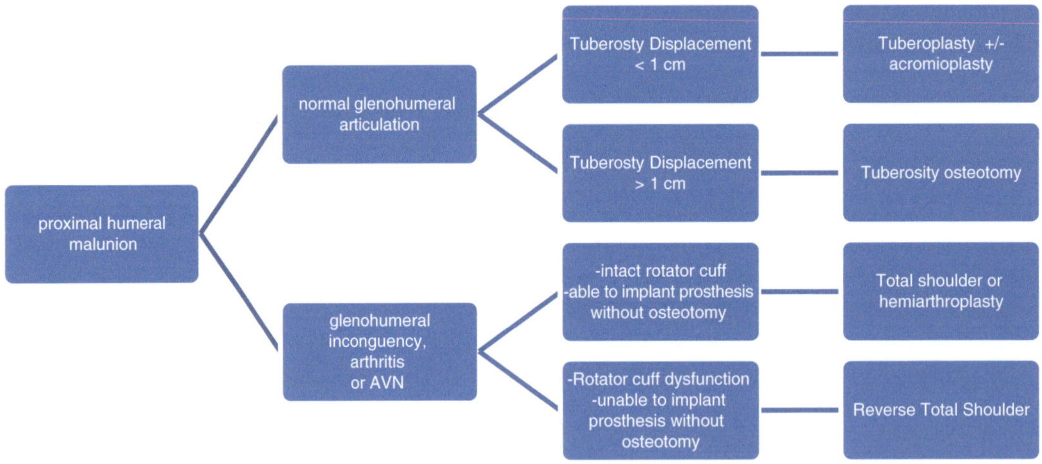

Summary

The sequelae of proximal humeral fractures, including fracture non-union and malunion, are relatively uncommon, but challenging to manage. A complete evaluation of these patients, including an investigation of the etiology, as well as the quality of the bone and soft tissues, will help to guide treatment. Multiple treatment options exist, including joint preservation techniques and arthroplasty options. Patients with good bone stock and no evidence of glenohumeral arthritis or avascular necrosis are good candidates for open reduction and internal fixation or osteotomy, while the presence of bone loss or articular pathology are indications for arthroplasty procedures. Limited data exists and good outcomes have been demonstrated in small series using all treatment options. Recent advances in surgical techniques and implants have shown promise in treating these challenging problems.

References

1. Iyengar JJ, Devcic Z, Sproul RC, Feeley BT. Nonoperative treatment of proximal humerus fractures: a systematic review. J Orthop Trauma. 2011;25(10):612–7.
2. Court-Brown CM, McQueen MM. Nonunions of the proximal humerus: their prevalence and functional outcome. J Trauma. 2008;64:1517–21.
3. Warner JJ, Coustouros JG, Gerber C. Fractures of the proximal humerus. In: Bucholz RW, Heckman JD, Court-Brown C, editors. Rockwood and Green's fractures in adults. 6th ed. Philadelphia: Lippincott, Williams and Wilkins; 2006. p. 1161–210.
4. Sudkamp N, et al. Open reduction and internal fixation of proximal humerus fractures with the use of the locking proximal humerus plate. J Bone Joint Surg. 2009;91:1320–8.
5. Fjalestad T, et al. Rotator cuff tears in proximal humeral fractures: an MRI cohort study in 76 patients. Arch Orthop Trauma Surg. 2010;130(5):575–81.
6. Brinker MR, O'Connor DP, Monla YT, Earthman T. Metabolic and endocrine abnormalities in patients with nonunions. J Orthop Trauma. 2007;21(8):557–70.
7. Dodson CC, et al. Propionibacterium acnes infection after shoulder arthroplasty: a diagnostic challenge. J Shoulder Elbow Surg. 2010;19(2):303–7.
8. Neer II CS. Displaced proximal humeral fractures. Part II. Treatment of three-part and four-part displacements. J Bone Joint Surg Am. 1970;52A:1090.
9. Nayak NK, Schickendantz MS, Regan WD, et al. Operative treatment of nonunion of surgical neck fractures of the humerus. Clin Orthop Relat Res. 1995;313:200–5.
10. Badman BL, Mighell M, Kalandiak S, Prasarn M. Proximal humeral nonunions treated with fixed-angle locked plating and an intramedullary strut allograft. J Orthop Trauma. 2009;23(3):173–9.
11. Walch G, Badet R, Nove-Josserand L, et al. Nonunions of the surgical neck of the humerus: surgical treatment with an intramedullary bone peg, internal fixation, and cancellous bone grafting. J Shoulder Elbow Surg. 1996;5:161–8.
12. Antuna SA, Sperling JW, Sanchez-Sotolo J, et al. Shoulder arthroplasty for proximal humeral nonunions. J Shoulder Elbow Surg. 2002;11:114–21.
13. Duquin TR, Jacobson JA, Sanchez-Sotelo J, Sperling JW, Cofield RH. Unconstrained shoulder arthroplasty for treatment of proximal humeral nonunions. J Bone Joint Surg Am. 2012;94:1610–7.
14. Martin TG, Iannotti JP. Reverse total shoulder arthroplasty for acute fractures and failed management after proximal humeral fractures. Orthop Clin North Am. 2008;39:45–457.
15. Beredjiklian PK, Iannotti JP, Norris TR, Williams GR. Operative treatment of malunion of a fracture of the proximal aspect of the humerus. J Bone Joint Surg Am. 1998;80:1484–97.
16. Ladermann A, Denard PJ, Burkhart SS. Arthroscopic management of proximal humerus malunion with tuberoplasty and rotator cuff retensioning. Arthroscopy. 2012;28(9):1220–9.
17. Kim SH, Ha KI. Arthroscopic treatment of symptomatic shoulders with minimally displaced greater tuberosity fracture. Arthroscopy. 2000;16:695–700.
18. Benegas E, Zoppi Filho A, Ferreira Filho AA, Ferreira Neto AA, Negri JH, Prada FS, et al. Surgical treatment of varus malunion of the proximal humerus with valgus osteotomy. J Shoulder Elbow Surg. 2007;16:55–9.
19. Antuna SA, Sperling JW, Sanchez-Sotelo J, Cofield RH. Shoulder arthroplasty for proximal humeral malunions: long-term results. J Shoulder Elbow Surg. 2002;11:122–9.
20. Boileau P, Chuinard C, Le Huec JC, Walch G, Trojani C. Proximal humerus fracture sequelae: impact of a new radiographic classification on arthroplasty. Clin Orthop Relat Res. 2006;442:121–30.
21. Boileau P, Trojani C, Walch G, Krishnan SG, Romeo A, Sinnerton R. Shoulder arthroplasty for the treatment of the sequelae of fractures of the proximal humerus. J Shoulder Elbow Surg. 2001;10:299–308.
22. Mansat P, Guity MR, Bellumore Y, Mansat M. Shoulder arthroplasty for late sequelae of proximal humeral fractures. J Shoulder Elbow Surg. 2004;13:305–12.
23. Radnay CS, et al. Total shoulder replacement compared with humeral head replacement for the treatment of primary glenohumeral osteoarthritis: a systematic review. J Shoulder Elbow Surg. 2007;16(4):396–402.

Complication Management: Stiffness

24

Ernst Wiedemann

Introduction

Any type of fracture of the humeral head irrespective of conservative or surgical therapy usually ends in some kind of restricted mobility of the shoulder joint in terms of stiffness of different extent. In the society of shoulder experts there exists no distinct differentiation between the degree of stiffness possibly considered as "normal" since it is related to the physiological processes necessary for healing in general, and the degree of stiffness exceeding these "normal" limits. Depending on the type of fracture and the chosen treatment, the injured shoulder is in general immobilised for a certain time period. In most cases physiotherapy and self-mobilisation is already initiated during this period of immobilisation and continued after immobilisation has been terminated. No later than after immobilisation had been terminated, but also sometimes already during the period of immobilisation, limited mobility of the shoulder in terms of stiffness occurs, since the treating shoulder specialist should have an idea of the range of motion of the shoulder joint during the entire time period after it had been fractured. If the range of motion of the affected shoulder joint differs too much from what is considered as "normal" at any point during the posttraumatic time phase, the shoulder joint is regarded as "stiff" in terms of restricted mobility associated with pain of different degree.

E. Wiedemann
Shoulder and Elbow Surgery,
OCM Clinic, Munich, Germany
e-mail: Ernst.Wiedemann@gmx.de

Definition

Stiffness of the shoulder joint is equivalent to a limitation in the passive range of motion. Taking the non-affected contralateral shoulder joint in account, the limitation in range of motion may be calculated as the difference in the range of motion of both sides. In these cases stiffness may even be expressed as percentage, e.g. passive external rotation might account for 60 % of the contralateral, non-affected side. Thus, the limitation in range of motion may be quantified independently from the actual range of motion of the opposite shoulder joint varying depending on training status, handedness, age, sex, as well as other factors influencing the motion of the shoulder joint. Some shoulder specialists do not regard the contralateral non-affected shoulder joint as possible reasonable benchmark. Consecutively, these colleagues calculate stiffness by comparing the passive range of motion of the injured shoulder to tables providing standard values.

Stiffness may affect only one or two directions of movement. If at least three directions of motion are involved, the restriction of movement in terms of stiffness is considered as global. At the initial stage of humeral head fractures such global

P. Biberthaler et al. (eds.), *Fractures of the Proximal Humerus*, Strategies in Fracture Treatments,
DOI 10.1007/978-3-319-20300-3_24

stiffness typically occurs. One year after treatment or even later, stiffness may concern only one or two directions of motion. Characteristically, these late occurring limitations of motion are in those directions initially affected by the distinct fracture fragments. For example in case of an isolated fracture of the major tuberosity late-onset stiffness affects abduction and external rotation, typically, whereas internal rotation stays within normal range. Multiple fragment humeral head fractures present with a higher tendency to develop global stiffness of the shoulder joint, also in late stages after fracture treatment.

Any limitation in active range of motion of an injured shoulder may envelop the actual symptom of stiffness, if the passive range of motion is also limited. Therefore it is of utmost importance to assess at any follow-up exam active as well as passive range of motion in at least three directions (see below). Any active range of motion being more restricted than passively assessed may not be explained by stiffness, however, but by a pseudo-paralysis or paralysis resulting from missing or displaced bony fragments, additional rotator cuff injuries or posttraumatic neurological disorders. Missing or displaced bony fragments may create stiffness by themselves as well, but this stiffness is always related to limitations in passive range of motion and does not lead to additional limitations in active range of motion.

Prevalence

As already described in the introduction any type of fracture of the humeral head usually ends in some kind of restricted mobility of the shoulder joint in terms of stiffness of different extent. There is no clear differentiation between "normal" and pathological stiffness. Nevertheless pathologic stiffness is considered as one of the most common complications following humeral head fractures. Contributing factors include the severity of the initial injury, duration of the immobilization, malunion of the articular surface, and patient non-compliance towards rehabilitation [14].

Pathology

In general several reasons for shoulder stiffness related to proximal humeral fractures exist. In comparison to the elbow joint, which is even more prone to posttraumatic stiffness, these are categorized in intra- or extraarticular reasons (see Table 24.1).

Intraarticular reasons for stiffness are first of all asperity of the articulating surfaces such as regional flat areas of the humeral head following posttraumatic necrosis or bony defects of the glenoid due to screw cut-out of locking plates, etc. However, stiffness of the shoulder joint is significantly more caused by surrounding soft tissue problems especially regarding the capsule. The capsule might show inflammatory changes, might be thickened, scarred, and rigid preventing movements in the corresponding direction. Especially the inferior portion of the capsule connecting the inferior glenoid and the inferior anatomical humeral neck may present a diameter of 1 cm or even more resulting in very effectively blocked elevation and rotation.

There are numerous extraarticular reasons for stiffness of the shoulder joint, such as scars and adhesions within the subacromial and subdeltoid space. For fractures involving the minor tuberosity scar formation and adhesions between the posterior portion of the short flexor muscles originating from the tip of the coracoid and the anterior surface of the subscapularis muscle are quite typical. In addition, the superior surface of the coracoid is covered by the coracohumeral ligament spreading out into the rotator cuff interval. In this context Mengiardi et al. [9] reported

Table 24.1 Reasons for stiffness

Intraarticular	Extraarticular
Asperity of articulating surfaces (humeral head/glenoid)	Adhesions in subacromial space
Rigid capsule	Adhesions in subcoracoidal space
	Tight coracohumeral ligament
	Non-anatomic healing of fragments
	Atrophy, fatty degeneration, and rigidity of rotator cuff muscles

on a 59 % sensitivity and a 95 % specificity in patients suffering from a frozen shoulder syndrome in case the coracohumeral ligament reached a diameter greater than 4 mm, nicely demonstrated on sagittal MR images. In conclusion the described high specificity of a thickened coracohumeral ligament might presumably be true also for cases of posttraumatic shoulder joint stiffness.

In case a more or less dislocated fracture of the greater or minor tuberosity occurs this fracture might not necessarily heal physiologically in its original anatomical position.

As long as the dislocated fragments are within the course of the force vector of the respective tuberosity, only active motion exerted by that tuberosity is limited, but does not influence the passive range of motion. A typical example is the case of a formally dislocated fracture of the greater tuberosity being healed but not in its correct or adequate anatomical position but distinctly medially dislocated in refer to its original anatomy however still connected to the humeral head.

The scenario changes quite dramatically if the fragment is displaced in an inferior direction meaning that the major or minor tuberosity is healed in a non-anatomical position inferior to the surgical neck of the proximal humerus. Any other but anatomic positioning of the tuberosities is disadvantageous since the malpositioning does not only limit rotation but especially elevation due to the passive adductive force deriving from the tuberosity displaced in this way.

The intra- as well as extraarticular reasons for posttraumatic stiffness discussed so far have the distinct advantage of being treatable in one way or the other. However, there exists another extraarticular reason for stiffness of great importance, but very difficult to treat regarding changes of the rotator cuff muscles and also the deltoid muscle in terms of atrophy, fatty degeneration, and rigidity. Up to date it is still not quite understood, why this type of stiffness occurs very often in case of humeral head fractures. The definitely necessary immobilisation of the shoulder in the course of fracture treatment certainly favours atrophy and/ or inactivity of these muscles although this explanation presents only a part of the truth, however. From several studies [2] in the literature it is known that up to 30 % of all cases with humeral head fractures cause dysfunction of the axillary nerve as well as of the plexus, which may be another explanation for the disorders of the muscles involved, and it may also explain why treatment takes longer than in simple proximal humeral fractures.

Clinical Findings

In order to assess patients suffering from posttraumatic stiffness, fracture anamnesis and the treatment performed have to be evaluated. For the further clinical evaluation active and passive range of motion in external and internal rotation, abduction and flexion need to be assessed. In addition, active and passive external and internal rotation in 90° abduction of both shoulders should be tested for comparison reasons.

However, it is not only important to be able to define the extent of limited motion, but also important to get an idea whether these limits are reached abruptly with hard impact or gradually with a smooth end-point. The latter mentioned type is better tolerated by the patients, possibly resulting from scars, which can resolve in the course of time and appropriate conservative treatment. Another point of utmost importance is the fact that stiffness mostly does not only stand for restricted passive range of motion, but also for a painful restriction of motion. In this context it should be mentioned that many patients tolerate a global restriction of their shoulder motion quite well as long as it is painless, but even moderate stiffness is not well tolerated, if associated with pain.

The shape of the humeral head as well as of the glenoid is easily evaluated on radiographs possibly performed in three directions in terms of true a.p., transscapular, and axial. If 90° abduction can not be performed by the patient due to pain, adequate axial radiographs can not be assessed so that the so-called Velpeau view presents an option. If these x-rays are not conclusive or if there are decisions to take regarding therapy, a ct scan is mandatory including 3D-reconstructions. If the bony anatomy turns out to be normal using these imaging techniques, a MR exam may be useful in order to assess the rotator cuff including the condition of the respective muscles. In addition, thickened parts of the capsule and ligaments may be identified especially if contrast agent is administered either in terms of intravenously or intraarticularly [9].

Treatment

The very best treatment of shoulder joint stiffness following humeral head fractures is to avoid it from the very beginning. However, this presents a challenge, since not all factors contributing to stiffness are known [14], and factors like the severity of the initial injury cannot be controlled. Another factor at least difficult to influence is the compliance of the patient regarding rehabilitation, physiotherapy and self-mobilisation. One very important factor and probably the only one easily managed by the treating surgeon, however, is the duration of immobilisation, also presenting the principal consideration provided by the AO (Arbeitsgemeinschaft Osteosynthesis) in their recommendations to reduce risk of stiffness [6]:

- immobilisation should be discarded as soon as possible in a progressive way beginning with eliminating the swath (circumferential bandage) during day time and encouraging pendulum exercises.
- sling-usage on a part-time basis as soon as appropriate.
- physical therapy should be considered for any patient with non-improving range of motion as expected.

However, a shortening of the duration of immobilisation always threatens the stability of the fracture. If the immobilisation phase is chosen too short, the risk of secondary fracture displacement increases, as well as the risk for pseudoarthrosis development. Therefore the treating surgeon has to create individual treating concepts with a distinct description of which movements in which direction are allowed at what time point always taking fracture stability in account. The individual treatment plan is the basis on which the physiotherapist as well as the patient himself has to rely on. The stability of the fracture needs to be re-evaluated every week, and treatment may accordingly be modified or even changed from conservative to operative treatment depending on the progress of fracture healing.

In case the prophylactic measures were not effective and the shoulder became stiff despite, the treatment to be performed depends on the underlying pathology described previously (see Table 24.1). However, even considerable amount of stiffness does not necessarily enforce surgery, as long as the patient still achieves improvement in motion. In this context the problem of differentiating stiffness due to underlying pathology from stiffness with chances of dissolving with time and patience needs to be mentioned. Nevertheless, there are also patients with failed conservative treatment, long-term residual pain and limited range of motion [1]. These individuals may benefit from operative intervention. There are no generally accepted rules on how to manage operative intervention of shoulder stiffness so that the author's preferred decision making in shoulder stiffness treatment is described:

- patients with proximal humeral fractures treated conservatively or surgically with intact articular surfaces and non-displaced fragments should undergo a minimum of 6 months of rehabilitation. In this context it should be mentioned that it is better evaluated if fragments are displaced in the area of the surgical neck of the proximal humerus compared to both tuberosities. Especially the major tuberosity is crucial, where displacement of more than 3 mm may be too much to be compensated for.
- considerable limitation of passive range of motion >20 % as compared to the opposite side or to normal values the patient is not willing to accept.
- no improvement in range of motion during 2 months despite of continued rehabilitation.

Regarding surgery, the role of arthroscopy is obviously more important regarding intraarticular pathologies, whereas extraarticular pathologies are traditionally treated by open surgery. Nowadays in the surgically treatment of shoulder stiffness several changes happened, since depending on the experience of the treating surgeon extraarticular pathologies may at least to a certain extent be also treated arthroscopically. This concept has been promoted for arthroscopic-assisted removal of hardware, especial following ORIF (open reduction internal fixation) using locking plates. Joint mobilisation under anaesthesia does not play a significant role regarding treatment, since a contracted, thickened capsule and severe extraarticular adhesions may not be disrupted by blunt force without putting the shoulder itself at risk for substantial damage [5].

Regarding bony anatomy of the proximal humerus special attention needs to be paid to the position of both tuberosities [14]. According to Moineau et al. [10] fracture sequelae type 1 may be treated conservatively as long as the patient tolerates the pain.

In case of persisting stiffness despite soft tissue release bony deformities within the articular surface have to be considered. Depending on the individual situation they should be solved by an arthroplastic procedure using either conventional stemmed, metaphyseal anchored stemless or even arthroscopically implanted partial surface prosthesis.

Arthroscopic capsulotomy was first described by Ogilvie-Harris et al. in 1995 [11] as treatment on cases of persisting frozen shoulder. Nowadays it presents the treatment of choice for cases with stiff and retracted capsule also posttraumatically and postoperatively [5]. This procedure is also possible to be performed if a prosthesis has been implanted before. Initially the arthroscope is placed in a standard posterior-superior portal. After release of the rotator interval, the anterior capsule is cut mid-way between its origin and insertion until the fibres of the subscapularis muscle are identified. In stiff shoulders, the anterior capsule may have a diameter of up to 8 mm [1].

During the capsule release the change of passive external rotation needs to be checked repeatedly. If external rotation does not improve during the performed release, it might be the case that the subscapularis tendon is scarred. Consecutively, its upper edge underneath the coracoid is cleared from the surrounding tissue as performed for arthroscopic repair of the subscapularis tendon. In addition, the anterior surface of the subscapularis muscle may be scarred to the short flexor muscles. Retracted subscapularis muscle may be treated by lengthening incision in the muculotendinous transition performed with caution not to damage the muscle and other soft tissue. It is however very rarely necessary. In case of persisting external rotation deficit despite extended anterior arthroscopial capsulotomy and subscapularis release surgery needs to be converted to an open procedure using an deltoideo-pectoral approach allowing for a release if scarring of the anterior surface of the subscapularis to the conjoint tendon is present.

For persisting loss of passive internal rotation even after the anterior capsular is released, the arthroscopy is moved to a standard anterior-superior portal and the posterior capsule is cut, also mid-way between its origin and insertion.

Regarding adhesions in the inferior axillary pouch it often can not be reached from the anterior as well as posterior standard portals. There are two solutions for this problem: in case the remaining inferior portion of the capsule is not too thick, the remaining bridge left after cutting the anterior as well as the posterior portion may be disrupted by gentle manipulation. If the remaining capsule is found to be too strong, however, an additional postero-inferior portal may be used to divide the remaining capsule. Radiofrequency electrical tool should be used for that purpose to be alarmed if coming closer to the axillary nerve. In this context a rule should be mentioned that the axillary nerve is accompanied by the subscapularis muscle forming a layer between the capsule and the nerve [13].

Though the arthroscopic technique has the advantage to be a less invasive approach, the capsulotomy may also be performed as open preferably using a deltoideo-pectoral approach following the guidelines for implantation of prostheses. After the subscapularis tendon has been divided or osteotomy of the minor tuberosity has been performed, the subscapularis muscle may be lifted medially. Consecutively, the anterior capsule needs to be cut in three planes in order to be able to remove it, at the anatomic neck of the humerus, at the glenoid close to the labrum, and at the inner border of the subscapularis muscle leaving a stump of 1 cm at the lateral edge of the subscapularis tendon in order to preserve the tendon as strong as possible. Thus the antero-inferior part of the capsule may be removed entirely. The resection may be continued to the posterior parts of the capsule by pulling the humeral head laterally creating a work window. However, the question whether a removal of the capsule is superior to only cutting it still remains unanswered.

Regarding extraarticular pathologies, signs of subacromial bursitis requires in most patients arthroscopic bursectomy. This is probably due to a non-outlet impingement caused by a contracted and stiff posterior capsule translating the center of rotation posteriorly and forces the humeral head in an upward direction during attempted elevation [12]. Additional scars and adhesions in the bursae around the humeral head may be removed arthroscopically as well. Also the coraco-humeral ligament can be assessed arthroscopically and divided starting at the tip of the coracoid. This procedure is part of the arthroscopic mobilisation of the suprapinatus tendon and performed on a regular basis. In case of subacromial impingement caused by a major tuberosity fracture healed in an unphysiological superior position, or by an acromion hooked at its tip additional subacromial bony decompression may be necessary.

Intra- or postoperatively an interscalene catheter should be implanted for postoperative pain management by the anesthesiologist and left for 2–4 days.

Immediately after arthroscopic or open capsular and scar release surgery postoperative rehabilitation should be started. According to the author's experience it is of crucial importance to release the mental block of the patients and to increase their motivation by demonstrating them the intraoperatively assessed range of motion. Physiotherapy and self-mobilisation concentrate on passive range of motion exercises. A shoulder cpm device assists to keep the intraoperatively assessed range of motion exercising only 15 min three to four times a day. Also cryotherapy devices can be helpful and used during this early phase of treatment to reduce pain and swelling.

Treatment Results

Regarding the timing of rehabilitation and physiotherapy, Koval and colleagues [7] studied the outcome of 104 patients with minimally displaced fractures of the humeral head. The authors describe at a mean follow-up of 41 months that patients who started a physical therapy program at a maximum of 2 weeks after trauma presented significantly better results in terms of forward flexion, external rotation, pain compared to those patients who started later. In this context the work of Hodgson et al. [4] should be mentioned focusing on two-part proximal humerus fractures who described similar findings. Patients with immobilisation times of more than 3 weeks presented with prolonged recovery times (2 years vs. 1 year).

Gerber and colleagues [3] studied the role of arthroscopy in treating shoulder stiffness in 45 patients. The authors found that 9 patients with idiopathic frozen shoulder presented better results than 21 cases of postoperative stiffness, whereas 15 out of these 21 posttraumatic patients were least favourable. Both groups revealed however no significant difference in comparing preoperative state and follow-up findings. All groups improved significantly and to a similar degree, whereas the final outcome was related to the initial degree of disability. Levy et al. [8] found quite similar results in a group of 21 posttraumatic patients with 14 patients suffering from a humeral head fracture. Elhassan et al. [1] however, published a study on 115 patients suffering from shoulder stiffness. The authors found no statistical significant difference between 41 patients with idiopathic and 26 patients with posttraumatic stiffness whereas only 7 patients suffered from a humeral head fracture. The Constant score was significantly lower in 48 patients suffering from postsurgical stiffness. In this series, 7 of the enrolled 115 patients (6 %) had recurrent shoulder stiffness requiring revision surgery.

Summary

Stiffness of the shoulder joint following fractures of the proximal humerus is a common problem. Correspondingly passive range of motion is limited in one or more directions whereas the reasons for stiffness can be divided in intra- as well as extraarticular pathologies. Intraarticular pathologies comprise of bony deformities of the humeral head or the glenoid, that may be treated by arthroplasty, as well as of thickening and retraction of the capsule possibly treated by arthroscopic or open capsulotomy or capsulectomy. Extra-articular pathologies comprise of scars and adhesions around the humeral head that may be treated by arthroscopic sectioning these adhesions. Scars and adhesions between the short flexor muscles and the subscapularis muscle are easier to remove via an open deltoideo-pectoral incision.

References

1. Elhassan B, Ozbaydar M, Massimini D, Higgins L, Warner JJ. Arthroscopic capsular release for refractory shoulder stiffness: a critical analysis of effectiveness in specific etiologies. J Shoulder Elbow Surg. 2010;19:580–7.
2. Fjalestad T, Hole M, Hovden IAH, Blücher J, Strømsøe K. Surgical treatment with an angular stable plate for complex displaced proximal humeral fractures in elderly patients: a randomized controlled trial. J Orthop Trauma. 2012;26:98–106.
3. Gerber C, Espinosa N, Perren TG. Arthroscopic treatment of shoulder stiffness. Clin Orthop Relat Res. 2004;390:119–28.
4. Hodgson SA, Mawson SJ, Saxton JM, Stanley D. Rehabilitation of two-part fractures of the neck of the humerus (two-year follow-up). J Shoulder Elbow Surg. 2007;16:143–5.
5. Holloway GB, Schenk T, Williams GR, Ramsey ML, Iannotti JP. Arthroscopic capsular release for the treatment of refractory postoperative or post-fracture shoulder stiffness. J Bone Joint Surg Am. 2004;83:1682–7.
6. Jaeger M, Leung F, Li W. Proximal humerus 11-A1.3 Nonoperative treatment. 2011. https://www2.aofoundation.org/wps/portal/surgery?showPage=redfix&bone=Humerus&segment=Proximal&classification=11A1.3&treatment&method=Nonoperative+treatment&implantstype&redfix_url=1301988687624#stepUnit-12.
7. Koval KJ, Gallagher MA, Marsicano JG, Cuomo F, McShinawy A, Zuckerman JD. Functional outcome after minimally displaced fractures of the proximal part of the humerus. J Bone Joint Surg Am. 1997;79:203–7.
8. Levy O, Webb M, Even T, Venkateswaran B, Funk L, Copeland SA. Arthroscopic capsular release for posttraumatic shoulder stiffness. J Shoulder Elbow Surg. 2008;17:410–3.
9. Mengiardi B, Pfirrmann CW, Gerber C, Hodler J, Zanetti M. Frozen shoulder: MR arthrographic findings. Radiology. 2004;233:486–92.
10. Moineau G, McClelland Jr WB, Trojani C, Rumian A, Walch G, Boileau P. Prognostic factors and limitations of anatomic shoulder arthroplasty for the treatment of posttraumatic cephalic collapse or necrosis (type-1 proximal humeral fracture sequelae). J Bone Joint Surg Am. 2012;23:2186–94.
11. Ogilvie-Harris DJ, Biggs DJ, Fitsialos DP, MacKay M. The resistant frozen shoulder. Manipulation versus arthroscopic release. Clin Orthop Relat Res. 1995;319:238–48.
12. Romeo AA, Loutzenheiser T, Rhee YG, Sidles JA, Harryman II DT, Matsen III FA. The humeroscapular motion interface. Clin Orthop Relat Res. 1998;350:120–7.
13. Warner JP, Allen A, Marks PH, Wong P. Arthroscopic release of post operative capsular contracture of the shoulder. J Bone Joint Surg Am. 1997;79:1151–87.
14. Wirth MA. Late sequelae of proximal humerus fractures. In: Wirth MA, editor. Proximal humerus fractures. Chicago: American Academy of Orthopaedic Surgeons; 2005. p. 49–55.

Complication Management (AVN)

25

Stefan Greiner

Introduction

Posttraumatic avascular necrosis of the humeral head (AVN) can lead to joint destruction with persistent pain and functional limitation. Fractures of the proximal humerus can proceed with disruption of the blood supply of the humeral head and then frequently lead to osteonecrosis and destruction of the humeral head's surface. The risk of AVN after proximal humeral fractures has been described to depend on the type of the fracture. After 3-part fractures according to Neer [14] the incidence has been described to be 3–14 % and after 4- part fractures from 13 up to 34 % [5]. If the congruency of the joint is lost, destruction of the entire joint may follow and surgical treatment is frequently necessary [16].

In general AVN may occur up to 5 years after the injury or the surgical intervention [5, 7]. Moreover, criticism on open reduction and internal fixation has often focused on the problem of extensile exposure and open fracture manipulation for implant positioning and its risk for iatrogenic damage of the humeral blood supply [6, 10, 12, 17, 18].

Implants with rigid fixation of head screws may potentially cause a cutout of sharp screws' tips with possible damage of the glenoid bone stock in the case of cephalic collapse due to AVN [15] (see Fig. 25.1a–c).

In a retrospective study on 48 patients treated with open reduction and angular stable plate fixation after proximal humeral fractures, our work group was able to show that after 1 year the incidence of AVN had been more than doubled at 45 months follow up [7]. The fact that AVN may occur also in the mid- and long-term follow-up shows the importance of a regular follow-up exceeding a 12 months period after fracture in order to react on developing necrosis of the humeral head, especially if the implant is left in place.

Management of AVN

Conservative and operative therapy of AVN is determined by several factors. The type of previous treatment (conservative/operative) and if surgical treatment was performed the type of the used implant (angular stable plate, intramedullary nail, screws, K-wires, etc.) and whether the implant is still in place are important factors to consider. Bedsides these factors it is important to know whether the fracture is healed in an anatomic or nearly anatomic position or if mal-or non-union is present.

In a retrospective study on 121 patients who sustained angular stable plating for proximal humeral fractures and were referred for further

S. Greiner
Shoulder and Elbow Surgery,
Sporthopaedicum, Regensburg, Germany
e-mail: greiner@sporthopaedicum.de

P. Biberthaler et al. (eds.), *Fractures of the Proximal Humerus*, Strategies in Fracture Treatments,
DOI 10.1007/978-3-319-20300-3_25

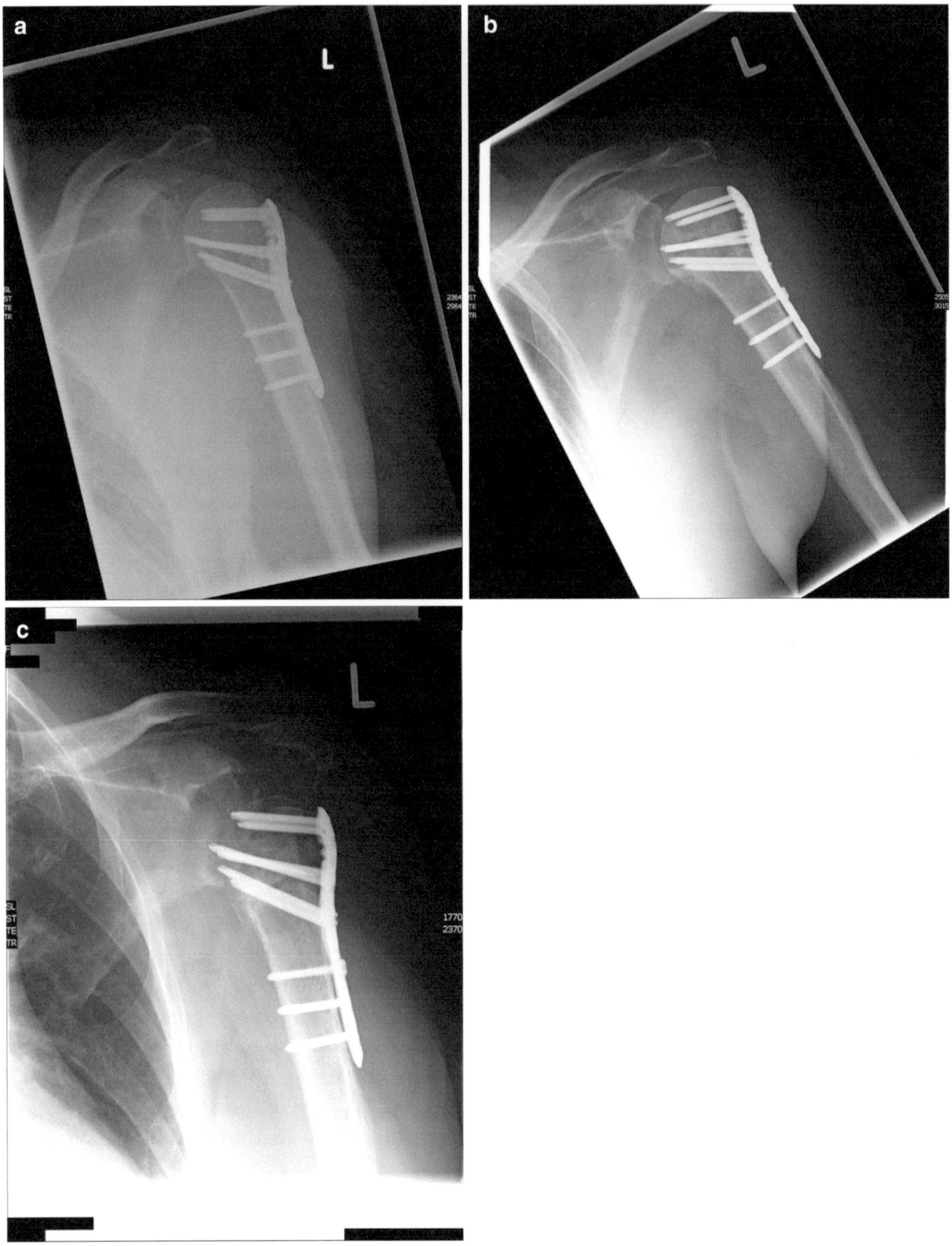

Fig. 25.1 (**a**) AP X-ray of a right shoulder after ORIF of a 3 part fracture of a 65 year old woman. (**b**) AP X-ray of the same patient 5 months later. Secondary screw perforation is already present. (**c**) AP X-ray at 10 months follow up with collapse of the humeral head and secondary glenoid erosion due to screw perforation

treatment due to complications, AVN was the major complication in 68 % (82 cases) [10]. The majority of cases were associated with other complications like non-union, mal-union or loss of reduction. Only in 33 cases AVN developed as result after an anatomic reduction. Thirty-seven of these cases were initially malreduced, 13 cases showed secondary loss of reduction and in 9 cases non-union was present whereas in 59 of these cases a secondary screw cut out was recognizable [10].

These fracture sequelae are best described using the Boileau classification system [1]. The authors were the first to report about a classification system of proximal humeral fracture sequelae. They divided the classification in two surgically important parts according to the need of performing an osteotomy of the greater tuberosity in case of an operative revision using an anatomic shoulder prosthesis was necessary. Accordingly, category 1 describes intra-capsular impacted fracture sequelae with a non- or only minimally displaced greater tuberosity and no need for an osteotomy including AVN and cephalic collapse of the humeral head. In contrast category 2 describes extra-capsular, non-impacted fragments with the need of performing an osteotomy or refixation of the greater tuberosity. Again both categories are divided in two types of fracture sequelae resulting in a total of four types as follows: type 1 shows a cephalic collapse or necrosis of the humeral head, for type 2 a locked dislocation or fracture dislocation (category 1) is described, type 3 shows a surgical non-union of the humeral neck and type 4 presents with a severe malunion of the tuberosity (category 4). In all of these cases AVN may be also associated. I did not find percentages in the literature.

Moreover in a recent study of Moineau et al. a sub-classification system of proximal humeral fracture sequelae type 1 was published. The sub-classification comprised either the absence (types 1A and 1B) or the presence (types 1C and 1D) of osseous deformation of the proximal humerus whereas type 1A represents a cephalic collapse of the proximal humerus, type 1B is associated with gleno-humeral osteoarthritis and type 1C comes along with valgus malunion and type 1D with varus malunion [13].

Conservative Therapy

Conservative therapy of an AVN may be indicated if the patient is not severely disabled due to the AVN or if there are risk factors present making surgical treatment impossible. Gerber et al. reviewed a total of 25 patients with posttraumatic AVN at a mean of 7.5 years after the fracture. Nineteen patients presented with a complete collapse of the humeral head and six cases with partial AVN. The subjective result was excellent or good in 67 % of the patients with partial AVN, whereas only 32 % good or excellent results were reported when the entire humeral head was involved [5].

If there has been previous operative treatment and the implant is left in place the risk of further damage of the glenoidal surface should be determined and taken into account when deciding for conservative treatment. If there is no such risk one should take into account that AVN may develop only in a part of the humeral head, leaving the patient with acceptable function and limited complaints. In any case, every patient should be closely followed with regular x-ray controls in order to determine whether the necrosis progresses or not.

Operative Therapy

Arthroscopy

Shoulder arthroscopy and arthroscopic assisted core decompression has been described for treating AVN caused by other factors than trauma [2, 4, 9]. Jost et al. treated ten patients with proximal humeral fractures and locking plate osteosynthesis suffering from persistent pain and beginning AVN along with a screw cut out with shoulder arthroscopy, capsular release and subacromial decompression along with total or partial hardware removal. In three of the ten cases the AVN progressed and secondary arthroplasty was indicated. None of the ten enrolled patients treated with shoulder arthroscopy showed significant improvement in shoulder function and forward flexion [10].

Partial/Total Implant Removal

Implant removal is mandatory if there is an AVN present with the implant still in place and there is a risk of damage of the glenoidal surface due to the implant.

Especially using locking screws along with locking plates or intramedullary nails a rapid damage may happen to the glenoidal bone stock. This complication of posttraumatic AVN is clearly related to the use of locking implants whereas the frequency of glenoidal destruction due to sharp perforation of screw heads was previously unknown [7, 10, 15].

Removal of the implant may be a sufficient therapy if the fracture shows signs of healing in an anatomic or nearly anatomic position and the AVN is only present in parts of the humeral head. However, it remains difficult to predict whether the AVN will stop and whether this treatment will be sufficient enough also in the longterm. In their series on patients having sustained locking plating for proximal humeral fractures Jost et al. performed partial implant removal in 16 cases and total hardware removal in 41 cases mainly because of a present AVN and/or screw cut-out. After partial hardware removal only three patients did not need any further revision surgery whereas seven patients needed secondary shoulder arthroplasty. After total hardware removal also 20/41 cases needed additional revision surgery with 17 patients being treated by secondary shoulder arthroplasty [10].

Resurfacing Arthroplasty

AVN is a condition which primarily involves only the humeral head as long as there is no involvement of the glenoid due to implant cut-out or due to loss of joint congruency and development of secondary osteoarthritis of the glenoid. Therefore resurfacing of the humeral head may be a sufficient treatment option. However, AVN should only be present in a part of the humeral head and anatomic healing of the proximal humerus should be recognizable. If AVN exceeds 8–37 % of the humeral head, depending on the used implant secure fixation may be difficult and a replacement of the humeral head should be taken into account [11]. Indication for resurfacing arthroplasty or any other kind of hemiarthroplasty should be strictly limited to patients without any changes of the glenoid since secondary glenoidal erosions remain the major complication leading to potential revision surgery [13].

If there is mal-union of the tuberosities, it is rather recommended to accept the malunion than to perform an osteotomy of the tuberosities.

Humeral Head Replacement, Total Shoulder Replacement

In case of involvement of the glenoidal surface with posttraumatic osteoarthritis or glenoidal damage due to the implants, total shoulder replacement is the best therapeutic option. Anatomic or minor malunion of the proximal humerus may lead to the best clinical results. The goal should always be to place the humeral head at the level of the greater tuberosity or slightly higher [3, 13] (see Fig. 25.2a, b). As in resurfacing, acceptance of the distorted anatomy seems to be more reliable than performing an osteotomy of the tuberosities. Although glenoidal replacement is described also in Literature without resection of the humeral head, exposure of the glenoid for implantation of a glenoid component seems to be more reliable after resecting the humeral head.

According to the literature, best results for anatomic unconstrained total shoulder replacement for fracture sequelae are achieved in patients with minor distortion of the anatomy and continuity of the tuberosities and the diaphysis [1]. This holds certainly also true in the case of associated posttraumatic AVN.

The outcome of anatomic total shoulder arthroplasty for the treatment of AVN after proximal humeral fractures has been described in the literature to be very good. In a retrospective study Moineau et al evaluated 55 patients with posttraumatic cephalic collapse or necrosis of the humeral head. Patients significantly improved in Constant Score Values from a mean of 32 points to 69 points. The subjective shoulder value was 81 and 93 % with the patients being satisfied or very satisfied with the procedure at a mean of 52 months after the operation [13]. Preoperative fatty infiltration of the rotator cuff and varus malunion of the proximal humerus showed to be negative predictive factors. These patients had a mean Constant Score 10 points lower in comparison to the rest of the group [13].

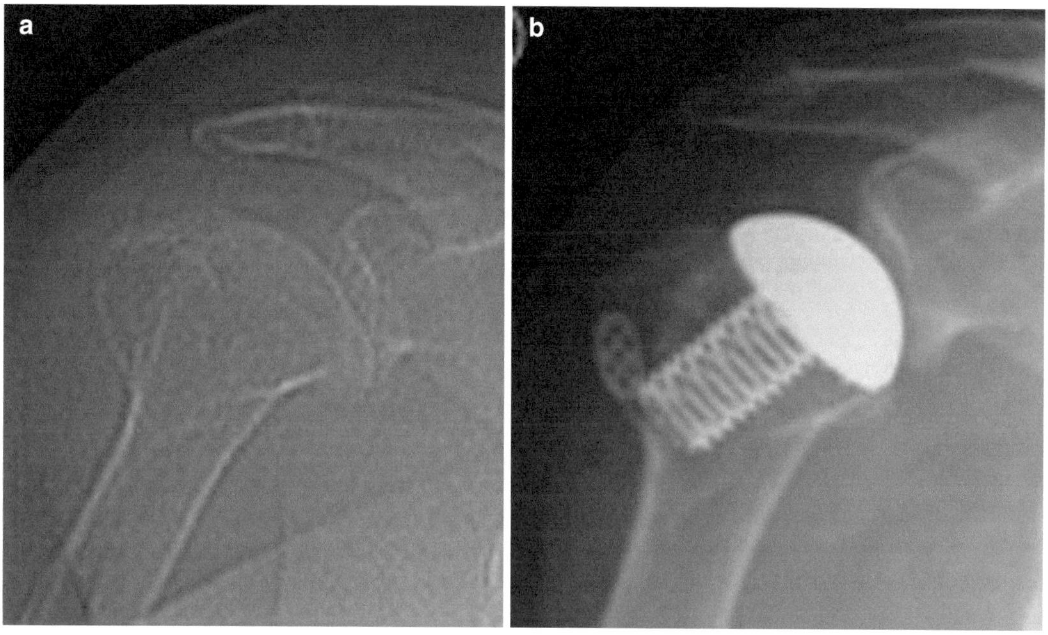

Fig. 25.2 (**a**) Type 1 fracture sequelae with posttraumatic cephalic collapse and limited anatomic distortion. (**b**) Humeral head replacement with Eclipse Prosthesis (Arthrex ®). Note that the top of the prosthetic head is placed slightly higher than the greater tuberosity

In posttraumatic cases with severe anatomic distortion and tuberosity malunion and/or discontinuity of the tuberosities and fatty infiltration of the rotator cuff reversed shoulder arthroplasty seems to be the most reliable option. In an own study on 32 patients with fracture sequelae after proximal humeral fractures we were able to treat 14 patients with an anatomic implant and 18 patients using a reversed implant. After a mean follow up of 24 months, both groups showed to be significantly improved with a Constant Score of 69 % in the anatomic group and 77 % in the reversed implant treated group [8].

Summary

AVN represents a major complication after proximal humeral fractures. Conservative treatment options are often limited. Operative treatment is challenging, especially since malunion, nonunion, soft tissue contracture and secondary glenoid erosion are frequently associated. Best results are achieved in anatomic shoulder replacement or resurfacing arthroplasty in cases with anatomic healing of the fracture. In cases with associated severe malunion or non-union of the tuberosities or degenerative cuff disease, reversed shoulder arthroplasty remains the more reliable option.

References

1. Boileau P, Trojani C, Chuinard C, Lehuec J-C, Walch G. Proximal humerus fracture sequelae. Clin Orthop Relat Res. 2006;442:121–30. doi:10.1097/01.blo.0000195679.87258.6e.
2. Chapman C, Mattern C, Levine WN. Arthroscopically assisted core decompression of the proximal humerus for avascular necrosis. Arthroscopy. 2004;20(9):1003–6. doi:10.1016/j.arthro.2004.07.003.
3. Demirhan M, Kilicoglu O, Altinel L, Eralp L, Akalin Y. Prognostic factors in prosthetic replacement for acute proximal humerus fractures. J Orthop Trauma. 2003;17(3):181–8; discussion 188–9.
4. Dines JS, Strauss EJ, Fealy S, Craig EV. Arthroscopic-assisted core decompression of the humeral head. Arthroscopy. 2007;23(1):103.e1–4. doi:10.1016/j.arthro.2006.07.011.
5. Gerber C, Hersche O, Berberat C. The clinical relevance of posttraumatic avascular necrosis of the humeral head. J Shoulder Elbow Surg. 1998;7(6):586–90.

6. Gerber C, Werner CML, Vienne P. Internal fixation of complex fractures of the proximal humerus. J Bone Joint Surg Br. 2004;86(6):848–55.
7. Greiner S, Kääb MJ, Haas NP, Bail HJ. Humeral head necrosis rate at mid-term follow-up after open reduction and angular stable plate fixation for proximal humeral fractures. Injury. 2009;40(2):186–91. doi:10.1016/j.injury.2008.05.030.
8. Greiner S, Schmidt C, Herrmann S, Perka C. Comparison of supply and time of implant used in the endoprosthetic treatment of proximal humeral fractures and their sequelae. Obere Extremität. 2012;704:210–5.
9. Hardy P, Decrette E, Jeanrot C, Colom A, Lortat-Jacob A, Benoit J. Arthroscopic treatment of bilateral humeral head osteonecrosis. Arthroscopy. 2000;16(3):332–5.
10. Jost B, Spross C, Grehn H, Gerber C. Locking plate fixation of fractures of the proximal humerus: analysis of complications, revision strategies and outcome. J Shoulder Elbow Surg. 2013;22(4):542–9. doi:10.1016/j.jse.2012.06.008.
11. Kasten P, Neubrech C, Raiss P, Nadorf J, Rickert M, Jakubowitz E. Humeral head resurfacing in central bone defects: in vitro stability of different implants with increasing defect size. J Orthop Res. 2012;30(8):1285–9. doi:10.1002/jor.22074.
12. Keener JD, Parsons BO, Flatow EL, Rogers K, Williams GR, Galatz LM. Outcomes after percutaneous reduction and fixation of proximal humeral fractures. J Shoulder Elbow Surg. 2007;16(3):330–8. doi:10.1016/j.jse.2006.09.006.
13. Moineau G, McClelland WB, Trojani C, Rumian A, Walch G, Boileau P. Prognostic factors and limitations of anatomic shoulder arthroplasty for the treatment of posttraumatic cephalic collapse or necrosis (type-1 proximal humeral fracture sequelae). J Bone Joint Surg. 2012;94(23):2186–94. doi:10.2106/JBJS.J.00412.
14. Neer CS. Displaced proximal humeral fractures. I. Classification and evaluation. J Bone Joint Surg Am. 1970;52(6):1077–89.
15. Owsley KC, Gorczyca JT. Fracture displacement and screw cutout after open reduction and locked plate fixation of proximal humeral fractures [corrected]. J Bone Joint Surg. 2008;90(2):233–40. doi:10.2106/JBJS.F.01351.
16. Raiss P, Kasten P, Baumann F, Moser M, Rickert M, Loew M. Treatment of osteonecrosis of the humeral head with cementless surface replacement arthroplasty. J Bone Joint Surg. 2009;91(2):340–9. doi:10.2106/JBJS.H.00560.
17. Schai P, Imhoff A, Preiss S. Comminuted humeral head fractures: a multicenter analysis. J Shoulder Elbow Surg. 1995;4(5):319–30.
18. Zyto K, Ahrengart L, Sperber A, Törnkvist H. Treatment of displaced proximal humeral fractures in elderly patients. J Bone Joint Surg Br. 1997;79(3):412–7.

Management of Vascular Lesions in Shoulder Trauma

26

Christian Reeps and Hans-Henning Eckstein

Introduction

Direct injuries or – far more often – concomitant injuries of the shoulder-arm-vessels close to the trunk (subclavian artery, axillary artery, proximal brachial artery) as complications of fractures or luxations near the shoulder joint are generally rather rare, due to the shielding bone and soft tissue mantle. Nevertheless, especially in case of severe and complex shoulder trauma the attending surgeon in particular should be always aware of vascular injuries in the area of the shoulder girdle, even if definitive diagnosis of these concomitant injuries is less frequent. However, in case of the potential consequences of vascular injuries on diagnostics, therapy and time management are enormous regarding the patients' treatment, as these may have a substantial impact on limb salvage and functionality or even survival.

Epidemiology

The true incidence of neurovascular injuries in case of trauma of the shoulder girdle is unknown. Penetrating sharp injuries due to violence are reported for the US [1, 2] & war zones [3] in 80–90 % as the predominant cause for vascular trauma of the upper extremities. In contrast, penetrating lesions of the arteries of the shoulder girdle and the proximal upper extremities are less common in Europe with an incidence of approx. 60 %. Comparably, closed concomitant vascular injuries as a consequence of blunt shoulder trauma e.g. by industrial or traffic accidents (40 %) are more common [4]. Thereby, central large vessels as subclavian artery, axillary artery and proximal brachial artery typically are less often affected than the more peripheral arteries of the arm and forearm. Naturally large central vessels lacerations are predominantly found in association with high speed or high energetic trauma, especially in multiple trauma patients with complex multiple injuries of the shoulder girdle (e.g. thoracoscapular dislocation). Then arterial or venous injuries are quite often combined with neural injuries such as the plexus and are accompanied with an considerable amputation rate [5]. In contrast, in isolated fractures or luxations injuries to the central arteries close to the trunk are extremely rare, however, with potentially fatal consequences for the patients. According to case studies, they occur in approx. 1 % of all dislocated fractures and/or luxations of the clavicle, the glenohumeral joint and the proximal humerus [6, 7] and are additionally combined frequently with neurologic complications in 20–40 % of cases [8].

C. Reeps (✉) • H.-H. Eckstein
Klinikum rechts der Isar, Technical
University of Munich, Munich, Germany
e-mail: christian.reeps@googlemail.com;
hh.eckstein@web.de

P. Biberthaler et al. (eds.), *Fractures of the Proximal Humerus*, Strategies in Fracture Treatments,
DOI 10.1007/978-3-319-20300-3_26

Anatomy and Pathomechanisms

Injuries of the vessels of the shoulder and shoulder girdle that are caused by accidents are rare due to the protected anatomic position. These injuries therefore mostly occur in highly energetic or unfortunate traumas with distinct dislocations. The subclavian artery (emanating directly from the aortic arch on the left side or from the brachiocephalic trunk on the right side) initially runs behind the sternum deeply inside the anterior mediastinum and moves up through the deep cervical and pectoral musculature (posterior scalenus gap) protected from anterior and posterior side. It then passes through the deep cervical fasciae, the prescalenic fat pads and the trapezius muscle to the rear side of the clavicle embedded between the subclavian muscle, the first rib and the ventrally running vein. There, the artery branches into various strong collateral vessels in intra-thoracic direction and towards the neck and shoulders. After traversing the first rib, the subclavian artery becomes the axillary artery, which runs into the armpit while being protected by the breast and shoulder muscles or thorax and soft tissue, respectively. At the teres major muscle, it merges into the brachial artery that runs inside the medial bicipital sulcus. The brachial artery also constantly emerges a large number of collateral branches. In relation to the minor pectoral muscle, three parts (Parts I, II, and III) are distinguished: the central, the retromuscular and the peripheral part. The axillary artery again has various collateral branches. The arteries of the shoulder girdle are accompanied ventrally or medially by their corresponding veins and the brachial plexus which initially runs in direct proximity behind the subclavian artery and entwines this artery in the area of the axillary artery.

As mentioned, due to the protected position of the subclavian artery, injuries are comparably rare, especially after blunt trauma because of their protected position. The fundamental mechanisms of vascular injury on the one hand are sharp injuries, i.e. perforating/penetrating trauma caused by stab or gun shot injuries or internal perforation by dislocated fracture ends. On the other hand, but less frequent vascular damages occur through blunt force such as distraction, compression or interposition [9]. The characteristic presentation of sharp penetrating injuries is a potentially life-threatening bleeding or a distinct pulsing hematoma (false aneurysm). Limb ischemia only results, if the arterial diameter is completely transected. In contrast, limb ischemia is the pathognomonic characteristic of blunt injuries, except in case of complete ruptures. Dissections of the intima, intramural hematoma and/or external compression are leading to artery occlusion with apposition thrombosis. Thereby arteriospasm, usually reversible after reposition has to be discriminated from real artery occlusions and taken into account in differential diagnosis. The third part of the axillary artery is a predilection site for (blunt/any) trauma. This is due to the narrow space between the clavicle and chest as well as the fixation by the circumflex artery around the humerus head [10], injuries therefore mostly occur there and are often accompanied by dislocated fractures.

The main pathomechanism of vascular injuries in these cases usually are punctual penetrations or complete transactions as well as interposition of the vessel. Due to the considerable mobility of the shoulder girdle and the rather central fixation of the vessels, injuries caused by mere shoulder luxations without fractures (mostly inferior-anterior ones) are quite rare, but if present are often extensive because of arterial distension with long segment dissection of the intima [6]. Patients older than 50 years are apparently more often affected by dissections, as they are predisposed for this type of injury due to beginning arteriosclerosis with diminished elasticity of the vessel walls [11].

Fortunately, most acute traumatic occlusions of the subclavian and axillary artery artery/vein are compensated due to the well developed preexisting collateral network in the area of the shoulder girdle [12]. Only in case of serious soft tissue damage, unfavorable localization (especially occlusions at the distal axillary artery after branching into the subscapular artery [13]) or in extensive lesions, severe limb-threatening ischemia can occur because of compromised collateral supply. In this situation further management of surgical treatment is predominantly defined by the ischemic conditions.

Fractures of the proximal humerus are accompanied in about 5 % by arterial lesions and can be revascularized or are treated conservatively (11 %). successfully in most cases. Nevertheless and despite of all revascularization attempts the amputation rate still amounts up to 21 % [11]. Moreover, concomitant nerve injuries have to be expected in up to 50 % of all cases, due to the close proximity of the vessels to the brachial plexus or by compressing hematoma [8, 14]. Therewith, clinical diagnosis and assessment of severe ischemia by sensory-motor function can be additionally impaired or obscured. Most common medium and long term consequences of untreated traumatic lesions are more or less collateralized occlusions with consecutive arm claudication or even rest pain and the development of false or pseudoaneurysms caused by incomplete or complete vessel wall damage. Potential complications thereby include tissue loss, compression syndromes [15], aneurysm ruptures and distal embolization [16, 17], as well as contractions after ischemic compartment syndrome.

Diagnosis

Due to their relative rareness, concealed symptoms and especially because of the potential severity of their complications, it is of utmost importance to exclude or verify vascular injuries in traumas of the shoulder girdle. In case of bleeding or severe ischemia, vascular injuries often determine the timing of surgical management and the prognosis for extremities and patients. Especially in case of overlooked, delayed diagnosed or secondary deteriorating vascular injuries of the shoulder griddle, amputation rates can therefore increase up to 50 % in the absence of proper monitoring [18]. Repetitive clinical examination of both sides of the upper extremities regarding skin temperature, complexion, filling of veins, sensorimotor function and particularly peripheral pulse status is therefore obligatory, but can be misleading due to associated neurologic injuries, pain limited function or good collateralization. In absence of confounding factors, the reduction of sensorimotor function of fingers and hand correlates well with the severity of ischemia and the threat toward limb loss (TASC II criteria for diagnostics of acute limb ischemia) [19]. In case of clinical suspicion an additional helpful tool for better orientation can be a simple CW Doppler examination or preferably a color-coded duplex sonography to verify or exclude vascular injury. In particular, the latter mentioned technique enables under adequate sonographic conditions experienced surgeons to detect and specify arterial as well as venous injuries, bleeding etc. [20] without any time delay and also helps to avoid radiation exposure. In case of unclear diagnostic results caused by inadequate sonographic conditions or suspicion towards central vascular lesions, immediate diagnostic CT angiography is clearly indicated, especially when a trauma CT is already conducted. The sensitivity and specificity of CTA for the detection of traumatic arterial vascular injury is high and reaches 90–95 % or 99–100 %, respectively [21]. CTA provides a good overview and valuable information on type, exact location and extent of vascular lesions as well as soft tissue damages or accompanying bone injury. Therefore, it is desirable for planning of any type of operative therapy, but its almost mandatory for endovascular procedure planning. Nowadays due to the better overview, the lesser invasiveness and quick performance, CTA therefore has to be preferred over catheter angiography, except simultaneous intervention is intended. The value of MR imaging in emergency diagnostics is limited because it takes considerable time – especially in cases of severe ischemia. This technique is particularly indicated when concomitant plexus lesions and posttraumatic compartment syndrome have to be evaluated beyond emergency treatment.

Therapy

As already mentioned, injuries of the arteries of the shoulder girdle and the proximal upper arm amount only 5–10 % of all vascular injuries, due to their anatomically protected position [22]. Therefore, especially proximal lesions are therefore difficult to access due to the surrounding neurovascular and bony structures. Attempting open surgical access considerable preparation is necessary and often accompanied by additional blood loss and damage of soft tissues, lymphatic and collateral vessels. In extreme cases, a complete exposition of the neurovascular bundle is necessary and only possible by sternotomy or osteotomy of the clavicle. In some cases the demanded surgical blood control can only be achieved with multiple accesses…. (e.g. brachial, axillary, infra- and supraclavicular) or auxiliary procedures as sternotomy or osteotomy of the clavicula. With this open surgical repair may cause significant additional traumatization of the patients [23] and mortality after open exposition for treatment of injuries of the subclavian or axillary arteries amounts between 5 and 30 % [24]. Thereby, following the damage control principle, the least invasive and shortest possible surgical procedure for stabilization of the seriously injured patient and to establish reperfusion of the extremity should be conducted. Bridging maneuvers, vessel ligatures or even primary amputations should be taken into consideration, but these procedures are rarely applied due to highly impaired quality of life after upper extremity amputations. Additionally, compared to the lower extremities revascularization of the arteries of the upper limbs can be much more technical demanding and problematic with poorer short- and long-term prognosis of the arterial reconstruction: central parts of the arteries are more difficult to expose, the arm muscles have low ischemic tolerance, the flow conditions are characterized by high peripheral resistance, vessels are small and fragile with an strong tendency towards arteriospasms.

Central issues considering the management and urgency of the treatment of traumatic lesions of the shoulder girdle arteries certainly are type, location and severity of injury. Active bleedings have to be treated immediately and in most cases at the same time or even before any other surgical procedure. In case of relevant extravasate in central intra-thoracic locations, transluminal balloon catheter occlusions can often be used successfully as an alternative to open operative central bleeding control and therefore minimize the additional trauma by sternotomy. In addition, severe ischemia can also determine sequence and timing of operative treatment of traumas of the extremities, as the interval for successful revascularization is limited [25]. Therefore, primary time-consuming surgical stabilization of the unstable shoulder girdle is not always viable prior to vessel reconstruction Thus secondary treatment by means of reposition maneuvers with torsions and length corrections can endanger the previous reconstructed sites. In rare cases, temporary reperfusion via an alloplastic shunt can be used to bridge arterial defects [26]. In contrast, in non-limb threatening ischemia, initial stabilization by trauma surgical procedures is initially an viable option when the patient is monitored accordingly. Further important issues of open operative peri-traumatic treatment of vascular injuries of the shoulder girdle arise from the increased risk of infection and low flow rates in the arms. Because of resistance against infection and better long-term outcomes, autologous reconstructions should always be preferred prior to alloplastic vascular replacement in case of sufficient congruence and time frame [27] and should be considered in planning of the surgery (access cover of a donor leg for the great saphenous vein). Depending on type location and extent of injury, available options in case of small injuries include simple stitching, direct suture, patch plasty and partial vascular resections with tension less end-to-end reanastomosis – following successful desobliteration or thrombectomy and bleeding control. Long segment arterial injuries or blood flow limiting dissections usually require the creation of an interposition or bypass ideally using autologous material. Thereby patency rates in the area of the shoulder girdle vary from 75 to 100 % after 2–5 years [22, 28, 29] as reported by mostly non-representative small cohort studies.

Due to the significantly improved catheter materials, technical simplicity and swiftness, relative resistance against infections and above all because of the significantly reduced additional traumatization induced by surgery, endovascular therapies have also been established in the management of vascular injuries of the shoulder girdle in the last few years [30]. Especially in emergencies with injuries of the subclavian artery and the proximal axillary artery – that are larger and difficult to access in open surgery – this approach is being used more and more in favor of the patients. Particularly central and short segment injuries with massive bleedings sometimes can be managed much less invasively by implantation of balloon expanding or better self-expanding and highly flexible covered stent grafts without any additional sternotomy. Besides thrombotic vascular obliterations caused by traumatic dissection or fracture compression can also be treated by a hybrid interventional technique. A semi-closed procedure using an open access at another site while the actual lesion is not exposed and treated by ove-the-wire thrombectomy combined with angioplasty and/or stenting. According to small case control studies the initial success rate of such endovascular interventions achieves up to 96 % and helps to minimize blood loss, operation time, neurologic complications and the duration of hospital stays [31, 32], but does not seem to have an influence on overall mortality [33]. Interestingly, patency rates after treatment with stent grafts seem to be comparable to open operative procedures in the short-term and the long-term course [24, 31]. Compared to the central large supra aortic vessels indication for endovascular treatment of the arteries in the motor segment, i.e. in the area of the medial and distal axillary artery and the proximal brachial artery, is much more limited and has to be considered with caution because strong flection forces and reduced vessel caliber increase the risk of stent fractures or stent thrombosis with a high risk of reocclusion. Furthermore, open operative restoration in this area with autologous replacement material is easier due to better accessibility and potentially has better long-term results.

Post-therapeutical Management and Outcome

The outcome after successful surgical or endovascular therapy of traumatic lesions of the arteries of the shoulder girdle naturally differs greatly and is particularly dependent on concomitant traumatic, bone, fascia and nerve injuries. Due to the anatomical proximity accompanied by distension, hematoma compression and surgical trauma, coincident injuries of the brachial plexus are quite common with an incidence of up to 50 % [8, 14]. Thus the presence of vessel-specific complications is quite variable. Attention should be directed to post-ischemic compartment syndrome and reperfusion syndrome, as these can be influenced therapeutically and possibly bear inherent complications. The time frame for a functionally successful revascularization following severe complete ischemia (TASC IIb – III) is very short and only amounts 3–4 h. After this, there is danger of exponentially increasing incidences of myonecroses and local malmetabolism with post-ischemic compartment and reperfusion syndromes [25]. These syndromes can determine both the prognosis for limb salvage and patient survival – depending on extent and the severity of ischemic damaged tissue. Especially the musculature of the upper extremities is more sensitive and therefore young, male muscular patients are predisposed for such complications [34]. After delayed revascularization of severe complete ischemia the mortality by reperfusion syndrome of the upper extremity can reach 5–15 % induced by systemic liberation of toxic anaerobic metabolites [35]. Especially in cases of obviously established ischemia or when the outcome of revascularization is doubtful, the surgeon has to take primary amputation into consideration to prevent further endangerment of the patient. Unfortunately in many situations the sensorimotor function and consequently the severity of ischemia can be judged only to a limited extent as e.g. in intubated patients or because of concomitant nervous injuries. Thus, the indication for complete surgical, prophylactic fasciotomy should be confirmed liberally in case of an overall duration of ischemia of more than 3–4 h, to avoid additional injury to the patients [34]. In doubt, at least close monitoring under conservative compartment therapy is advisable. With this under optimal management, the amputation rates after vascular injuries of the upper extremity are low with 1.3 % and are mostly determined by the severity of the overall tissue trauma [36]. After successful, open operative or endovascular treatment of a traumatic arterial lesion, therapy for such patients is however not finished yet. Depending on the risk of bleedings of the concomitant injuries, a therapy with ASS that inhibits the aggregation of thrombocytes should be initiated as soon as possible. In case of a treatment with a small caliber stent graft or an alloplastic bypass smaller than 6–7 mm, a prolonged treatment with antiplatelet drugs should be performed or at least considered to avoid graft thrombosis. Some authors advocate long-term oral anti-coagulation with coumarin derivatives particularly in case of venous reconstructions. However, the evidence for coagulation therapies to improve the patency of arterial reconstructions in the area of the shoulder girdle is completely uncertain.

In addition to anti-thrombotic or anticoagulatory therapy close post operative surveillance, because of possible restenoses or anastomotic aneurysms, is mandatory. The patient should present routinely for clinical follow-ups with duplex sonography after 6 weeks, 6 months, 12 months and afterwards in intervals of at least 2 years.

Summary

Direct injuries or concomitant injuries of the proximal shoulder-arm-vessels as complications of fractures or luxations near the shoulder joint in generally are rather rare, due to the shielding bone and soft tissue mantle, but in case of, they can have potentially fatal consequences for limb function and salvage or even general patients prognosis. Therefore, they often determine the diagnostic pathways and surgical management. Relevant arterial injuries typically present sometimes with life threatening bleeding with pulsating hematoma after perforating or penetrating trauma or otherwise by vessel occlusion consecutive limb ischemia after interposition, compression or distension with dissection. For clinical orientation and confirmation of diagnosis, lesion localization and therapy planning of more peripheral vascular lesions color coded duplex sonography is extremely helpful while CT-angiography is first line diagnostic and essential for evaluation of central large vessel injuries or in concomitant complex multiple trauma. In modern surgical management of acute vascular injuries of the shoulder girdle in addition to the established conventionally open surgical procedures, nowadays much less invasive and traumatic endovascular or hybrid techniques gain more and more relevance for bleeding control and revascularization in feasible cases, with short-term benefit for the patient and with presumably comparable long-term results. Thereby, in the postoperative course and nonetheless despite of initially successful therapy the attending surgeon must be aware of secondary complications as reperfusion- or compartment syndrome, restenosis, pseudoaneurysms witch may jeopardize the surgical results. Therefore close perioperative and later patient surveillance are mandatory.

References

1. Cikrit DF, Dalsing MC, Bryant BJ, Lalka SG, Sawchuk AP, Schulz JE. An experience with upper-extremity vascular trauma. Am J Surg. 1990;160(2):229–33.
2. Hardin Jr WD, O'Connell RC, Adinolfi MF, Kerstein MD. Traumatic arterial injuries of the upper extremity: determinants of disability. Am J Surg. 1985;150(2):266–70.
3. Clouse WD, Rasmussen TE, Perlstein J, Sutherland MJ, Peck MA, Eliason JL, Jazerevic S, Jenkins DH. Upper extremity vascular injury: a current in-theater wartime report from Operation Iraqi Freedom. Ann Vasc Surg. 2006;20(4):429–34.
4. Franz RW, Goodwin RB, Hartman JF, Wright ML. Management of upper extremity arterial injuries at an urban level I trauma center. Ann Vasc Surg. 2009;23(1):8–16.
5. Richter A, Silbernik D, Oestreich K, Karaorman M, Storz LW. Peripheral vascular injuries in polytrauma. Unfallchirurg. 1995;98(9):464–7.

6. Sparks SR, DeLaRosa J, Bergan JJ, Hoyt DB, Owens EL. Arterial injury in uncomplicated upper extremity dislocations. Ann Vasc Surg. 2000;14(2):110–3.
7. Matheï J, Depuydt P, Parmentier L, Olivie F, Harake R, Janssen A. Injury of the axillary artery after a proximal humeral fracture: a case report and overview of the literature. Acta Chir Belg. 2008;108(5):625–7.
8. Adovasio R, Visintin E, Sgardi G. Arterial injury of the axilla: an unusual case after blunt trauma of the shoulder. J Trauma. 1996;41:754–6.
9. Heberer G, Becker HM, Dittmer H, Stelter WJM. Vascular injuries in polytrauma. World J Surg. 1983;7(1):68–79.
10. Gates JD, Knox JB. Axillary artery injury secondary to anterior dislocation of the shoulder. J Trauma. 1995;39:58–63.
11. Mc Laughlin J, Light R, Lustrin I. Axillary artery injury as a com-plication of proximal humerus fractures. J Shoulder Elbow Surg. 1998;7:292–4.
12. Henson GF. Vascular complications of shoulder injuries: a report of two cases. J Bone Joint Surg. 1956;38-B:528–31.
13. Moore KI. Clinical oriented anatomy. Baltimore: Williams and Wilkins; 1980. p. 707–9.
14. Kendall KM, Burton JH, Cushing B. Fatal subclavian artery transection from isolated clavicle fracture. J Trauma. 2000;48(2):316–8.
15. Jeganathan R, Harkin DW, Lowry P, Lee B. Iatrogenic subclavian artery pseudoaneurysm causing airway compromise: treatment with percutaneous thrombin injection. J Vasc Surg. 2004;40(2):371–4.
16. Heffernan EJ, Keaveny TV. Pathological fracture of the clavicle causing subclavian pseudoaneurysm formation. Ir Med J. 2008;101(6):184–5.
17. Barra JA, Le Saout J, Gaultier Y. Late signs of vascular complications of closed trauma of the shoulder. J Chir. 1978;115(3):151–7.
18. Sathyarup D, Huilgol AK, Iyer KM. Axillary artery thrombosis following a fracture of the neck of the humerus. Injury. 1988;19(1):45–7.
19. Norgren L, Hiatt WR, Dormandy JA, Nehler MR, Harris KA, Fowkes FG; TASC II Working Group, Bell K, Caporusso J, Durand-Zaleski I, Komori K, Lammer J, Liapis C, Novo S, Razavi M, Robbs J, Schaper N, Shigematsu H, Sapoval M, White C, White J, Clement D, Creager M, Jaff M, Mohler E 3rd, Rutherford RB, Sheehan P, Sillesen H, Rosenfield K. Inter-society consensus for the management of peripheral arterial disease (TASC II). Eur J Vasc Endovasc Surg. 2007;33(Suppl 1):S1–75.
20. Gullo J, Singletary EM, Larese S. Emergency bedside sonographic diagnosis of subclavian artery pseudoaneurysm with brachial plexopathy after clavicle fracture. Ann Emerg Med. 2013;61:204–6.
21. Miller-Thomas MM, West OC, Cohen AM. Diagnosing traumatic arterial injury in the extremities with CT angiography: pearls and pitfalls. Radiographics. 2005;25 Suppl 1:S133–42.
22. Ender TA, Nesimi EM. Management of axillo-subclavian arterial injuries and predictors of outcome. Minerva Chir. 2011;66(4):307–15.
23. Loeprecht H. Chronische Verschlussprozesse der Arterien der oberen Extremitäten. In: Heberer Van Dongen editors. Gefäßchirurgie. Berlin/Heidelberg: Springer. 1 Auflage; 1987–2004. p. 545–54.
24. Xenos E, Freeman M, Stevens S, Cassada D, Pacanowski J, Goldman M. Covered stents for injuries of subclavian and axillary arteries. J Vasc Surg. 2003;38(3):451–4.
25. Labbe R, Lindsay T, Walker PM. The extent and distribution of skeletal muscle necrosis after graded periods of complete ischemia. J Vasc Surg. 1987;6(2):152–7.
26. Rasmussen TE, Clouse WD, Jenkins DH, et al. The use of temporary vascular shunts as a damage control adjunct in the management of war time vascular injury. J Trauma. 2006;60(2):432–42.
27. Mesh CL, McCarthy WJ, Pearce WH, Flinn WR, Shireman PK, Yao JS. Upper extremity bypass grafting. A 15-year experience. Arch Surg. 1993;128(7):795–801.
28. Hudorovic N, Lovricevic I, Ahel Z. In situ cephalic vein bypasses from axillary to the brachial artery after catheterization injuries. Interact Cardiovasc Thorac Surg. 2010;11(1):103–5.
29. Perkins JM, Magee TR, Hands LJ, Collin J, Morris PJ. The long-term outcome after axillo-axillary bypass grafting for proximal subclavian artery disease. Eur J Vasc Endovasc Surg. 2000;19(1):52–5.
30. Shalhub S, Starnes BW, Hatsukami TS, Karmy-Jones R, Tran NT. Repair of blunt thoracic outlet arterial injuries: an evolution from open to endovascular approach. J Trauma. 2011;71(5):E114–21.
31. DuBose JJ, Rajani R, Gilani R, Arthurs ZA, Morrison JJ, Clouse WD, Rasmussen TE. Endovascular management of axillo-subclavian arterial injury: a review of published experience. Injury. 2012;43(11):1785–92.
32. Mousa A, Chong B, Aburahma AF. Endovascular repair of subclavian/axillary artery injury with a covered stent. A case report and review of literature. Vascular. 2013 [Epub ahead of print].
33. Sinha S, Patterson BO, Ma J, Holt PJ, Thompson MM, Carrell T, Tai N, Loosemore TM, London Trauma Network. Systematic review and meta-analysis of open surgical and endovascular management of thoracic outlet vascular injuries. J Vasc Surg. 2013;57(2):547–67.
34. Blaisdell FW. The pathophysiology of skeletal muscle ischemia and the reperfusion syndrome: a review. Cardiovasc Surg. 2002;10(6):620–30.
35. Blaisdell FW, Steele M, Allen RE. Management of acute lower extremity arterial ischemia due to embolism and thrombosis. Surgery. 1978;84(6):822–34.
36. Tan TW, Joglar FL, Hamburg NM, Eberhardt RT, Shaw PM, Rybin D, Doros G, Farber A. Limb outcome and mortality in lower and upper extremity arterial injury: a comparison using the National Trauma Data Bank. Vasc Endovascular Surg. 2011;45(7):592–7.

27 Nerve Injury During Treatment of the Proximal Humerus Fracture

Dominik Pförringer

Introduction

Nerve injuries, next to vascular lesions pose one of the major surgical risks in any operative procedure. While damage to minor and micro nerves cannot be avoided by the surgeon, large neurological structures by exact knowledge of their anatomical position and their potential variations can be protected. Planning of the surgical approach in accordance to the anatomic landmarks may help the surgeon in avoiding a large variety of foreseeable risks. However nerve lesions do occur and even the most diligent operating skills will never be able to rule out 100 % of the risk. Nerve lesions can be evaluated electrophysiologically or clinically. Most nerve lesions after humeral neck fracture have proven to be temporary with a high chance of full recovery [1]. Early detection as well as appropriate countermeasures have proven to have the most significant influence on the long term outcome. It is important to realize that, in both conservative and operative treatment of proximal humeral fractures, a paresis due to nerve injury can affect the restoration of shoulder motions [2].

By **pathomechanism of lesion**, one needs to differentiate the following types of lesions:

- Lesions during fracture caused by sharp bone fragments
- Compartmental lesions, inflicted by pressure within the surrounding tissue
- Approach/instrument lesions: scalpell, hooks…
- Drilling lesions
- Screw/wire lesions

The above described can be clustered into surgically avoidable and non-avoidable harm.

General **types of nerve lesions** may be found in Table 27.2 [3, 4].

One can also classify the neurological lesions according to the involved major **nerves of the shoulder region**:

- Plexus brachialis
- Fasciculus lateralis, medialis, posterior
- Nervus axillaris
- Nervus medianus
- Nervus musculocutaneus
- Nervus radialis
- Nervus subscapularis
- Nervus suprascapularis
- Nervus thoracicus longus
- Nervus thoracodorsalis
- Nervus ulnaris

One may classify in reference to the **therapeutic approach** chosen:

D. Pförringer
Department of Trauma Surgery, Klinikum rechts der Isar, Technical University of Munich, Munich, Germany
e-mail: dominik@pfoerringer.de

P. Biberthaler et al. (eds.), *Fractures of the Proximal Humerus*, Strategies in Fracture Treatments,
DOI 10.1007/978-3-319-20300-3_27

- Conservative (without surgical approach)
  - In a sling
  - In a cast
- K-wire fixation only (mostly children)
- Plate and screw fixation
- Humeral nail with locking screws

Affected Nerves

A prospective study of Cornelis et al. has shown that anatomically, the nerves most frequently involved are the axillary nerve [58 %] and the suprascapular nerve [48 %]. Frequently a combination of nerve lesions was seen. The mean number of nerves involved for all patients with nerve injury was 2.8 nerves [2]. See Table 27.1 for detailed examination of lesion locations.

Most literature describes Nervus radialis lesions. De Franco et al. state that in general a radial nerve palsy may be defined as partial or complete. Complete motor loss occurs in approximately 50–68 % of cases [5] and [6]. Primary nerve palsies identified during the initial evaluation of the fracture occur at the time of the injury. Ten percent to 20 % of nerve palsies develop during the course of treatment. These are referred to as secondary radial nerve palsies [7, 8]. The extent of injury to peripheral nerves can be defined using Seddon's classification system [4] (Table 27.2).

The classification of a radial nerve injury as primary or secondary is useful in determining the prognosis for recovery. Shaw and Sakellarides [9] reported spontaneous recovery in only 40 % of patients with primary paralysis and in all patients with secondary paralysis after closed or open reduction and internal fixation [3].

Garcia and Maeck found that radial nerve palsies occurred in 11.7 % of their patients with humeral shaft fractures. Among the patients who had immediate radial nerve palsies and who underwent surgery on or shortly after admission, only 1 of them had a radial nerve that was severed. Complete recovery occurred in 18 of the 23 patients who underwent surgery. The 1 patient

Table 27.1 Percentual nerve lesions in proximal humerus fracture. Details of 142 patients with 143 fractures of proximal humerus

Characteristics	Data
Absolute No.	
Fractures	143
Sex	
Men	21
Women	122
Side	
Left	75
Right	68
Nerve injury	96
Men	15
Women	81
Type of fracture (Neer class)	
I	93
II	1
IIIA	12
IIIB	9
IIIC	7
IV2	5
IV3	4
IV4	3
V2	1
VI2A	2
VI4A	2
Caput	4
Means	
All fractures (n = 143)	
Age (years) (95 % CI)	68.8 (65.7, 71.9)
Range	5–92
Men	56.5
Women	71
With nerve injury (n = 96)	
Age (years) (95 % CI)	70.1 (68.0, 73.2)
Range	13–91
Men	53.9
Women	73.1
Nerves involved[a]	
Mean No. (95 % CI)	2.8 (2.5, 3.1)
Mean maximum severity (95 % CI)	1.8 (1.6, 2.0)
Mean severity/nerve (95 % CI)	1.6 (1.5, 1.7)

With the permission [2]

[a]Calculated per patient in 96 patients with nerve lesions

Table 27.2 Principal types of nerve injury [3, 4]

	Neurotmesis	Axonotmesis	Neuropraxia
Pathologic			
Anatomic continuity	May be lost	Preserved	Preserved
Essential damage			
Clinical			
Motorparalysis	Complete	Complete	Complete
Sensory paralysis	Complete	Complete	Usually much sparing
Sympathetic paralysis	Complete	Complete	Usually much sparing
Reaction of degeneration	Present	Present	Absent
Nerve conduction below lesion	Lost	Lost	Preserved
Muscle atrophy	Progressive	Progressive	Preserved
Recovery			
Surgical repair	Essential	Not necessary	Not necessary
Rate of recovery	1–2 mm/day after repair	1–2 mm/day	Rapid: days or weeks
March of recovery	According to order of innervation	According to order of innervation	No order
Quality	Always imperfect	Perfect	Perfect
Sunderland classification	V	II	I

Modified with permission from [3]

with a severed radial nerve recovered completely after primary repair of the nerve. Three of the patients had residual, incomplete deficits. The authors concluded that severity of injury defined at the time of surgery correlated with recovery and that there was no constant relationship between operative findings and rate of return of sensation and motor power [3, 6].

Detection and Examination of Potential Nerve Lesions

Electromyography is method of choice, while ultrasound may be helpful in detecting potential nerve lesions. However most results of US evaluations are based on humeral shaft fractures [10].

Injury Mechanism

Injury Through the Trauma

Transverse and spiral fractures were more likely to be associated with radial nerve palsy than oblique and comminuted patterns of fracture ($p<0.001$) [11].

De Franco et al. have described that several researchers have suggested a correlation between the fracture level and the incidence of radial nerve injury. For example Bostman et al. [7] reported an equal number of radial nerve injuries in fractures of the middle and distal humerus. Pollock et al. [5] however, have shown that there is a higher likelihood of neurovascular injuries in the middle third of the humerus whereas Garcia and Maeck [6] found fractures of the distal third of the humerus to have a higher incidence of concomitant neurovascular injury. Although radial nerve palsies are associated most commonly with spiral fracture patterns they also occur with transverse and oblique fractures.

Injury Within the Operation

Rasool et al. have conducted a study regarding the intraoperative nerve lesion in K-wire fixation showing that six cases of ulnar nerve injury resulted from crossed K-wire fixation of displaced supracondylar humeral fractures in children. The age ranged between 4 and 10 years. Pain on extension of the little and ring fingers and early clawing were important post operative signs of ulnar nerve involvement. Early exploration of all six cases revealed medial pin placement in the cubital tunnel in five cases. In two of these, the nerve was directly penetrated, and in three, it was constricted by the cubital tunnel retinaculum. In the case 6, the nerve was hypermobile and found to be fixed anterior to its groove over the medial epicondyle. The nerve was decompressed in all cases, and the wire was repositioned. Follow-up ranged from 4 to 14 months. Full nerve recovery occurred in three cases, partial in two, and no recovery in one. Early exploration rather than simple pin removal is safer and diagnostic of the mechanism of injury [12].

Treatment of Nerve Lesions

De Franco et al. have described The controversy and resultant strategy surrounding the management of a humeral shaft fracture with a radial nerve injury can be divided into three categories: no exploration, early exploration, and late exploration. The first reports [13] and [14] on this injury pattern in the literature recommended surgical fracture management and nerve exploration [3].

Subsequently satisfactory results were obtained with expectant management, especially among patients with a primary radial nerve palsy [15] and [5]. With regard to secondary nerve palsies, the treatment approach varies among surgeons. Most researchers advise early exploration because of the high frequency of nerve entrapment after manipulation [3, 14, 16, 17].

Shao et al. in 2005 for the radial nerve palsy have described an overall rate of recovery of 88.1 % (921 of 1045), with spontaneous recovery reaching 70.7 % (411 of 581) in patients treated conservatively [11].

So comprehensively it can be stated that the degree as well as the etiology of the nerve lesion is pivotal for its outcome.

Long Term Outcome

Shao et al. described no significant difference in the final results when comparing groups which were initially managed expectantly with those explored early, suggesting that the initial expectant treatment did not affect the extent of nerve recovery adversely and would avoid many unnecessary operations [11].

Summary

Nerve lesions pose a common risk in humeral neck fractures. In our increasingly ageing population we assume a rise in total figure of fractures and in logical consequence a rise in nerve lesions associated to these fractures. Nerve lesions, when detected early and addressed appropriately display a high chance of full recovery, while most studies show a positive outcome with conservative treatment.

References

1. de Laat EA, et al. Nerve lesions in primary shoulder dislocations and humeral neck fractures. A prospective clinical and EMG study. J Bone Joint Surg Br. 1994;76(3):381–3.
2. Visser CP, et al. Nerve lesions in proximal humeral fractures. J Shoulder Elbow Surg. 2001;10(5):421–7.
3. DeFranco MJ, Lawton JN. Radial nerve injuries associated with humeral fractures. J Hand Surg Am. 2006;31(4):655–63.
4. Seddon HJ. Nerve lesions complicating certain closed bone injuries. J Am Med Assoc. 1947;135(11):691–4.
5. Pollock FH, et al. Treatment of radial neuropathy associated with fractures of the humerus. J Bone Joint Surg Am. 1981;63(2):239–43.
6. Garcia Jr A, Maeck Jr BH. Radial nerve injuries in fractures of the shaft of the humerus. Am J Surg. 1960;99:625–7.
7. Bostman O, et al. Radial palsy in shaft fracture of the humerus. Acta Orthop Scand. 1986;57(4):316–9.
8. Kettelkamp DB, Alexander H. Clinical review of radial nerve injury. J Trauma. 1967;7(3):424–32.
9. Shaw JL, Sakellarides H. Radial-nerve paralysis associated with fractures of the humerus. A review of forty-five cases. J Bone Joint Surg Am. 1967;49(5):899–902.
10. Bodner G, et al. Radial nerve palsy associated with humeral shaft fracture: evaluation with US—initial experience. Radiology. 2001;219(3):811–6.
11. Shao YC, et al. Radial nerve palsy associated with fractures of the shaft of the humerus: a systematic review. J Bone Joint Surg Br. 2005;87(12):1647–52.
12. Rasool MN. Ulnar nerve injury after K-wire fixation of supracondylar humerus fractures in children. J Pediatr Orthop. 1998;18(5):686–90.

13. Holstein A, Lewis GM. Fractures of the humerus with radial-nerve paralysis. J Bone Joint Surg Am. 1963;45:1382–8.
14. Packer JW, et al. The humeral fracture with radial nerve palsy: is exploration warranted? Clin Orthop Relat Res. 1972;88:34–8.
15. Mast JW, et al. Fractures of the humeral shaft: a retrospective study of 240 adult fractures. Clin Orthop Relat Res. 1975;112:254–62.
16. Bleeker WA, Nijsten MW, ten Duis HJ. Treatment of humeral shaft fractures related to associated injuries. A retrospective study of 237 patients. Acta Orthop Scand. 1991;62(2):148–53.
17. Klenerman L. Fractures of the shaft of the humerus. J Bone Joint Surg Br. 1966;48(1):105–11.

Periprosthetic Complications

28

Peter Michael Prodinger and Rüdiger von Eisenhart-Rothe

With the advancing age of the population, acute fractures of the proximal humerus have reached importance and are currently the third most frequent fracture of the elderly, accounting for up to 10 % of all fractures [39]. It is estimated that the incidence will rise up to three times in the next decades [55]. Though many of these patients are treated by open reduction, a significant percentage will require arthroplasty if the fracture displacement, a high risk of fixation loss, mal-union, non-union, or avascular necrosis will not allow for a preservation of the humeral head [82]. Hemiarthroplasty has traditionally been the treatment of choice advocated as the gold standard by Neer in patients with complex 3- and 4-part fractures with poor bone stock inapproachable to reconstruction [51, 52]. Reported results remain heterogenous and depend majorly on the fate of the tuberosities with mal- or non-union rates between 39 and 50 % [7, 82]. In consequence, proximal migration of the implant will occur and has been confirmed in multiple surveys [7, 57]. This leads to a relatively high incidence of poor results, with a surgical complication rate of up to 50 % requiring reoperations in more than 10 % and up to 62 % of not satisfied patients [7, 65].

P.M. Prodinger (✉) • R. von Eisenhart-Rothe
Division for Orthopedic Surgery,
Klinikum rechts der Isar,
Technical University of Munich,
Munich, Germany
e-mail: peter.prodinger@tum.de;
ortho@mri.tum.de

Reverse shoulder arthroplasty reveals a newer treatment option, originally indicated and designed for patients suffering from rotator cuff arthropathy [41]. In cases of a non-functional rotator cuff due to chronic fracture sequelae with non-union or resorption of mainly the greater tuberosity, the reverse shoulder arthroplasty has been introduced in trauma surgery with predictable and reproducible results [8, 41, 78]. Consequently, surgeons have been encouraged to adopt this option for acute fractures with favorable short- and mid-term outcome [11, 14, 21, 35, 43, 73, 82].

With the evolution regarding the surgical technique and increasing traumatic or post-traumatic shoulder replacements, specific complications concerning the stability of the implant, the loosening of the components, dislocation of the prosthesis, periprosthetic fractures and infections have become more evident and are progressively enhancing the need for revision surgery. Despite the increase in the annual volume of performed procedures, the data furthermore suggests that three of four operations are still performed by surgeons who do less than two shoulder replacements per year [5, 27, 28]. As the favorability of the clinical outcome as well as the decision to proceed with a total shoulder replacement instead of a hemiarthroplasty have been shown to depend on the surgeons' experience and hospital volume, complication rates might be linked to this fact [27, 28, 30, 31, 42].

P. Biberthaler et al. (eds.), *Fractures of the Proximal Humerus*, Strategies in Fracture Treatments,
DOI 10.1007/978-3-319-20300-3_28

The largest, recent meta-analysis summarizing 2810 shoulder replacements (predominantly glenohumeral osteoarthritis) revealed 414 complication-events associated with the surgery (rate of 14.7 %) [5]. These findings are in line with previous work reporting complication rates between 12 and 14 % [17, 80]. According to Kalandiak et al. the reasons for a failure of arthroplasties can be grouped into three broad categories. Primarily these causes involving soft tissue, such as instability, stiffness, tuberosity nonunion or rotator cuff tears, secondarily those involving the glenoid component and finally those reasons involving the humeral component [32]. Most complications remain multifactorial. In the current literature the rates of patients actually needing revision surgery vary between 5 and 42 % for both – constrained (reversed) and unconstrained (anatomical) prosthetic implants [5].

Fracture arthroplasty in particular seems to be associated with higher complication rates than elective shoulder replacement irrespective of the causative pathology [57]. Furthermore, the patterns of failure are different and arise mainly in the challenging reconstruction of the destructed anatomy lacking important landmarks, length and orientation. Most complications linked to fracture arthroplasty develop intraoperatively and reach clinical significance in the short-term. Malpositioning of the arthroplasty components is a frequent problem (around 39 % [76]) leading to postoperative instability and prosthetic dislocation. Intraoperative, periprosthetic fractures frequently occur and demand specific treatment. Of those, especially primary or secondary involvement of the tuberosities (about 30 % of all complications in fracture arthroplasty [76]) draws impact on the faith of the prosthesis. Lastly, typical long-term complications such as loosening of the components or prosthetic infections will occur and will demand specific treatment, though the relative proportion of those patients is smaller compared to elective shoulder replacement surgery.

Malpositioning of the Components and Instability

Shoulder arthroplasty alters the complex interactions of capsulolabral, bone- and soft-tissue structures which warrant the function of the glenohumeral joint, making soft-tissue tensioning and component positioning critical in preventing postoperative instability. Deficiencies might thus lead to glenohumeral instability requiring surgical revision.

Glenohumeral instability is the second most common cause of complications associated with total shoulder arthroplasty in general (about 30% of all complications), with a reported prevalence of 4 % [5]. It is especially frequent in fracture arthroplasty and was reported to affect up to 15 % of all reconstructed patients. The lack of anatomical landmarks after complex fractures of the proximal humerus impedes proper orientation i.e. retroversion of the humeral makes no sence component thus promoting the risk of malpositioning. Contradictory to former considerations, the suitability to position the implant along the bicipital sulcus was challenged because of large interindividual differences and an anatomical tendency regarding a medialisation of its distal parts [29]. In consequence, the humeral retroversion should be determined using the epicondylar axis with the recommendation of approximately 20° retroversion [26]. Excessive retroversion (>20°) would provoke a dislocation of the re-adapted greater tuberosity during internal rotation and should therefore be avoided [26]. Especially problematic and demanding in fracture arthroplasty is the restoration of the proper length of the humerus. Murachovsky et al. demonstrated, that the distance between the cranial edge of the M. pectoralis major insertion and the most cranial point of the humeral head measures relatively constant 5.6 ± 0.5 cm, which could serve the surgeon as landmark in restoring physiological anatomy [49].

The etiology of anterior instability in fracture-arthroplasty is multifactorial and mostly involves a combination of soft-tissue failure and

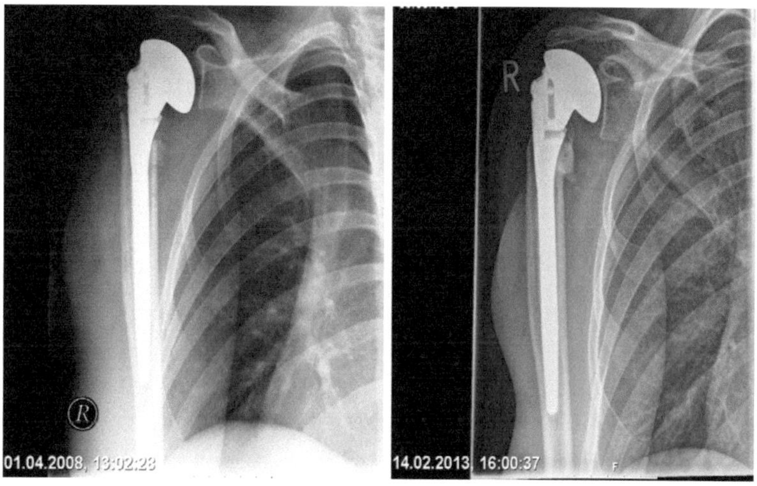

Fig. 28.1 The *left* image shows radiographic results 3 months after shoulder arthroplasty. The *right* radiograph of the right shoulder 5 years post surgery shows a high non-anatomical seat of the anatomical implant compared to the postoperative image. Clinically the rotator cuff was found to be insufficient with a resulting superior instability as functional correlate of the picture

mal-positioning of the implant. In detail it could be associated with an anteversion of the humeral component, anterior glenoid deficiency, dysfunction of the anterior parts of the deltoid muscle or failure of the subscapularis tendon and the anterior capsule [79, 80]. As described before, posterior instability has been attributed to excessive retroversion of the components [79]. Furthermore posterior glenoid erosion and soft-tissue imbalance have been implicated in the development of posterior instability [5].

Irrespective of the direction of the instability, a detailed analysis of the underlying origin has to precede revision surgery to address the causative pathology. Malrotation of the components, either of the humerus or the glenoid, will generally require reorientation. In case of excessive humeral ante- or retroversion the restoration of normal retroversion of the humeral component is technically easier than glenoid reorientation and feasible by performing an exchange of the component. Newer, modular implants offer the possibility of retaining a fixed stem. If a glenoid component has been used, glenoid reorientation on the other hand is a demanding procedure often requiring excentrical glenoid reaming or bone grafting [50, 79]. Soft tissue failure leading to anterior instability is generally due to tears of the subscapularis tendon. It first of all represents a function of operative technique or insufficient refixation and bad tissue quality [5]. Moreover inappropriate physical treatment and oversized components can result in a subscapularis tendon rupture and instability. In these cases the muscular integrity has to be restored, eventually by the use of tendon-allografts or muscle transfers [1, 60]. Posterior laxity demands posterior capsulorhaphy [50].

Superior instability after anatomical shoulder replacement (total or hemi-arthroplasty) is generally caused by muscular imbalance between the (torn) rotator cuff and the deltoid muscle (Fig. 28.1). In consequence, the eccentric loading forces on the glenoid, if applied, provoke accelerated wear and loosening of the prosthesis expressed in the typical, clinical picture of the patient suffering from severe pain and functional deficits due to the destabilization of the rotational center [75]. The first step in the treatment of superior instability would be the identification of patients at high risk for developing superior instability after fracture-arthroplasty. Thus, the desired treatment should implement a preexisting cuff-arthropathy especially in elderly patients and primary treatment with a reversed total shoulder arthroplasty should be considered [4, 22]. Similarly, reversed shoulder replacements may be used in patients in whom a total shoulder arthroplasty has failed secondary to rotator cuff dysfunction with or without a symptomatic loosened glenoid component [4].

Inferior instability is a rare problem though closely related to fracture and tumor arthroplasty. It results from failure of restoring the original length of the humerus. Affected patients lack the ability to abduct the arm above the horizontal plane due to poor deltoid muscle tensioning. If first line physiotherapeutic treatment and strengthening of the abductor muscles fail, surgical therapy is recommended demanding a restoration of the proper length of the humerus [60, 80].

Periprosthetic Fractures

In general, periprosthetic fractures in shoulder arthroplasty are majorly a problem of the humeral component. Their incidence ranges between 0.6 and 3 % and they account for approximately 20 % of all complications associated with total shoulder arthroplasty [17, 38, 61, 67, 81]. Most of the fractures occur intraoperatively, more frequent during total than during hemi-arthroplasty. This may be attributed to the difficulty in gaining access to the glenoid during total shoulder arthroplasty [67]. Furthermore, periprosthetic humerus fractures are more common during revision than primary surgery.

According to Wright and Cofield, periprosthetic fractures of the humeral shaft can be classified in three types relative to the tip of the humeral prosthesis: Type A fractures extend proximally to the tip of the stem, type B fractures involve the tip with a variable amount of extension distally and type C fractures are located distal to the tip of the stem (Fig. 28.2) [81]. In general a differentiation between intraoperative and postoperative fractures is made drawing impact on surgical or conservative treatment options.

Treatment of periprosthetic humeral fractures is complicated due to higher non-union rates when an implant is present [67]. Whenever a prosthesis is involved, the force transmission goes preferentially through the fracture site if the patient moves the shoulder or the elbow [9]. The disruption of the endosteal blood supply is a contributing factor as well, finally resulting in delayed fracture healing. Additionally, the prosthetic stem tip may cause distraction at the fracture site in case of diaphyseal fractures [9, 67]. Concomitant host factors such as osteopenia, female sex, rheumatoid arthritis and medical comorbidities in the elderly patient may also result in delayed healing and poor functional outcome [9, 61]. The fracture pattern and the amount of displacement in periprosthetic humerus fractures have a significant effect on union. A higher incidence of non-unions has been reported in transverse and short oblique fractures of the shaft compared to long spiral fractures [81]. Fractures with more than 2 mm residual displacement take significantly more time to union regardless of the type [12].

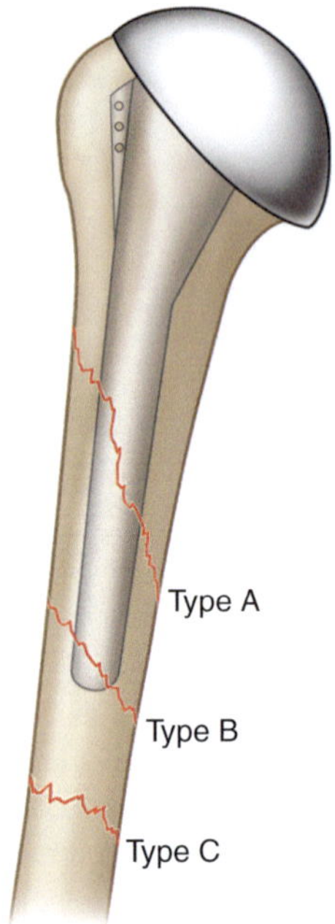

Fig. 28.2 The Wright and Cofield classification of periprosthetic humerus fractures [81]. A *type A* fracture is affects the stem and extends proximally. *Type B* is centered at the tip of the stem and extends distally. *Type C* is located distal to the tip of the stem

The healing of the fracture, pain relief and restoration of function are the major goals of treatment. Maintaining the glenohumeral function however has limited perspective of success [67]. Because of the sparse, preexisting literature concerning the treatment of periprosthetic fractures in shoulder arthroplasty, current treatment concepts refer closely to experience in the treatment of periprosthetic hip fractures [67]. Principally, conservative and surgical concepts are available.

Intraoperative Fractures of the Humerus Diaphysis

Intraoperative fractures of the humeral shaft are closely associated with failure of the surgical technique such as inadvertent reaming, harsh impaction or inadequate manipulation of the arm during glenoid exposure [45, 80]. Spiral fractures are often caused by substantial torsional forces generated during external rotation of the shoulder. Inappropriate placement of the prosthesis or the reamer may finally result in a cortical perforation, most likely if the initial reamer or trial stem is not eccentrically positioned in the superolateral aspect of the proximal humerus [45, 80]. The presence of soft-tissue contracture as well as the necessity to remove a well-fixed cemented prosthesis for revision arthroplasty present challenges and may also result in intraoperative fracture [67].

In general, surgery is the management of intraoperative fractures of the humeral shaft. Simple cerclage wiring has been advocated for fractures proximal to the tip of the implant (Type A). If the tip of a standard prosthesis does not span the fracture site at least two to three cortical diameters, the implantation of a long-stemmed prosthesis is recommended [5, 80]. Similarly, intraoperative type B fractures should be treated with a long-stem prosthesis that spans the fracture site by two to three cortical diameters with the option of cement augmentation. Care should be taken to avoid extrusion of cement into the fracture site as this would impede healing [67]. Cerclages might be an option to augment fixation, especially in case of inferior bone quality (Fig. 28.3). Most periprosthetic fractures require at least extension of the deltopectoral approach to provide sufficient exposure of the fracture site. Fractures distal to the implant tip (Type C) warrant a long stemmed prosthesis placed through a combined deltopectoral and anterolateral humeral approach [80], alternatively plating could be an option. The distance of the fracture to the fossa olecrani is crucial and might prevent from sufficient stabilization using a long stem prosthesis. In case of very distal humeral shaft fractures additional plate fixation and/or cerclages should be considered. In patients in whom a standard cemented stem prosthesis has already been placed before recognition or generation of an intraoperative fracture, removal of the stem would risk extension of the fracture or nerve injury. In these cases, plate-and-screw and/or cerclage wire fixation adjacent to the stem is a viable option as well [67].

Postoperative Fractures of the Humerus

Postoperative fractures of the proximal humerus provide the option of non surgical treatment by bracing if they are minimally or non-displaced and if the component is well fixed [12]. Though, time to consolidation might be protracted and counts for an average of 180 days [38]. Postoperative type C fractures can be seen (and treated) as routine humeral shaft fractures which implements the possibility of a conservative regime in case of satisfactory alignment.

Loosening of the humeral stem would generally dispose the patient to surgical treatment and revision by long-stem implants. Both, cemented and non-cemented stems have been used in type A and B fractures in small case series and have shown satisfactory union rates [38, 81]. In case of a substantial overlap between the fracture length and a well fixed humeral stem (especially in type A fractures), as well as in case of a displacement of more than 2 mm and angulation greater than 20° in any plane, those fractures will preferably be treated as if the humeral component was loose [67]. Revision to a long-stem prosthesis is advised to bypass the fracture by at least two cortical diameters and fixation by cerclages should be supplemented distally. If necessary, plates and screws may afford torsional rigidity [67]. A displaced or unstable type B fracture with a well-fixed humeral stem is preferentially managed by plating. Recently, the locking compression plate (LCP) has been used

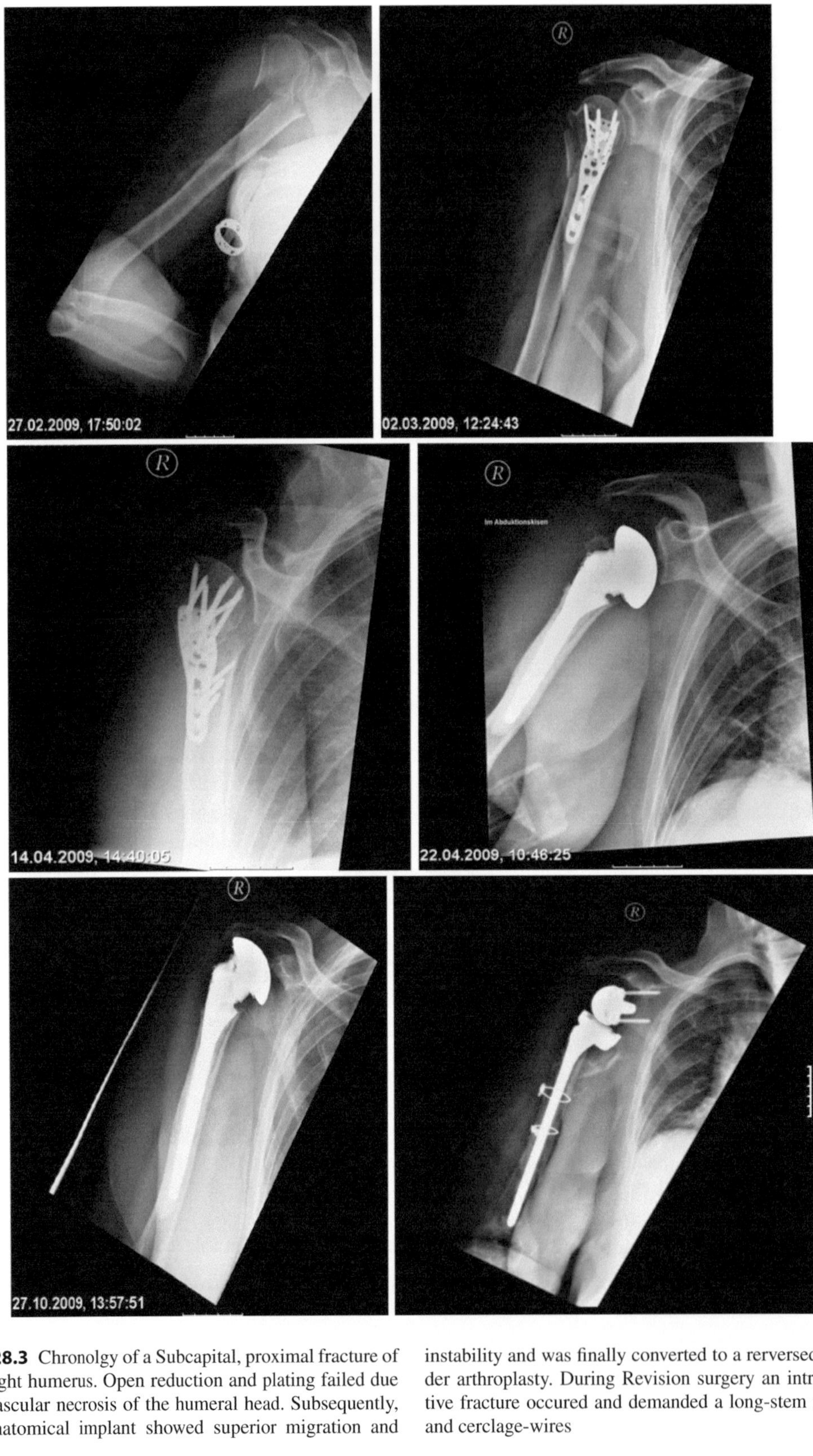

Fig. 28.3 Chronolgy of a Subcapital, proximal fracture of the right humerus. Open reduction and plating failed due to avascular necrosis of the humeral head. Subsequently, an anatomical implant showed superior migration and instability and was finally converted to a rerversed shoulder arthroplasty. During Revision surgery an intraoperative fracture occured and demanded a long-stem implant and cerclage-wires

with favorable outcome offering the possibility to combine wire-cerclages with plating, at least eight cortices should secure stability distal to the fracture [34]. Patients suffering from osteoporotic bone might benefit from additional use of allograft strut constructs [67]. Open reduction and internal fixation is recommended for fractures distal to the stem tip (Type C) without signs of healing after at least 3 months showing a well fixed stem, whereas revision with a long stem should be done for similar fractures associated with a loose humeral component [38].

Fractures and Fixation of the Tuberosities

The success of fracture-arthroplasty relies closely and more frequently than in elective surgery in the integrity of the tuberosities. Their acute dislocation or nonunion cause about 30 % of all complications in fracture arthroplasty and are one of the leading issues for revision surgery [76].

Fractures or involvement of the tuberosities may be treated by additional transosseous repair using non-absorbable sutures to secure the rotator cuff attachments [67], correct positioning of the fragments is crucial to achieve good and stable long-term results. Fixation of the greater tuberosity more than 2 cm distal to the apical circumference of the humeral head leads to overstuffing and deficient, functional results [48], whereas a cranialisation might cause subacromial impingement with limited function mostly in terms of limited abduction.

Only a stable and tension-free repair of the tuberosities will facilitate reintegration. Several prosthetic designs have been developed especially for fracture arthroplasty providing a better integration of the bony fragments in terms of the tuberosities and allowing for functional treatment postoperatively achieved either by a broad proximal shaping of the prosthesis enabling large interaction with the tuberosities or by the slim, so called "open stem design" offering multiple opportunities for transosseous suturing and good interfragmentary contact favoring ingrowth of the implant [76].

In the current literature it is stated that in primary fracture arthroplasty around 37 % of re-fixed tuberosities will reintegrate with a dislocation smaller than 5 mm, 17 % show more than 5 mm dislocation and the vast majority (46 %) will result in mal-positioning, non-union or bone resorption [37]. So the rate of expected complications and the need for revision-surgery because of fracture-involvement or intraoperative fracture of the tuberosities is imminent. Reintegration of the major tuberosity fragment has significant impact on the functional outcome, since more than 90 % of all patients presenting with less than 5 mm dislocation and adequate bone healing are satisfied with the surgical treatment result [37]. Furthermore, it has been proven that the patient's age, the type of the implant and the total number of surgical procedures have a significant impact on the faith of the tuberosities, whereas the type of fixation seems negligible [37].

Once a fracture arthroplasty has failed because of dislocation of a reintegrated greater tuberosity (more than 5 mm), a corrective osteotomy should be considered [10]. In case of non-union, resorption or a non-functional rotator-cuff, a conversion to reversed shoulder-arthroplasty is recommendable, though the results are known to be inferior to primary reversed arthroplasty [10].

Fractures of the Glenoid

Glenoid fractures occur almost only during surgery, mostly during the preparation of the bonestock preceding the implantation of the glenoid-component. These fractures may compromise stability of the component, especially when involving the scapular neck and may lead to early, symptomatic loosening of the prosthesis. As these conditions are very unfavorable, the situation of a fractured glenoid might easier be avoided than managed. Glenoid resurfacing is not advocated when bone support is questionable. As a salvage step, the remaining intact glenoid can be sculpted with a hand burr or glenoid reamer to match the radius of curvature of the humeral head component [46, 80]. In case of an intraoperative fracture, bone-grafting combined with a revision (metal back) glenoid component with wedge reinforcement and screws may be employed to restore stability of the bone and the implant [46, 80].

Loosening of the Components

Loosening of the glenoid or humeral component is the most common long term complication associated with shoulder replacement surgery accounting for about 40 % [5]. In more than 80 % the glenoid component is involved. Although glenoid components are less commonly used in fracture arthroplasty than in primary shoulder arthroplasty, treatment strategies are presented in the following.

Glenoid

Achieving secure long term fixation of the glenoid component is the primary goal in total shoulder arthroplasty. In this context, the low strength and the small volume of bone of the glenoid vault are critical factors to secure fixation and finally limit the long term "survival" of the implant [54]. To date, the most common mid and long-term complication of total shoulder replacement is glenoid loosening causing postoperative pain, limited function, and the potential need for revision surgery [69].

The reported prevalence of radiolucencies at the cement-bone interface of the glenoid component ranges from 0 to 100 % and increases with time. Ten years after surgery most authors observe radiolucency in terms of radiographic signs of loosening in at least 80 % of the cases standing for migration, tilting or shifting of the component in 34 % [33, 66, 83]. Though, only a small fraction with radiologic signs of loosened glenoid components needs revision surgery (7 % after 13 years [5], 9 % after 10 years [83]). Efforts have been made to improve long term stability, including the preservation of the subchondral plate, concentric reaming of the glenoid, selected biomaterials and advanced prosthetic design [44, 69, 77]. Cemented pegged components were most commonly used and supposed to provide the most predictable fixation. In the current literature, pegged designs showed advantages in terms of better implant-seating and less signs of radiolucencies, finally leading to lower implant-loosening rates [23]. Furthermore curved back glenoids turned out to be beneficial concerning malpositioning-related failure however leading to higher mid- and long-term failure [71]. The technique and mode of cementation has significant impact on implant stability whereas a uniform cement mantle of 1 mm and implementation of a so called pressurization-technique show the best results [36, 72]. Non-cemented glenoid components on the other hand rely upon mechanical interlock and biologic integration, typically by screw fixation or a combination of screws and press-fit pegs, to achieve sufficient initial fixation facilitating bone in-growth. Although non-cemented glenoids offer many theoretical advantages compared to cemented glenoids, they have been associated with higher complication rates due to increased ultra-highmolecular-weight polyethylene (UHMWPE) wear and to joint-overstuffing [6]. Boileau et al. identified two major causes of metal-back glenoid loosening as follows: primarily the mechanical failure arising from a lack of initial stability and secondly osteolysis caused by PE and metal wear. In accordance, the four primary failure modes of metal-back glenoids were summarized as: (1) insufficient polyethylene thickness (4 mm instead of 5 mm); (2) Excessive thickness of the component (7 mm) with massive stressing of the rotator cuff; (3) Rigidity of the metal-back component accelerating polyethylene wear and stress-shields bone; and (4) Posterior i.e. eccentric loads on the glenoid leading to polyethylene disassociation [6]. For these reasons, Boileau et al. concluded that the fixation of metal-back glenoids is inferior to that of cemented glenoids which is also confirmed by other authors in the literature [44, 68]. Resent trends follow a combination of the two strategies entitled as minimally cemented glenoids [69].

The common opinion about the mechanism of glenoid loosening is a repetitive, eccentric load of the humeral head onto the glenoid, commonly called "rocking horse" phenomenon. This eccentric or edge loading conditions produce a torque on the fixation surface inducing tensile stress at the bone-implant or bone-cement-implant interface, potentially causing interfacial failure and glenoid disassociation [69]. When the glenoid is resurfaced using conforming implants, eccentric loading is enhanced because of the inability of the artificial surface (PE) to mimic viscoelastic properties of the former cartilage and labrum as essentials of the physiologic glenohumeral motion. Eccentric loading might also result from glenoid mal-positioning or seating and humeral mal-positioning, all finally leading to implant-failure. The radial mismatch has been introduced to cope this problem, showing the ideal compromise between stability and native kinematics with a mismatch of 6–7 mm [77]. Finally an intact rotator-cuff preserves the artificial joint, because the magnitude of eccentric loading increases with weakness or insufficiency of the rotator cuff.

If a loose glenoid-component has to be revised there are strong arguments pointing towards a re-resurfacing of the glenoid [3, 15, 20]. Three retrospective surveys by Antuna et al., Deutsch et al. and Cheung et al. compared the functional and subjective outcome of revision-procedures with and without glenoid reimplantation. All uniformly described a better symptomatic and functional outcome for the patient group with reimplanted glenoids [3, 15, 20]. It is important to note, however, that these findings may include a selection bias, since patients in whom a glenoid implant was possible had a better bone stock and soft tissue situation than those patients being revised with a hemiarthroplasty.

The glenoid bone stock is crucial when considering re-resurfacing after aseptic loosening. As in primary surgery, attention should be drawn to a correct orientation of the glenoid component which can be achieved by eccentric reaming. Though, the limits of correction are even smaller than in primary resurfacing. Gillespie et al. conducted a cadaveric analysis on eight specimens to evaluate the degree of glenoid retroversion that can be corrected with eccentric reaming in primary gleno-humeral arthritis. They reported that an anterior correction of 10° resulted in a significant decrease of the glenoid width, 15° anterior correction resulted in an inability to seat the glenoid in 50 % of the tested specimens due to an inadequate bone stock, and 20° anterior correction resulted in an inability to seat the glenoid in 75 % of the tested specimens [25]. These results led the authors to suppose that 10° of anterior correction may be the limit. Beyond these findings, bone grafting should also be considered. Accordingly, treatment strategies for glenoid revision should include bone grafting to improve the glenoid bone stock. In these cases reversed shoulder arthroplasty represents a reliable therapeutic option providing the benefit of glenoid bone stock reconstruction by fixing the bone graft with a baseplate and screws and of solving the immanent problem of soft tissue insufficiency and prosthetic instability [4, 47]. Patients, in whom intraoperative findings preclude immediate component reimplantation would be candidates for singular bone grafting. Repeated revision with a glenoid component after graft consolidation should be considered for patients with continuous pain during shoulder activity after component removal and grafting [3, 56].

Humerus

Aseptic loosening of the humeral component, despite its rare occurrence, accounts however for approximately 7 % of all reported complications in refer to shoulder arthroplasty [5]. Similar to loosening of the glenoid component, radiolucent lines on radiographs are the first indicator of ongoing disintegration of the implant. Recent reports have indicated a higher frequency when press-fit humeral stems were used [45]. Thus, humeral component survival was supposed to be affected by the chosen type of fixation and the biologic response to wear particles. Changes at the periprosthetic humeral interface in the presence of a glenoid component raised concern about osteolysis and the potential for symptomatic loosening [59]. Sperling et al. defined humeral components at risk if they showed radiographic evidence of subsidence, tilting or lucent lines of more than 2 mm around the implant [66].

Male gender, younger age (>65 years) and acute fracture or posttraumatic arthritis have been associated with an increased risk of revision surgery due to loosening of the humeral component [18]. Besides, the survival of the humeral component (cemented or press-fit) seems significantly decreased in prosthetic settings using metal-back glenoid components [18]. These findings are in accordance with biomechanical studies reporting high stress within the polyethylene of metal-backed glenoid components, with the implication that these components have inferior wear properties [70].

If a humeral component is loose it might be revised by either standard or long-stem implants. In cases with poor bone-quality the revision with a long-stem component is recommended. Bone insufficiency might additionally require the use of allografts or extension towards tumor-prosthetic reconstructions, both procedures highly associated with a poor clinical and functional outcome [2, 13].

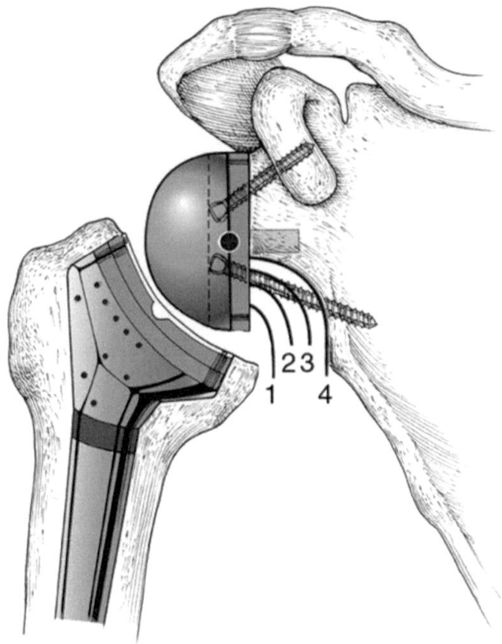

Fig. 28.4 This figure demonstrates the classification of scapular notching as described by Sirveaux et al. [64] Grade *1* defects are confined to the pillar. Grade *2* defects extend to the lower screw. Grade *3* defects encompass the lower screw. Grade *4* defects extend under the baseplate, which leads to loosening (Reprinted with permission from Cheung et al. [16])

Scapular Notching

The most frequent complication after reversed shoulder arthroplasty is scapular notching. Since reversed arthroplasty for fracture treatment is increasingly performed in the elderly population, some basics on this complication will be presented in the following.

Scapular notching is defined as an erosion of the inferior glenoid neck caused by repetitive mechanical abutment of the humeral component with the inferior scapular neck and the so called biological notching caused by the resulting PE-wear [53, 64]. This complication typically occurs within the first months after surgery with an incidence ranging from 44 to 96 % in the literature [24]. Aside of patient related factors associated with the development of scapular notching, such as preoperative rotator cuff-arthropathy and glenoid erosion, the surgical approach and the positioning of the glenosphere seem to be crucial to avoid postoperative notching [53, 64]. Recent studies demonstrated, that notching can be progressive in the long-term and is associated with reduced range of motion, strength, poor clinical outcome, increased polyethylene-wear and loosening [62]. A classification was introduced according to Sirveaux et al. [64] (see Fig. 28.4).

Preoperatively, the diagnosis of rotator cuff arthropathy should prompt the surgeon to evaluate the condition of the glenoid looking for evidence of superior defects and the condition of especially the patient's infraspinatus tendon should be evaluated on MRI [53]. As the antero-superior approach seems to be associated with higher notching rates it should be avoided in cases where the preoperative workup indicates potential for scapular notching [40]. Instead, the delto-pectoral approach may be warranted to ensure appropriate implant positioning [53]. Intraoperatively, efforts should be done to ensure that the glenosphere baseplate is implanted as inferior on the native glenoid as possible to foster an inferior overhang. Superior glenoid wear can be visually confirmed and preferentially reaming can be performed to promote a slight inferior tilt of the implanted glenosphere. Superior defects remaining after reaming can be bone grafted to avoid superior tilting of the baseplate.

Periprosthetic Infection

Prevalence of infection following primary total shoulder arthroplasty accounts for 0.6–2.4 % of all procedures, thus with more than 10 % of all complications revealing number four in the ranking why shoulder-replacements needs to be revised [5, 58, 63, 74]. In fracture arthroplasty, infection rates are even higher and account for up to 6 % overall [76].

Though not very common, infection after shoulder arthroplasty remains a devastating complication often requiring two-stage exchange of the prosthesis [58]. The majority of cases are related to immunosuppression secondary to host-related factors such as diabetes, rheumatoid arthritis or other rheumatoid illnesses, and systemic therapy with corticosteroids or cytotoxic agents. Previous surgery and repeated intraarticular steroid injections are the most common predispositions for intraarticular infection [46].

Common isolates in periprosthetic infections of the shoulder are Staphylococcus aureus, coagulase-negative Staphylococci and Propionibacterium acnes [5, 63]. According to the clinical appearance of the infection, it may be classified as acute (presenting symptoms less than 3 months after arthroplasty), subacute (presenting 3 months to 1 year after surgery), or late (presenting symptoms more than 1 year after surgery) [19, 84]. Periprosthetic infections show a broad range of clinical presentation. Highly purulent, acute infections with septic temperatures are rare. Most patients show nonspecific symptoms like prolonged pain or discomfort in combination with slightly elevated leucocyte-count or C-reactive protein blood levels. Especially low-grade infections with subclinical appearance and without significant alteration of blood-parameters are a diagnostic dilemma demanding for multiple, microbiologic samples by puncture or biopsy. Differentiation between aseptic loosening and low-grade infections might thus be challenging [84].

Established treatment protocols relate closely to the treatment of periprosthetic infections of the hip and knee based on the concept provided by Zimmerli et al. [84]. If the onset of symptoms is within 3–6 weeks after surgery, the infection can be treated by irrigation, exchange of the mobile parts and specific antibiotic treatment. In all other cases, retaining of the implant is associated with high re-infection rates due to foreign-body adherence of the causative bacteria and demands exchange of the implant. Whether a one- or two stage procedure is done depends on the pathogen, the soft tissue and general conditions of the patient and is currently subject of discussion. As for the hip and knee joint, the soft-tissue sleeve of the shoulder must be maintained to minimize contractures. Some surgeons have advocated the use of antibiotic-impregnated cement spacers after implant removal. Several independent reports have indicated favorable outcomes after the use of anatomically designed polymethylmethacrylate spacers, allowing for delayed exchange or permanent placement [5, 58].

References

1. Abboud JA, Anakwenze OA, Hsu JE. Soft-tissue management in revision total shoulder arthroplasty. J Am Acad Orthop Surg. 2013;21:23–31.
2. Abdeen A, Healey JH. Allograft-prosthesis composite reconstruction of the proximal part of the humerus: surgical technique. J Bone Joint Surg Am. 2010;92(Suppl 1 Pt 2):188–96.
3. Antuna SA, Sperling JW, Cofield RH, Rowland CM. Glenoid revision surgery after total shoulder arthroplasty. J Shoulder Elbow Surg. 2001;10:217–24.
4. Austin L, Zmistowski B, Chang ES, Williams Jr GR. Is reverse shoulder arthroplasty a reasonable alternative for revision arthroplasty? Clin Orthop Relat Res. 2011;469:2531–7.
5. Bohsali KI, Wirth MA, Rockwood Jr CA. Complications of total shoulder arthroplasty. J Bone Joint Surg Am. 2006;88:2279–92.
6. Boileau P, Avidor C, Krishnan SG, Walch G, Kempf JF, Mole D. Cemented polyethylene versus uncemented metal-backed glenoid components in total shoulder arthroplasty: a prospective, double-blind, randomized study. J Shoulder Elbow Surg. 2002;11:351–9.

7. Boileau P, Krishnan SG, Tinsi L, Walch G, Coste JS, Mole D. Tuberosity malposition and migration: reasons for poor outcomes after hemiarthroplasty for displaced fractures of the proximal humerus. J Shoulder Elbow Surg. 2002;11:401–12.
8. Boileau P, Watkinson D, Hatzidakis AM, Hovorka I. Neer Award 2005: The Grammont reverse shoulder prosthesis: results in cuff tear arthritis, fracture sequelae, and revision arthroplasty. J Shoulder Elbow Surg. 2006;15:527–40.
9. Boyd Jr AD, Thornhill TS, Barnes CL. Fractures adjacent to humeral prostheses. J Bone Joint Surg Am. 1992;74:1498–504.
10. Brunner U, Kohler S. Shoulder arthroplasty for treatment of the sequelae of proximal humerus fractures. Orthopade. 2007;36:1037–49.
11. Bufquin T, Hersan A, Hubert L, Massin P. Reverse shoulder arthroplasty for the treatment of three- and four-part fractures of the proximal humerus in the elderly: a prospective review of 43 cases with a short-term follow-up. J Bone Joint Surg Br. 2007;89:516–20.
12. Campbell JT, Moore RS, Iannotti JP, Norris TR, Williams GR. Periprosthetic humeral fractures: mechanisms of fracture and treatment options. J Shoulder Elbow Surg. 1998;7:406–13.
13. Cannon CP, Paraliticci GU, Lin PP, Lewis VO, Yasko AW. Functional outcome following endoprosthetic reconstruction of the proximal humerus. J Shoulder Elbow Surg. 2009;18:705–10.
14. Cazeneuve JF, Cristofari DJ. The reverse shoulder prosthesis in the treatment of fractures of the proximal humerus in the elderly. J Bone Joint Surg Br. 2010;92:535–9.
15. Cheung EV, Sperling JW, Cofield RH. Revision shoulder arthroplasty for glenoid component loosening. J Shoulder Elbow Surg. 2008;17:371–5.
16. Cheung E, Willis M, Walker M, Clark R, Frankle MA. Complications in reverse total shoulder arthroplasty. J Am Acad Orthop Surg. 2011;19(7):439–49.
17. Chin PY, Sperling JW, Cofield RH, Schleck C. Complications of total shoulder arthroplasty: are they fewer or different? J Shoulder Elbow Surg. 2006;15:19–22.
18. Cil A, Veillette CJ, Sanchez-Sotelo J, Sperling JW, Schleck CD, Cofield RH. Survivorship of the humeral component in shoulder arthroplasty. J Shoulder Elbow Surg. 2010;19:143–50.
19. Coste JS, Reig S, Trojani C, Berg M, Walch G, Boileau P. The management of infection in arthroplasty of the shoulder. J Bone Joint Surg Br. 2004;86:65–9.
20. Deutsch A, Abboud JA, Kelly J, Mody M, Norris T, Ramsey ML, Iannotti JP, Williams GR. Clinical results of revision shoulder arthroplasty for glenoid component loosening. J Shoulder Elbow Surg. 2007;16:706–16.
21. Gallinet D, Clappaz P, Garbuio P, Tropet Y, Obert L. Three or four parts complex proximal humerus fractures: hemiarthroplasty versus reverse prosthesis: a comparative study of 40 cases. Orthop Traumatol Surg Res. 2009;95:48–55.
22. Garrigues GE, Johnston PS, Pepe MD, Tucker BS, Ramsey ML, Austin LS. Hemiarthroplasty versus reverse total shoulder arthroplasty for acute proximal humerus fractures in elderly patients. Orthopedics. 2012;35:e703–8.
23. Gartsman GM, Elkousy HA, Warnock KM, Edwards TB, O'Connor DP. Radiographic comparison of pegged and keeled glenoid components. J Shoulder Elbow Surg. 2005;14:252–7.
24. Gerber C, Pennington SD, Nyffeler RW. Reverse total shoulder arthroplasty. J Am Acad Orthop Surg. 2009;17:284–95.
25. Gillespie R, Lyons R, Lazarus M. Eccentric reaming in total shoulder arthroplasty: a cadaveric study. Orthopedics. 2009;32:21.
26. Habermeyer P, Magosch P. Frakturendoprothetik. In: Lill H, editor. Die proximale Humerusfraktur. Stuttgart/New York: Thieme; 2006. p. 135–62.
27. Hammond JW, Queale WS, Kim TK, McFarland EG. Surgeon experience and clinical and economic outcomes for shoulder arthroplasty. J Bone Joint Surg Am. 2003;85-A:2318–24.
28. Hasan SS, Leith JM, Smith KL, Matsen 3rd FA. The distribution of shoulder replacement among surgeons and hospitals is significantly different than that of hip or knee replacement. J Shoulder Elbow Surg. 2003;12:164–9.
29. Hempfing A, Leunig M, Ballmer FT, Hertel R. Surgical landmarks to determine humeral head retrotorsion for hemiarthroplasty in fractures. J Shoulder Elbow Surg. 2001;10:460–3.
30. Jain NB, Hocker S, Pietrobon R, Guller U, Bathia N, Higgins LD. Total arthroplasty versus hemiarthroplasty for glenohumeral osteoarthritis: role of provider volume. J Shoulder Elbow Surg. 2005;14:361–7.
31. Jain N, Pietrobon R, Hocker S, Guller U, Shankar A, Higgins LD. The relationship between surgeon and hospital volume and outcomes for shoulder arthroplasty. J Bone Joint Surg Am. 2004;86-A:496–505.
32. Kalandiak S, Wirth MA, Rockwood Jr CA. Complications of shoulder arthroplasty. In: Williams GR, Yamaguchi K, Ramsey ML, Galatz LM, editors. Shoulder and elbow arthroplasty. Philadelphia: Lippincott Williams and Wilkins; 2005. p. 229–49.
33. Kasten P, Pape G, Raiss P, Bruckner T, Rickert M, Zeifang F, Loew M. Mid-term survivorship analysis of a shoulder replacement with a keeled glenoid and a modern cementing technique. J Bone Joint Surg Br. 2010;92:387–92.
34. Kent ME, Sinopidis C, Brown DJ, Frostick SP. The locking compression plate in periprosthetic humeral fractures a review of two cases. Injury. 2005;36:1241–5.
35. Klein M, Juschka M, Hinkenjann B, Scherger B, Ostermann PA. Treatment of comminuted fractures of the proximal humerus in elderly patients with the Delta III reverse shoulder prosthesis. J Orthop Trauma. 2008;22:698–704.
36. Klepps S, Chiang AS, Miller S, Jiang CY, Hazrati Y, Flatow EL. Incidence of early radiolucent glenoid

lines in patients having total shoulder replacements. Clin Orthop Relat Res. 2005;(435):118–25.
37. Kralinger F, Schwaiger R, Wambacher M, Farrell E, Menth-Chiari W, Lajtai G, Hubner C, Resch H. Outcome after primary hemiarthroplasty for fracture of the head of the humerus. A retrospective multicentre study of 167 patients. J Bone Joint Surg Br. 2004;86:217–9.
38. Kumar S, Sperling JW, Haidukewych GH, Cofield RH. Periprosthetic humeral fractures after shoulder arthroplasty. J Bone Joint Surg Am. 2004;86-A:680–9.
39. Lanting B, MacDermid J, Drosdowech D, Faber KJ. Proximal humeral fractures: a systematic review of treatment modalities. J Shoulder Elbow Surg. 2008;17:42–54.
40. Levigne C, Boileau P, Favard L, Garaud P, Mole D, Sirveaux F, Walch G. Scapular notching in reverse shoulder arthroplasty. In: Walch G, Boileau P, Mole D, Favard L, Levigne C, Sirveaux F, editors. Reverse shoulder arthroplasty: clinical results, complications, revision. Montpellier: Sauramps Medical; 2006. p. 353–72.
41. Levy J, Frankle M, Mighell M, Pupello D. The use of the reverse shoulder prosthesis for the treatment of failed hemiarthroplasty for proximal humeral fracture. J Bone Joint Surg Am. 2007;89:292–300.
42. Lyman S, Jones EC, Bach PB, Peterson MG, Marx RG. The association between hospital volume and total shoulder arthroplasty outcomes. Clin Orthop Relat Res. 2005;(232):132–7.
43. Martin TG, Iannotti JP. Reverse total shoulder arthroplasty for acute fractures and failed management after proximal humeral fractures. Orthop Clin North Am. 2008;39:451–7.
44. Martin SD, Zurakowski D, Thornhill TS. Uncemented glenoid component in total shoulder arthroplasty. Survivorship and outcomes. J Bone Joint Surg Am. 2005;87:1284–92.
45. Matsen 3rd FA, Iannotti JP, Rockwood Jr CA. Humeral fixation by press-fitting of a tapered metaphyseal stem: a prospective radiographic study. J Bone Joint Surg Am. 2003;85-A:304–8.
46. Matsen FA III, Rockwood CJ, Wirth MA, Lippitt SB, Parsons M. Glenohumeral -arthritis and its management. In: Rockwood Jr CA, Matsen FA III, Wirth MA, Lippitt SB, editors. The shoulder. 3rd ed. Philadelphia: WB Saunders; 2004. p. 879–1008.
47. Melis B, Bonnevialle N, Neyton L, Levigne C, Favard L, Walch G, Boileau P. Glenoid loosening and failure in anatomical total shoulder arthroplasty: is revision with a reverse shoulder arthroplasty a reliable option? J Shoulder Elbow Surg. 2012;21:342–9.
48. Mighell MA, Kolm GP, Collinge CA, Frankle MA. Outcomes of hemiarthroplasty for fractures of the proximal humerus. J Shoulder Elbow Surg. 2003;12:569–77.
49. Murachovsky J, Ikemoto RY, Nascimento LG, Fujiki EN, Milani C, Warner JJ. Pectoralis major tendon reference (PMT): a new method for accurate restoration of humeral length with hemiarthroplasty for fracture. J Shoulder Elbow Surg. 2006;15:675–8.
50. Namba RS, Thornhill TS. Posterior capsulorrhaphy in total shoulder arthroplasty. A case report. Clin Orthop Relat Res. 1995;(435):135–9.
51. Neer 2nd CS. Displaced proximal humeral fractures. I. Classification and evaluation. J Bone Joint Surg Am. 1970;52:1077–89.
52. Neer 2nd CS. Displaced proximal humeral fractures. II. Treatment of three-part and four-part displacement. J Bone Joint Surg Am. 1970;52:1090–103.
53. Nicholson GP, Strauss EJ, Sherman SL. Scapular notching: recognition and strategies to minimize clinical impact. Clin Orthop Relat Res. 2011;469:2521–30.
54. Orr TE, Carter DR, Schurman DJ. Stress analyses of glenoid component designs. Clin Orthop Relat Res. 1988; (232):217–24.
55. Palvanen M, Kannus P, Niemi S, Parkkari J. Update in the epidemiology of proximal humeral fractures. Clin Orthop Relat Res. 2006;442:87–92.
56. Phipatanakul WP, Norris TR. Treatment of glenoid loosening and bone loss due to osteolysis with glenoid bone grafting. J Shoulder Elbow Surg. 2006;15:84–7.
57. Plausinis D, Kwon YW, Zuckerman JD. Complications of humeral head replacement for proximal humeral fractures. Instr Course Lect. 2005;54:371–80.
58. Sabesan VJ, Ho JC, Kovacevic D, Iannotti JP. Two-stage reimplantation for treating prosthetic shoulder infections. Clin Orthop Relat Res. 2011;469:2538–43.
59. Sanchez-Sotelo J, O'Driscoll SW, Torchia ME, Cofield RH, Rowland CM. Radiographic assessment of cemented humeral components in shoulder arthroplasty. J Shoulder Elbow Surg. 2001;10:526–31.
60. Sanchez-Sotelo J, Sperling JW, Rowland CM, Cofield RH. Instability after shoulder arthroplasty: results of surgical treatment. J Bone Joint Surg Am. 2003;85-A:622–31.
61. Sewell MD, Kang SN, Al-Hadithy N, Higgs DS, Bayley I, Falworth M, Lambert SM. Management of peri-prosthetic fracture of the humerus with severe bone loss and loosening of the humeral component after total shoulder replacement. J Bone Joint Surg Br. 2012;94:1382–9.
62. Simovitch RW, Zumstein MA, Lohri E, Helmy N, Gerber C. Predictors of scapular notching in patients managed with the Delta III reverse total shoulder replacement. J Bone Joint Surg Am. 2007;89:588–600.
63. Singh JA, Sperling JW, Schleck C, Harmsen WS, Cofield RH. Periprosthetic infections after total shoulder arthroplasty: a 33-year perspective. J Shoulder Elbow Surg. 2012;21:1534–41.
64. Sirveaux F, Favard L, Oudet D, Huquet D, Walch G, Mole D. Grammont inverted total shoulder arthroplasty in the treatment of glenohumeral osteoarthritis with massive rupture of the cuff. Results of a multicentre study of 80 shoulders. J Bone Joint Surg Br. 2004;86:388–95.
65. Smith AM, Mardones RM, Sperling JW, Cofield RH. Early complications of operatively treated proximal humeral fractures. J Shoulder Elbow Surg. 2007;16:14–24.
66. Sperling JW, Cofield RH, Rowland CM. Minimum fifteen-year follow-up of Neer hemiarthroplasty

and total shoulder arthroplasty in patients aged fifty years or younger. J Shoulder Elbow Surg. 2004; 13:604–13.
67. Steinmann SP, Cheung EV. Treatment of periprosthetic humerus fractures associated with shoulder arthroplasty. J Am Acad Orthop Surg. 2008;16:199–207.
68. Stone KD, Grabowski JJ, Cofield RH, Morrey BF, An KN. Stress analyses of glenoid components in total shoulder arthroplasty. J Shoulder Elbow Surg. 1999;8:151–8.
69. Strauss EJ, Roche C, Flurin PH, Wright T, Zuckerman JD. The glenoid in shoulder arthroplasty. J Shoulder Elbow Surg. 2009;18:819–33.
70. Swieszkowski W, Bednarz P, Prendergast PJ. Contact stresses in the glenoid component in total shoulder arthroplasty. Proc Inst Mech Eng H. 2003;217:49–57.
71. Szabo I, Buscayret F, Edwards TB, Nemoz C, Boileau P, Walch G. Radiographic comparison of flat-back and convex-back glenoid components in total shoulder arthroplasty. J Shoulder Elbow Surg. 2005;14:636–42.
72. Terrier A, Buchler P, Farron A. Bone-cement interface of the glenoid component: stress analysis for varying cement thickness. Clin Biomech (Bristol, Avon). 2005;20:710–7.
73. Tischer T, Rose T, Imhoff AB. The reverse shoulder prosthesis for primary and secondary treatment of proximal humeral fractures: a case report. Arch Orthop Trauma Surg. 2008;128:973–8.
74. Trappey GJ, O'Connor DP, Edwards TB. What are the instability and infection rates after reverse shoulder arthroplasty? Clin Orthop Relat Res. 2011;469:2505–11.
75. Visotsky JL, Basamania C, Seebauer L, Rockwood CA, Jensen KL. Cuff tear arthropathy: pathogenesis, classification, and algorithm for treatment. J Bone Joint Surg Am. 2004;86-A Suppl 2:35–40.
76. Voigt C, Lill H. Primary hemiarthroplasty in proximal humerus fractures. Orthopade. 2007;36:1002–12.
77. Walch G, Edwards TB, Boulahia A, Boileau P, Mole D, Adeleine P. The influence of glenohumeral prosthetic mismatch on glenoid radiolucent lines: results of a multicenter study. J Bone Joint Surg Am. 2002;84-A:2186–91.
78. Wall B, Walch G. Reverse shoulder arthroplasty for the treatment of proximal humeral fractures. Hand Clin. 2007;23:425–30.
79. Warren RF, Coleman SH, Dines JS. Instability after arthroplasty: the shoulder. J Arthroplasty. 2002;17:28–31.
80. Wirth MA, Rockwood CA Jr. Complications of shoulder arthroplasty. Clin Orthop Relat Res. 1994;(307): 47–69.
81. Wright TW, Cofield RH. Humeral fractures after shoulder arthroplasty. J Bone Joint Surg Am. 1995;77: 1340–6.
82. Young SW, Segal BS, Turner PC, Poon PC. Comparison of functional outcomes of reverse shoulder arthroplasty versus hemiarthroplasty in the primary treatment of acute proximal humerus fracture. ANZ J Surg. 2010;80:789–93.
83. Young A, Walch G, Boileau P, Favard L, Gohlke F, Loew M, Mole D. A multicentre study of the long-term results of using a flat-back polyethylene glenoid component in shoulder replacement for primary osteoarthritis. J Bone Joint Surg Br. 2011;93:210–6.
84. Zimmerli W, Trampuz A, Ochsner PE. Prosthetic-joint infections. N Engl J Med. 2004;351:1645–54.

Part VIII

Fracture Management in Children

29 Fracture Management in Children

Andrew W. Howard and Mohamed Kenawey

Introduction

The proximal humerus is an uncommon location for children to fracture. Full functional recovery is common after closed treatment, even when anatomic reduction is not attained, due to rapid physeal growth and remodeling, and proximity to a universal joint. The older literature emphasizes complications of surgery and recommends closed treatment for all ages. More recent literature promotes anatomic reduction and internal fixation, particularly if little growth remains. The most commonly reported internal fixation techniques include percutaneous pinning, or intramedullary nailing, each with closed and possibly open reduction. There is currently little comparative literature or high quality evidence, leaving the surgeon and patient able to select from all options.

A.W. Howard (✉)
Division of Orthopaedic Surgery, Hospital for Sick Children, Toronto, ON, Canada

Departments of Surgery and Health Policy, Management and Evaluation, University of Toronto, Toronto, ON, Canada
e-mail: andrew.howard@sickkids.ca

M. Kenawey
Lecturer and Consultant of Orthopaedic Surgery, Orthopaedic Surgery Department Faculty of Medicine, Sohag University, Sohag, 82524, Egypt

Growth and Development of the Proximal Humerus

From the paediatric orthopaedic perspective, it is always essential to know the sequence of development of secondary ossification centers at each bony end and to have an idea about the relative growth contribution of each physeal plate. This knowledge is important in the initial assessment of paediatric trauma cases to distinguish proper physeal/epiphyseal injuries from the normally developing secondary ossification centers as well as in the follow up of such injuries and management of resultant growth disturbances.

The paediatric proximal humerus has two main secondary ossification centers, the capital humeral ossification center and that of the greater tuberosity. The ossification center of the capital humerus can be present at birth but is more frequently seen 2–3 months postnatally [1]. By the 7th month of age, the secondary ossification center of the greater tuberosity is present on radiographs. Both ossification centers start to fuse with each other by the age of 3 years to form a single epiphyseal ossification center for the proximal humerus and this fusion is complete by the age of 5–7 years. By 10 years of age, the dense metaphyseal cortex is becoming more mature and extending closer to the physis more laterally than medially. This might be a factor in the tendency to have a large medial fragment in the Salter-Harris type II injuries commonly seen in

P. Biberthaler et al. (eds.), *Fractures of the Proximal Humerus*, Strategies in Fracture Treatments,
DOI 10.1007/978-3-319-20300-3_29

older children (Thurston – Holland fragment). Finally, fusion of the combined ossification centers to the metaphysis may be as late as 18 and 20 years for females and males respectively (typically 14 in girls and 16–18 in boys).

The proximal humeral physeal plate accounts for most of the humeral growth in length. Pritchett used the extension of the nutrient canal into the middle of the medulla as a fixed point of measurement in each of the upper extremity bones to quantify the contribution of each physeal plate to the longitudinal growth of the studied bone [2]. The proximal humeral growth plate was found to contribute to 80–90 % of the humeral growth and 40 % of the total length of the upper extremity while the distal growth plate contributes to 20 % of the total length of the humerus and 10 % of the total length of the upper extremity. In the forearm, the distal growth plates of the radius and ulna account for 75 and 85 % of the longitudinal radial and ulnar growth respectively and they account for 39–40 % of the total length of the upper extremity. This explains the high remodeling activity of the proximal humerus.

Incidence of Proximal Humeral Fractures in Paediatric Population

The incidence of fractures in children is almost twice that in adults. The overall incidence of paediatric fractures varies from 20 to 40 fractures/1000/year. There is a slight male predominance (60 % of paediatric fractures). Fractures of the upper extremities account for 82 % of fractures in children while 17 % are in the lower limbs and 0.5 % of paediatric fractures are in the pelvis and spine. Only 0.7 % of fractures are open and 15–30 % are physeal injuries.

The most common fractures in childhood are those of the distal radius and metacarpals, which represent 57.1 % of all paediatric fractures. Proximal humeral fractures are not common injuries in paediatric population and they represent about 2 % of all paediatric fractures. Physeal injuries of the proximal humerus represent 1.9–3.1 % of all long bone physeal injuries. Proximal humeral fractures are commonly metaphyseal in about 64 % of cases while physeal fractures represent 36 % of all proximal humeral fractures.

Physeal injuries of the proximal humerus are commonly Salter-Harris types I and II injuries. Salter-Harris types III and IV injuries are rarely encountered. Salter-Harris type II fractures are the commonest proximal humeral physeal injuries, accounting for 58–88 % of all proximal humeral physeal injuries and 1.4 % of all paediatric physeal injuries. They usually do take place in older children and their peak is in boys aged 12 years and girls aged 11 years. Salter-Harris type I physeal separations are usually encountered in younger children, younger than 5 years of age, when the physis is growing rapidly. However, this theory couldn't be supported by Peterson et al who reported a peak for Salter-Harris type I fractures around the age of 14 and 12 years in boys and girls respectively [3]. Salter-Harris type III and IV are rarely reported in the area of the proximal humerus and they can be associated with glenohumeral dislocation. Binder et al. reported 4 patients with Salter-Harris type III and 3 patients with Salter-Harris type IV injuries in 72 proximal humeral physeal fractures (6 and 4 % respectively) [4]. Peterson et al described a modification for Salter-Harris classification where a Peterson type A is metaphyseal fracture with linear longitudinal component extending down to the physis but not along the physis. In their article studying the epidemiology of paediatric long bone physeal fractures in Olmsted County, Minnesota, they reported one Peterson type A proximal humeral physeal injury among 951 physeal injuries (0.1 %).

Mechanism of Injury

Paediatric proximal humeral fractures are commonly caused by sports related activities, motor vehicle accidents or uncommonly due to child abuse or birth trauma. Common reported mechanism of injuries are fall, snow boarding, skiing, football, biking, pedestrian struck by motor vehicle, basketball, hockey, wrestling, horseback riding, motocross or soccer. The main described mechanism of injury is a fall on extended, abducted and externally rotated arm, often as a result of extending the arm to protect against a backwards fall. This causes a metaphyseal lesion in toddlers and an epiphyseal lesion in children and adolescents. The second commonest mechanism constitutes a direct trauma caused by a fall on the shoulder, causing a direct injury of the physis, epiphysis, or the metaphysis. According to Kohler, the main mechanism of injury in proximal humeral fractures is adduction and extension, causing varus and apex anterior angulation [5].

An interesting article by David Williams speculated on arm position and mechanism in the pathogenesis of paediatric proximal humeral physeal injuries. It is impossible to abduct the arm beyond 90° without external rotation or adduct it beyond neutral without external or internal rotation. He believes that proximal humeral injuries are mainly caused by one or more of four basic forces: (1) forced extension, (2) forced flexion, (3) forced internal rotation or (4) forced external rotation. Six combinations are clinically relevant: (1) forced external rotation and extension, (2) forced internal rotation and flexion, (3) forced internal rotation and extension, (4) pure extension, (5) pure flexion, (6) forced external rotation and flexion. He stressed that fact that the identification of the mechanism of injury would help predict the most suitable manipulation technique, which is to reverse the mechanism of trauma. The mechanism of injury can be sought by combining injury history, physical examination of bony fragments and bruising, and evaluation of radiographs in two planes at 90° to each other. In his article, he presented four cases as examples for the combinations of different forces that cause proximal humeral fractures and implications for closed reduction.

1. Forced external rotation and extension, which will be presented by abduction and extension deformity of the arm with anteromedial displacement of the proximal end of the humeral metaphysis. Fracture reduction is by hyperextension, traction, flexion and internal rotation.
2. Forced internal rotation and flexion will cause posterolateral bruising and displacement of the proximal metaphysis of the humerus. Manipulation technique will be mainly by traction, external rotation and extension.
3. Forced internal rotation with extension will be associated with anterolateral displacement of the proximal metaphysis of the humerus and therefore, an anterolateral swelling and bruising. The upper metaphysis pierces the deltoid muscle anteriorly. Manipulation is mainly by traction, external rotation and flexion.
4. Pure extension injury will cause an anterior arm swelling and bruising due to anterior displacement of the proximal humeral metaphysis and radiographs will show pure anterior translation or angulation with no medial or lateral displacement. Reduction maneuver is mainly by traction and flexion.

Birth trauma can be also a cause of proximal humeral epiphysiolysis which is almost exclusively a Salter-Harris type I injury. There is one reported case in the literature of Salter-Harris type II proximal humeral fracture due to birth trauma. Because of the lack of the ossific nucleus of the proximal humerus at birth, displacement of the proximal metaphysis in relation to the glenoid may be the only radiographic finding. With follow up radiographs, callus is usually seen within 5–7 days. In such situations, ultrasound, arthrography or even MRI examination may help in diagnosis.

It is important as well to distinguish accidental injuries from child abuse. Fractures from abuse predominantly take place in infant and toddler age groups, mostly under the age of 18 months [6, 7]. Definite abuse is diagnosed with positive skeletal survey of multiple recent fractures or fractures of various stages of healing not consistent with the history, multiple internal injuries or physical findings suggestive of abuse like bruises or suspicious unexplained burns or scars. A history suggestive of abuse might be no eyewitness, history of no sufficient injury for this kind of trauma or a history of injury which is not consistent between different family members.

Finally, pathological fractures of the proximal humerus are not uncommon in paediatric patients and are usually secondary to simple bone cysts in that common location. The history is often of minimal trauma and it is essential to distinguish these cases for subsequent management and follow up.

Classifications

Paediatric proximal humeral fractures can be classified into those involving the growth plate (physeal injuries) versus the metaphyseal fractures. Physeal fractures are commonly described by Salter-Harris classification system while metaphyseal fractures are grouped according to their location, degree of angulation and displacement.

The Salter-Harris classification has been criticized by Peterson et al and others [3]. One of the reported limitations is that type V injuries are virtually not existent in multiple large studies which looked at the epidemiology of physeal fractures. Another limitation is that large number of fractures didn't fit into the classification. Peterson et al in their study of the epidemiology of physeal fractures in Olmsted County, Minnesota 1979–1988, described two new patterns of physeal injuries (type A and type B) which didn't fit into Salter-Harris system and which were fairly common injuries constituting almost 15.7 % of all physeal injuries in this study. The Peterson type A pattern is a metaphyseal fracture with linear longitudinal component extending to the physis but not along the physis. The Peterson type B is a fracture in which part or all of the physis is missing, and this injury is always an open injury. Peterson reported one proximal humeral physeal injury with pattern A fracture. Finally, Salter-Harris classification provides as well a limited prognostic ability for growth arrest following physeal injuries. Such growth disturbances and growth arrest are now believed to be related to a combination of factors, including the specific injured physis, the force of injury, the degree of displacement and comminution and age as well as fracture type.

In 1965, Neer and Horwitz described a grading system for proximal humeral physeal injuries according to the magnitude of displacement. Grade I fractures have less than 5 mm of displacement. Grade II fractures have displacement between 5 mm and one-third the diameter of the humeral shaft. Grade III fractures have displacement between one-third and two-thirds the diameter of the humeral shaft, and Grade IV fractures have displacement greater than two-thirds the diameter of the humeral shaft [8]. There is recently an increased interest and controversy in the management of severely displaced fractures (Neer-Horwitz grades III and IV) among older children and adolescents.

The Paediatric Expert Group of the AO Foundation in Collaboration With AO Clinical Investigation and Documentation and the International Association for Pediatric Traumatology has recently published the comprehensive AO Paediatric Classification of Long Bone Fractures. It is a numerical system, which is arranged by a bony code, segment code, fracture type, child code (child pattern), severity code and lastly exceptions or additional codes [9, 10].

They have followed the same rules of the numerical Müller-AO classification system for adults and the bones were similarly coded: 1 = humerus, 2 = radius/ulna, 3 = femur, 4 = tibia/fibula. The segments within each bone follow as well a similar coding scheme: 1 = proximal, 2 = diaphyseal and 3 = distal. However, from the anatomic and developmental point of view, paediatric long bones are divided into three segments: epiphysis, metaphysis and diaphysis. Consequently, each end or bony segment whether proximal or distal, would be subdivided into an epiphysis and metaphysis. Therefore, each bony segment can be further encoded into; 1 = proximal epiphysis and metaphysis and 3 = distal metaphysis and epiphysis. To define the extent of proximal and distal metaphyses of long bones, a square is drawn with one side over the growth plate and whose sides have the same length as the widest part of the physeal plate in question. For paired bones as radius/ulna and tibia/fibula, both bones must be included in the square (Fig. 29.1).

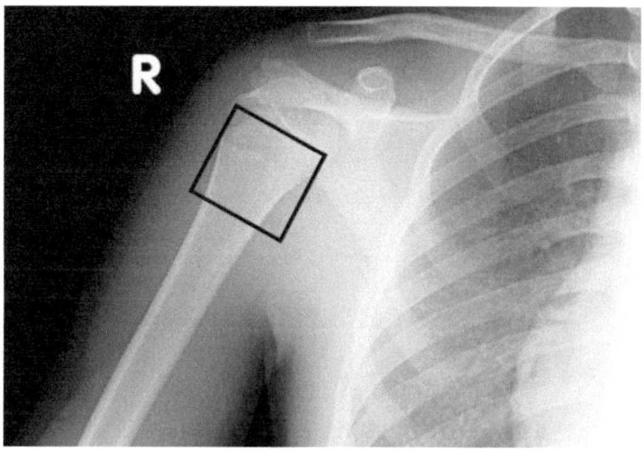

Fig. 29.1 The square method to identify the extent of the proximal humeral metaphyseal segment. The square is drawn with one of its side on the proximal humeral physeal plate and the length of its sides is the same as the width of the proximal humeral growth plate. The metaphyseal area will lie inside this square

The next step is to define the fracture type. In paediatric fractures, the most common fracture types are either shaft fractures (segment 2) or the epi-metaphyseal fractures (segment 1 and 3). Epiphyseal injuries are intra-articular by definition whereas metaphyseal fractures are extra-articular injuries identified with the square technique. Therefore, the original severity coding A-B-C used in adults was replaced by the location of fracture according to (E) epiphysis, (M) metaphysis or (D) diaphysis and this change would enable the users of this classification system to differentiate intra-articular versus extra-articular injuries.

As a result, paediatric proximal humeral fractures would be basically encoded as either 11-E or 11-M for epiphyseal or metaphyseal fractures respectively (Fig. 29.2). Then a child code, according to the fracture morphology is used for each specific fracture type E or M. Therefore, similar fracture morphology are given the same child code regardless the fracture type (Table 29.1). A fracture severity is used to distinguish simple 0.1, wedge 0.2 (partially unstable fracture with three fragments including a fully separated fragment), and complex 0.3 (totally unstable fracture with more than three fragments) (Table 29.2).

Interestingly, all previous classifications didn't describe separately fractures of the proximal humerus associated with glenohumeral dislocation, which is quite rare in paediatric population. Intrathoracic dislocation of the humeral head is also exceedingly rare. The only reported case in paediatric population was by Simpson et al who have described a young 14-year-old girl with intrathoracic dislocation of the humeral head [11]. She was hit from the left side by a speeding motor vehicle and she was thrown about 6 m landing on her right side. The right upper extremity was held in 80° of abduction and 70° of external rotation. Radiographic signs were: increase in the width of the intercostal space at the level at which the humeral head is seen on the initial radiograph of the chest (in this case was between 2nd and 3rd ribs) and outline of pleura around the humeral head. Fracture dislocation with intrathoracic displacement of the humeral head was then confirmed on CT examination. Reduction of the humeral head was achieved by gentle lateral traction and if difficult, manipulation of the humeral head through small thoracotomy can be performed.

Acute Complications

Brachial plexus and neurological complications following proximal humeral fractures are rare in skeletally immature patients. In the series of Hwang et al., 4 patients (0.7 %) of the 578 cases of proximal humerus fractures had concomitant brachial plexus and/or major peripheral nerve palsies [12]. Fractures that might cause neurovascular injury may be epiphyseal or metaphyseal and either radial, ulnar or median nerves can be affected. Medial translation and valgus angulation of the distal fracture fragment into the axilla is an important cause of neuropraxia or even axonotomesis of the brachial plexus. Full neurological recovery is expected with appropriate fracture care however, given the proximal location of these injuries, neurologic recovery may take up to 6–9 months. It is expected as well that those patients may complain of pain syndrome with dysesthesias and burning sensation, which completely resolve with neurologic recovery. They may benefit from drugs to treat neuropathic pain during this period.

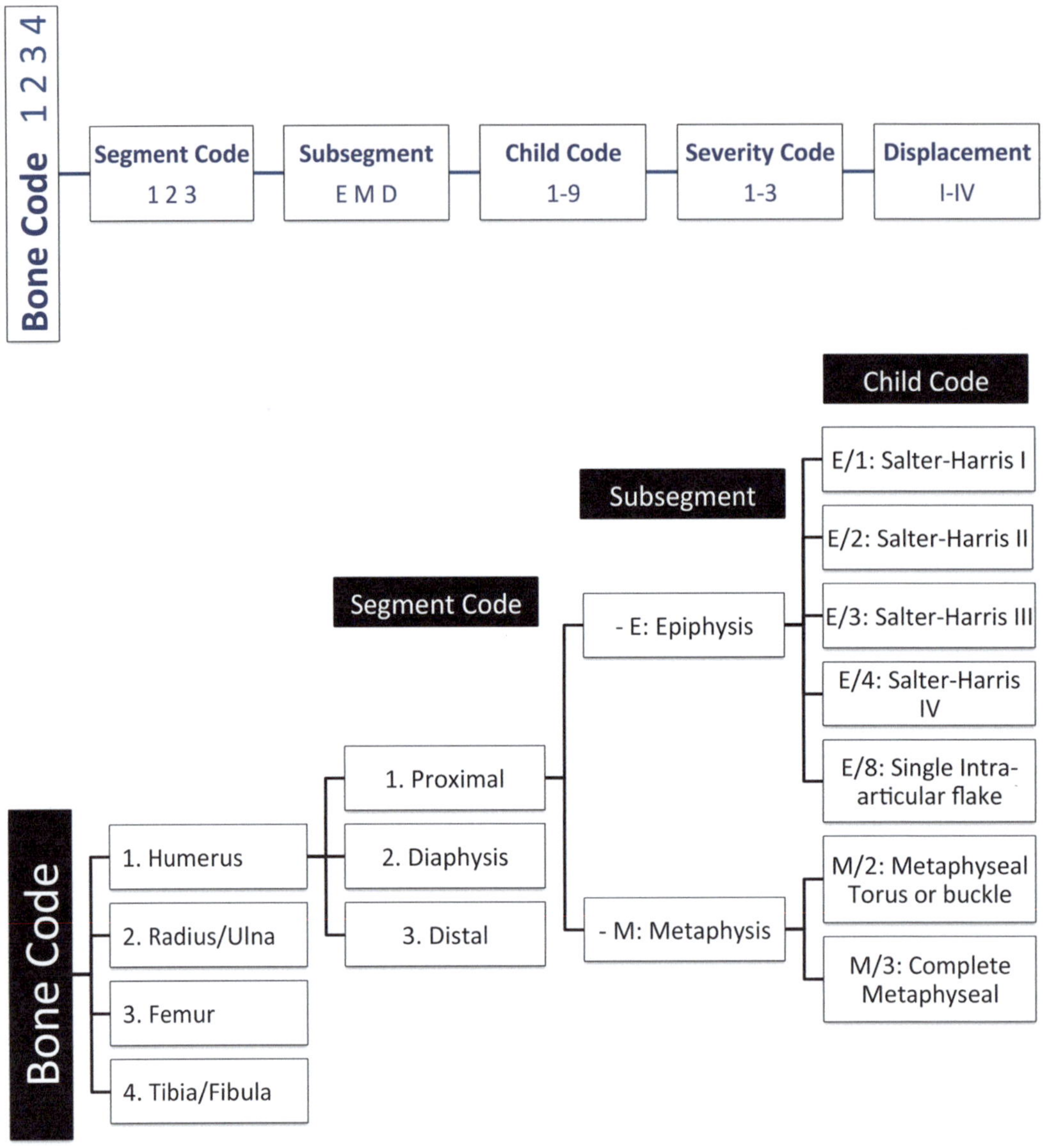

Fig. 29.2 The general outline of the AO Paediatric Comprehensive Classification of Long Bone Fractures and its specific use in the paediatric proximal humerus

Proximal humeral fractures may also cause axillary artery injury. Wera et al reported a case of displaced Salter-Harris type II proximal humeral fractures with absent distal pulses [13]. On exploration, the axillary artery was stretched and thrombosed. This was successfully managed with percutaneous pinning of the proximal humerus for stabilization and vascular reconstruction using reversed saphenous vein graft. Another case was reported in the series of Baxter and Wiley (one case out of 57) with interruption of the brachial artery in the axilla [14].

Treatment

The proximal humeral growth plate accounts for 80 % of the humeral growth and this explains the high remodeling capacity and the rationale for conservative treatment of virtually all proximal humeral fractures in children [2]. This high remodeling potential usually results in excellent functional outcomes in young children regardless of the amount of displacement or angulation. That is why Smith advocated *the leave it alone* treatment approach while Neer and Horwitz found that it is difficult to justify an operative treatment in the paediatric proximal humeral fractures [8]. However as early as 1969, it was clear that this remodeling potential is less powerful in older children and that angulations of more than 20° are partially corrected in children older than 11 years [15]. The only absolute indications for surgical treatment in younger (under 11) age groups would therefore be neurovascular injury, open fractures or severely displaced fractures where the metaphyseal fragment is tenting and endangering the integrity of the skin.

Table 29.1 Child codes according to different fracture types. Comprehensive AO Paediatric Classification of Long Bone Fractures

Type	Child codes	Description
E	/1	Salter-Harris I
	/2	Salter-Harris II
	/3	Salter-Harris III
	/4	Salter-Harris IV
	/5	Tillaux fracture (two plane)
	/6	Triplane fracture
	/7	Ligament avulsion
	/8	Flake fracture
	/9	Other epiphyseal injuries
M	/2	Green stick fracture
	/3	Complete fracture
	/7	Avulsion injuries
	/9	Others not-classified

Interestingly, articles published before 1990 uniformly advocated nonoperative treatment for all paediatric proximal humeral fractures, while after 2000, there are more recommendations for age and deformity specific treatment schemes [16]. This is mainly to achieve the goals of modern fracture treatment through stable anatomical reduction and healing without any residual deformity or functional deficit in ways that are appropriate for children. Multiple age and deformity specific protocols have been suggested, however, there is no universal agreement about age limits and deformity magnitude cutoffs which would define an unacceptable alignment and would be the bases of evidence based practice [16].

According to Beaty, acceptable proximal humeral alignment as well as the magnitude of displacement are age dependent and his recommendations were: (1) in children younger than 5 years, up to 70° of angulation and total displacement is acceptable; (2) in children 5–12 years, 40°–70° of angulation; and (3) in children older than 12 years, 40° of angulation and 50 % apposition would be the limit.

The summary of Dobbs et al provides slightly different figures: (1) in children younger than 7 years, 75° of angulation, (2) in children 8–11 years, 60° of angulation and (3) in children older

Table 29.2 Different patterns of paediatric proximal humeral fractures according to comprehensive AO Paediatric Classification of Long Bone Fractures

Simple fractures		Wedge/complex fractures	
Code	Description	Code	Description
11-E/1.1	Simple Salter-Harris type I (Simple epiphysiolysis)		
11-E/2.1	Simple Salter-Harris type II (Simple epiphysiolysis with metaphyseal wedge)	11-E/2.2	Epiphysiolysis with multifragmentary metaphyseal wedge
11-E/3.1	Simple Salter-Harris type III (Simple epiphyseal fracture)	11-E/3.2	Multifragmentary epiphyseal fracture
11-E/4.1	Simple Salter-Harris type IV (Simple epi-metaphyseal fracture)	11-E/4.2	Multifragmentary epimetaphyseal fracture
11-E/8.1	Single intraarticular flake fracture	11-E/8.2	Multiple intraarticular flake
11-M/2.1	Metaphyseal torus/buckle fracture		
11-M/3.1	Complete, simple metaphyseal	11-M/3.2	Complete, multifragmetary metaphyseal

than 11 years, 45° of angulation is maximum acceptable deformity [17].

On the other hand, according to the national German guidelines, nonoperative treatment is recommended in patients younger than 10 years for proximal humeral fractures with a total angulation of less than 60° and less than 10° valgus deformity. In adolescent patients older than 10 years, fractures with a displacement of less than 30° and a valgus deformity of less than 10° can be also treated nonoperatively. A surgical treatment is recommended in patients younger than 10 years with fractures that were angulated more than 60° or totally displaced. In patients older than 10 years with total displacement and/or an angulatory displacement of more than 30° and/or more than 10° valgus deformity, surgery is also advocated [18].

Pahlavan et al recommended as well another treatment protocol based on their systematic review of all articles published on the treatment paediatric proximal humeral fractures in the last 50 years (January 1960 to April 2010). They grouped children according to their age into three main groups: <10-year-old, 10–13 year-old and >13-year-old. Children <10 years of age can be treated nonoperatively due to the expected high remodeling. Those above 13 years of age with limited remodeling capacity should certainly be offered the choice of appropriate alignment and fixation and be allowed to come to an informed decision, provided the displacement of their fracture warrants it. The interim group should be treated on a case-to-case basis, including their gender, true bone age, and biological capacity to remodel [16].

As we see from these differing publications, no agreement on age limit or deformity parameters can be found. All of the aforementioned recommendations are based on level IV case series. Unfortunately, there are no randomized trials or prospective studies published in this area to try to validate these alignment and displacement limits as well as age specific decision making and to compare nonoperative and operative treatments and therefore the evidence in this area is inconclusive.

Treatment options can range from nonoperative treatment with an arm sling immobilization or collar and cuff for 3–4 weeks till the child is pain free and then progressive mobilization can be started to aggressive open reduction aiming at anatomical alignment and internal fixation. The recommended methods for conservative immobilization are collar and cuff, Gilchrist's bandage, Desault bandage, Mitella bandage, Velpeau sling, spica cast, hanging cast or traction. In cases of unacceptable alignment or displacement, closed reduction under general anaesthesia can be tried and then followed by either immobilization with one of the previously mentioned methods or by definitive internal fixation using percutaneous pinning or retrograde elastic stable intramedullar nailing. Open reduction is always reserved for cases with failure to achieve acceptable alignment with closed techniques. Open reduction is done through deltopectoral approach and then fixation can be achieved by percutaneous pinning, retrograde elastic stable intramedullary nailing, staples, screws or plates and screws.

The technique of closed reduction is by abduction of the arm greater than 90°, flexion and external rotation and then traction. Depending on the direction of fracture displacement, posterior or anterior pressure on the proximal shaft may be performed to reduce the distal fragment. Before any trial of closed reduction, it is necessary to study the plain radiographs and to define the direction of displacement and determine the injury mechanism. Closed reduction technique should reverse the injury mechanism as detailed by David Williams [19].

Bahr et al investigated the possible causes that might lead to failure of achieving satisfactory closed reduction of severely displaced proximal humeral fractures. They found soft tissue interposition in 53 % of cases. Long head of biceps and to a lesser degree entrapped periosteum were the offending structures [18]. An interesting study by Lucas et al. challenged the concept of the interposition of the long head of biceps as a cause of failure of closed reduction in severely displaced proximal humeral fractures. MRI of the shoulder joint was performed in four children with fully displaced proximal humeral fractures and none of them showed entrapment of the long head of biceps between fracture fragments despite failure of closed reduction in three children. Moreover, they tried to simulate a fully displaced proximal humeral fracture in a cadaveric situation and they failed to find any interposition of the long head of biceps in between fragments while displacing the distal fragment in different directions. They believe that failure of closed reduction is mainly related to the degree of displacement [20].

In cases of operative treatment of proximal humeral fractures in children and adolescents, the most common fixation devices are either percutaneous k-wires or retrograde elastic stable intramedullary nailing. Elastic nails can be inserted through a midline portal just superior to the olecranon fossa or through two drill holes made at the lateral supracondylar ridge (Figs. 29.3 and 29.4). Holes to insert these nails should be slightly larger than the diameter of the chosen nail. In this

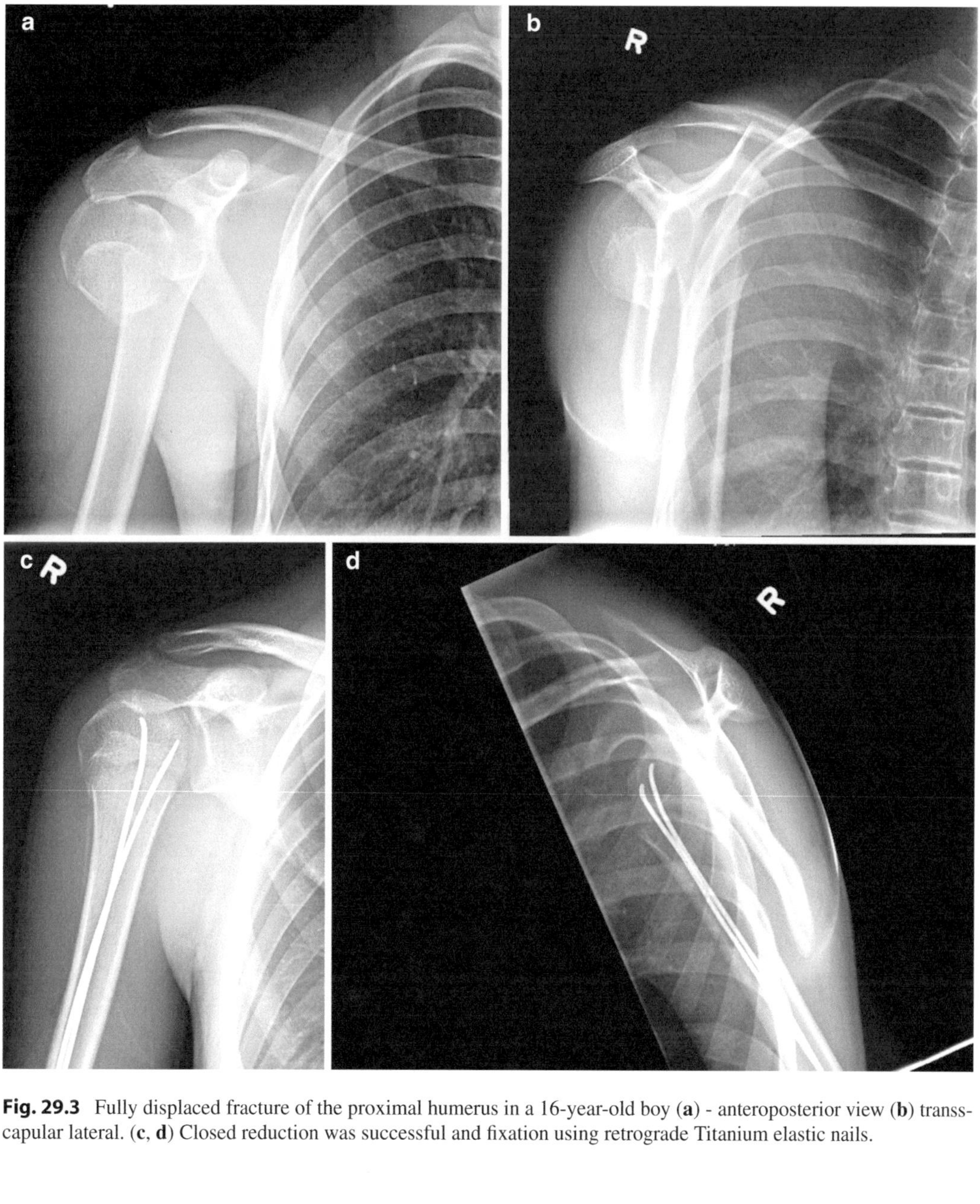

Fig. 29.3 Fully displaced fracture of the proximal humerus in a 16-year-old boy (**a**) - anteroposterior view (**b**) transscapular lateral. (**c**, **d**) Closed reduction was successful and fixation using retrograde Titanium elastic nails.

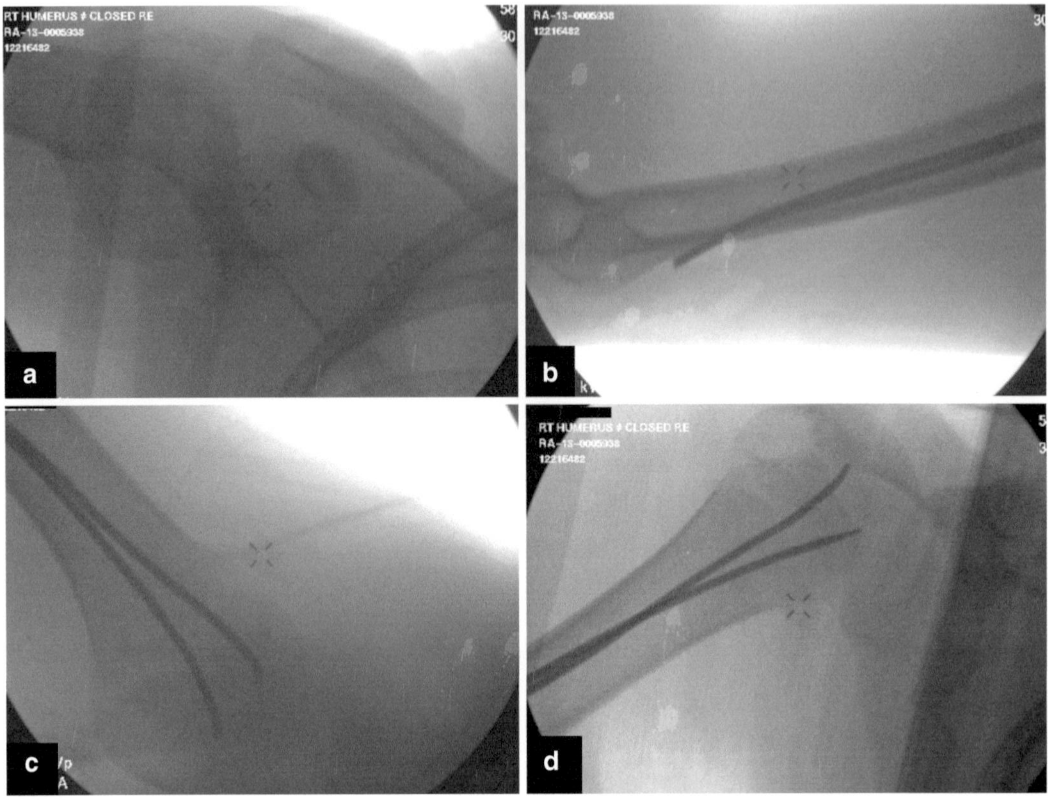

Fig. 29.4 Intraoperative C-Arm shots for the same patient in Fig. 29.3. (**a**) Closed reduction was successful in full abduction of the arm. (**b–d**) Fixation with Titanium elastic nails inserted proximal to the olecranon fossa

situation, there is a small risk of iatrogenic distal humeral fracture if the nails are inserted through the lateral supracondylar ridge, therefore another choice is to use a lateral and a medial supracondylar holes and a nail is inserted through each hole [21].

Percutaneous pinning is the other common fixation technique in both adult and paediatric proximal humeral fractures (Fig. 29.5). In order to fix the head fragment, the most commonly used technique is retrograde pinning from the humeral shaft up into the head. Two main configurations exist, either two retrograde anterolateral pins or retrograde anterolateral and anterior pins. The usual starting point for anterolateral pins is midway between the lateral and anterior surfaces of the arm above the insertion of the deltoid with pin angulation of 45° to the shaft in the coronal plane and 30° to the shaft in the sagittal plane. Humeral retroversion averages 19°, and percutaneous pins must be directed posteromedially to account for this angle. Structures at risk are mainly the radial and axillary nerves. The radial nerve is relatively protected if pins are kept above the deltoid insertion while the axillary nerve is usually located about 5 cm below the acromion. In selected cases, a third pin can be added in an antegrade fashion from the greater tuberosity down to the humeral shaft [4, 17, 22].

Review of Selected Literature

As early as 1969, Dameron and Reibel evaluated 46 patients with proximal humeral physeal fractures and noted poor outcomes in patients aged 14 years or older who lost fracture reduction during the treatment period [15]. Several authors have then tried to compare retrospectively the results of conservative treatment versus operative

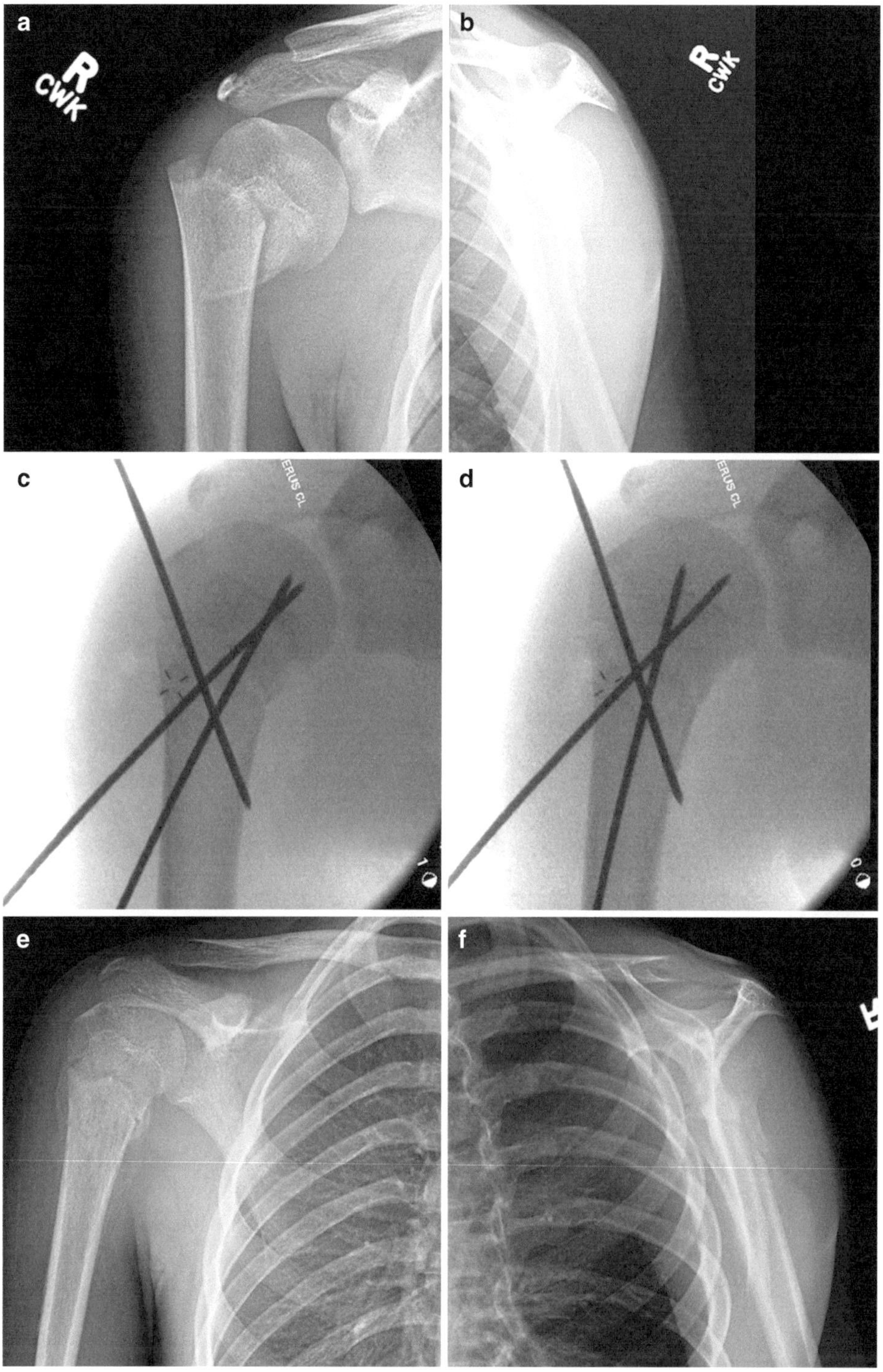

Fig. 29.5 Displaced fracture of the proximal humerus in a 14-year-old boy. (**a**, **b**) The distal fragment pierced the deltoid anteriorly and was felt subcutaneously. Trial of closed reduction was not successful and therefore we proceeded with open reduction. (**c**, **d**) Intraoperatively, the biceps tendon and the periosteum were interposed between fracture fragments and we had to dissect lateral to biceps tendon and open periosteum widely in order to reduce the fracture. Then fixation with percutaneous pinning was achieved. (**e**, **f**) radiographs following removal of the k-wires after weeks showed maintained correction and good early healing

intervention and the effect of age as well as fracture displacement and angulation on the final outcomes.

Baxter and Wiley reviewed 57 Salter-Harris type I and II proximal humeral physeal injuries (age range 8–15-years). Patients were divided into three groups according to treatment (no reduction, closed reduction or open reduction group). Closed or open reduction was done in half of Neer and Horowitz grade II, most patients with grade III (except one patient who was in the no reduction group) and all patients with grade IV displacement. Manipulation of the fracture, whether closed or open, improved the position in only one third of the patients. Interestingly, the final outcome was not better than those who healed with the same initial degree of displacement due to extensive remodeling of severely displaced injuries. Thirty percent of their patients had >1 cm of radiographic humeral shortening, however none was aware of any discrepancy. Therefore, no obvious advantage could be found with open reduction. The authors concluded that paediatric proximal humeral fractures should be always treated conservatively by simple arm sling and bandage till the patient is pain free and then mobilized early. The only exception of this rule would be fully displaced metaphyseal end, which pierced the deltoid muscle, tenting the skin with the risk of skin breakdown or in cases with neurovascular injury [14].

In another study by Binder et al, 72 paediatric proximal humeral fractures with mean age of 10 years were reviewed. Fifty-seven patients (79 %) were treated conservatively while 15 patients (21 %) underwent operative intervention (12 closed reductions and 3 open reductions) with fixation by percutaneous pinning. Operative treatment was indicated in patients with angular deformities greater than 30° and this group of patients had an average age of 11.8-years and all of them had anatomical reduction. Only 5.6 % of the patients had poor results reported. One patient had poor result due to persistent angular deformity of more than 20° following conservative treatment. Their final conclusion was that the patient's age has a major influence on the treatment of such injuries as the remodeling potential of the proximal humerus is considerable but related to age [4].

Beringer et al reviewed 48 children with average age of 13.5 years and all of them had Neer and Horwitz grade III or IV displacement (Salter-Harris type I in 6 and Salter-Harris type II in 42 patients). One half of the patients were 15 years or older. Thirty-nine patients had nonoperative management with closed reduction and then traction, sling immobilization, abduction bolster bracing, or shoulder spica casting. Operative intervention was done in 9 patients, 6 closed reduction and percutaneous pinning and 3 open reduction and internal fixation using screw, staples or plate. Closed reduction was less likely to be successful among patients with greater displacement. About two-thirds of patients with displacement ≥80 % remained malpositioned. No significant complications were recorded in the nonoperative group while the operative group had three complications and two of them were significant; one patient had osteomyelitis of the humerus with sequestrum following pin removal and in another patient, spiral fracture of the proximal shaft took place through a pin fixation site. From the functional point of view, no patient reported employment or activity restrictions caused by their injuries, and all described routine vigorous use of both shoulders and upper extremities. The authors concluded that the quality of reduction is not correlated with late functional outcome. Even in patients aged 15-years or older with inadequate reduction (defined by failure to achieve improvement of at least one Neer-Horwitz grade), greater proportion of minor clinical abnormalities, mostly mild loss of external rotation, could be identified but were not statistically significant. Therefore, the authors concluded that an attempt to achieve and maintain an anatomic reduction of severely displaced proximal humeral epiphyseal fractures was justified, especially in children 15 years and older [23].

Several authors have described their results with the use of specific fixation device and tried to compare the results of fixation using percutaneous pinning versus elastic nailing. Hutchinson et al reviewed 73 skeletally immature patients who underwent reduction and fixation using either intramedullary elastic stable nails or percutaneous k-wires. All of these fractures were displaced proximal humeral physeal or metaphyseal injuries deemed to be in unacceptable alignment given patient age and remodeling potential. The main indications of operative treatment were age of 12-years-old or more with Neer-Horwitz grade 4 fractures or angulation of 40° or more. They found that intramedullary nails had fewer complications, 4 % (one case of stitch abscess) versus 41 % in the percutaneous pinning group where most complications are pin tract infection or pin migration. In one case in the percutaneous pinning group, pin tract infection caused osteomyelitis. On the other hand, intramedullary nails were associated with longer operative time, higher blood loss and the need for second surgical procedure for removal. In the percutaneous pinning group, a second surgical procedure was needed for removal if the k-wires were buried under the skin. The final conclusion of this article was that both percutaneous pinning and elastic nailing have comparable short-term radiographic results although percutaneous pinning technique has higher rates of pin-related complications compared to intramedullary nails which generally require longer surgeries, greater blood loss, and higher rates of surgical implant removal [22].

According to the authors, both techniques can provide satisfactory results. The choice between either fixation method is mainly dependent on patient factors and surgeon factors. In case of difficult or unreliable regular follow-up, intramedullary nailing might be a better choice due to fewer hardware related complications while in reliable patients, percutaneous pinning is a good option if the ends of the pins are left outside the skin to avoid second anaethesia. On the other hand, surgeons who do more adult trauma are more familial with percutaneous pinning while paediatric orthopaedic surgeons have more experience with the use of elastic stable intramedullary nails in long bone fractures. Location of the fracture itself, whether epiphyseal or metaphyseal seems to play a less important role in implant choice. Other reported complications of intramedullary nail fixation include implant perforation and loss of position, misplaced nail, revision due to hematoma and difficulty removal of the nails.

Xie et al reported also their experience with Titanium elastic intramedullary nailing in 25 proximal humeral fractures in children. Their indications for surgical intervention were irreducible fractures (because of the "button-holing" phenomenon and/or interposition of the long head of the biceps), unstable fractures noted after closed reduction, open fractures, multitrauma, and patients older than 10 years with displacement of more than two-thirds of the diameter of the humerus and/or angulation of over 45° between fragments. All patients in this series were satisfied with the final outcome and the range of motion of the shoulder was full. There were only three minor complications in the form of skin irritation adjacent to the distal end of the nail and the nails were removed 3 weeks postoperatively in one patient and 6 months in the other two patients and this didn't seem to compromise the final functional outcome [24].

Dobbs et al reviewed their experience in the treatment of severely displaced humeral fractures (Neer-Horwitz grades III and IV) in older children, age range 5 16 years and 69 % of children were ≥15-year-old. All patients had an attempt at closed reduction under general anaesthesia then followed by immobilization or percutaneous pinning and in case of failure of closed reduction, open reduction through deltopectoral approach and fixation with percutaneous pinning or screws. Potential causes for failure of closed reduction were interposed periosteum, deltoid, capsule, or the long head of the biceps tendon. In all cases, displacement was reduced to Neer-Horwitz grades I or II. At the latest follow up, all patients were satisfied and non complained of any pain or functional deficit with near normal glenohumeral range of motion and full return to activities [17].

Conclusion

A rational approach to treating the proximal humerus fracture in a child begins with appreciating the biology of the fracture and the empirical results in the published literature, both of which favour nonoperative treatment. Operative reduction, with k-wire or elastic nail fixation, is currently promoted for severely displaced fractures among older children although no definite evidence or consensus has emerged regarding the exact indications for these techniques. Patient, fracture, surgeon, and setting factors must be taken into account when proposing operative care.

These are rare fractures so most surgeons will not have extensive specific experience. Operative closed reduction is not universally successful, and notable complications occur with both percutaneous pin fixation and intramedullary nailing techniques. Surgeons should consider their familiarity with these common paediatric fixation techniques for other more common fractures when choosing whether, or how, to treat any of these fractures operatively. An understanding of the biology and biomechanics, the excellent results of nonoperative management, and the potential difficulties with operative management will allow rational, individual decisions to be made while further evidence is sought to guide care.

References

1. Ogden JA, Conlogue GJ, Jensen P. Radiology of postnatal skeletal development: the proximal humerus. Skeletal Radiol. 1978;2(3):153–60.
2. Pritchett JW. Growth plate activity in the upper extremity. Clin Orthop Relat Res. 1991; 268:235–42.
3. Peterson HA, Madhok R, Benson JT, Ilstrup DM, Melton 3rd LJ. Physeal fractures: part 1. Epidemiology in Olmsted county, Minnesota, 1979–1988. J Pediatr Orthop. 1994;14(4):423–30.
4. Binder H, Schurz M, Aldrian S, Fialka C, Vecsei V. Physeal injuries of the proximal humerus: long-term results in seventy two patients. Int Orthop. 2011;35(10):1497–502.
5. Kohler R, Trillaud JM. Fracture and fracture separation of the proximal humerus in children: report of 136 cases. J Pediatr Orthop. 1983;3(3):326–32.
6. Thomas SA, Rosenfield NS, Leventhal JM, Markowitz RI. Long-bone fractures in young children: distinguishing accidental injuries from child abuse. Pediatrics. 1991;88(3):471–6.
7. Kemp AM, Dunstan F, Harrison S, Morris S, Mann M, Rolfe K, et al. Patterns of skeletal fractures in child abuse: systematic review. BMJ. 2008;337:a1518.
8. Neer 2nd CS, Horwitz BS. Fractures of the proximal humeral epiphysial plate. Clin Orthop Relat Res. 1965;41:24–31.
9. Slongo T, Audige L, Schlickewei W, Clavert JM, Hunter J, International Association for Pediatric Traumatology. Development and validation of the AO pediatric comprehensive classification of long bone fractures by the Pediatric Expert Group of the AO Foundation in collaboration with AO Clinical Investigation and Documentation and the International Association for Pediatric Traumatology. J Pediatr Orthop. 2006;26(1):43–9.
10. Slongo TF, Audige L, AO Pediatric Classification Group. Fracture and dislocation classification compendium for children: the AO pediatric comprehensive classification of long bone fractures (PCCF). J Orthop Trauma. 2007;21(10 Suppl):S135–60.
11. Simpson NS, Schwappach JR, Schwappach JR, Toby EB. Fracture-dislocation of the humerus with intrathoracic displacement of the humeral head. A case report. J Bone Joint Surg Am. 1998;80(6):889–91.
12. Hwang RW, Bae DS, Waters PM. Brachial plexus palsy following proximal humerus fracture in patients who are skeletally immature. J Orthop Trauma. 2008;22(4):286–90.
13. Wera GD, Wera GD, Friess DM, Friess DM, Getty PO, Getty PO. Fracture of the proximal humerus with injury to the axillary artery in a boy aged 13 years. J Bone Joint Surg Br. 2006;88(11):1521.
14. Baxter MP, Wiley JJ. Fractures of the proximal humeral epiphysis. Their influence on humeral growth. J Bone Joint Surg Br. 1986;68(4):570–3.
15. Dameron Jr TB, Reibel DB. Fractures involving the proximal humeral epiphyseal plate. J Bone Joint Surg Am. 1969;51(2):289–97.
16. Pahlavan S, Baldwin KD, Pandya NK, Namdari S, Hosalkar H. Proximal humerus fractures in the pediatric population: a systematic review. J Child Orthop. 2011;5(3):187–94.
17. Dobbs MB, Luhmann SL, Gordon JE, Strecker WB, Schoenecker PL. Severely displaced proximal humeral epiphyseal fractures. J Pediatr Orthop. 2003;23(2):208–15.
18. Bahrs C, Zipplies S, Ochs BG, Rether J, Oehm J, Eingartner C, et al. Proximal humeral fractures in children and adolescents. J Pediatr Orthop. 2009;29(3):238–42.
19. Williams DJ. The mechanisms producing fracture-separation of the proximal humeral epiphysis. J Bone Joint Surg Br. 1981;63-B(1):102–7.
20. Lucas JC, Mehlman CT, Laor T. The location of the biceps tendon in completely displaced proximal humerus fractures in children: a report of four cases with magnetic resonance imaging and cadaveric correlation. J Pediatr Orthop. 2004;24(3):249–53.
21. Fernandez FF, Eberhardt O, Langendorfer M, Wirth T. Treatment of severely displaced proximal humeral fractures in children with retrograde elastic stable intramedullary nailing. Injury. 2008;39(12):1453–9.
22. Hutchinson PH, Bae DS, Waters PM. Intramedullary nailing versus percutaneous pin fixation of pediatric proximal humerus fractures: a comparison of compli-

cations and early radiographic results. J Pediatr Orthop. 2011;31(6):617–22.

23. Beringer DC, Weiner DS, Noble JS, Bell RH. Severely displaced proximal humeral epiphyseal fractures: a follow-up study. J Pediatr Orthop. 1998;18(1):31–7.

24. Xie F, Wang S, Jiao Q, Shen Y, Ni XY, Ying H. Minimally invasive treatment for severely displaced proximal humeral fractures in children using titanium elastic nails. J Pediatr Orthop. 2011;31(8):839–46.

Index

P. Biberthaler et al. (eds.), *Fractures of the Proximal Humerus*, Strategies in Fracture Treatments,
DOI 10.1007/978-3-319-20300-3

MIX
Papier aus verantwortungsvollen Quellen
Paper from responsible sources
FSC® C105338

If you have any concerns about our products,
you can contact us on
ProductSafety@springernature.com

In case Publisher is established outside the EU,
the EU authorized representative is:
Springer Nature Customer Service Center GmbH
Europaplatz 3, 69115 Heidelberg, Germany

Printed by Libri Plureos GmbH
in Hamburg, Germany